Promoting Self-Change From Addictive Behaviors

Practical Implications for Policy, Prevention, and Treatment

Promoting Self-Change From Addictive Behaviors

Practical Implications for Policy, Prevention, and Treatment

Edited by

Harald Klingemann
University of Zurich
Zurich, Switzerland

Linda Carter Sobell
Nova Southeastern University
Fort Lauderdale, FL, USA

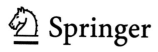

Harald Klingemann
University of Zurich
Zurich
Switzerland
harald.klingemann@suedhang.ch

Linda Carter Sobell
Nova Southeastern University
3301 College Avenue
Fort Lauderdale, FL 33314
USA
sobelll@nova.edu

Library of Congress Control Number: 2007924715

ISBN 978-0-387-71286-4
e-ISBN 978-0-387-71287-1

Printed on acid-free paper.

9 8 7 6 5 4 3 2 1

springer.com

Dedication

To my brother Hans-Dieter Klingemann, who has been supportive in times of change, on the occasion of his 70th birthday.

H. K.

To my father, Harold A. Carter, who has been a beacon of support over the years, and to my two daughters, Stacey Sobell Williams and Kimberly Allison Sobell, who are the joys of my life.

L. C. S.

Acknowledgments

We would like to thank all our colleagues who over the past several years have participated in the natural recovery conferences and related publications. Without their support and research, we would not have been able to prepare this book. As researchers, we believed that self-change was possible and sought to study the process. However, this would not have been possible without those individuals around the world who shared their stories with us. Thank you for giving your time and graciously consenting to be interviewed. We were willing to learn and you taught us more than we ever imagined.

In addition, we want to extend a very special thanks to Andrew Voluse and Kristen Harris who labored over every word in this book to insure that the final product was perfect. Lastly, we want to thank our publisher, Springer, who encouraged us to prepare this book.

Harald Klingemann
Linda Carter Sobell

Foreword

Considering the Unimaginable: Challenges to Accepting Self-Change or Natural Recovery from Addiction

Howard J. Shaffer
Harvard Medical School;
The Division on Addictions, The Cambridge Health Alliance[1,2]

> So thoroughly and sincerely are we compelled to live, reverencing our life, and denying the possibility of change. This is the only way, we say; but there are as many ways as there can be drawn radii from one centre. All change is a miracle to contemplate; but it is a miracle which is taking place every instant.
> —Henry David Thoreau, *WALDEN; Or, Life in the Woods* (1854, p.14)

> The great enemy of the truth is very often not the lie—deliberate, contrived, and dishonest—but the myth—persistent, persuasive, and unrealistic.
> —John F. Kennedy (Yale University Commencement Address, 1962)

During the middle 1980s, Stephanie Jones and I began to consider whether and how people might escape from cocaine addiction (Shaffer & Jones, 1989). During that time, cocaine misuse was a widespread and growing activity. There were many claims that even a single episode of cocaine use would lead to cocaine addiction. In the midst of this fervor, we speculated that many people would try this newly discovered drug, but that few would become addicted. We also suggested that among those who did become cocaine dependent, many more would stop using on their own than would seek treatment to help them stop. Our logic was that most people who stopped their nicotine dependence—another short-acting stimulant with many cocaine-like

---

[1] Please send correspondence to Howard J. Shaffer, Ph.D., Director, Division on Addictions, 101 Station Landing, Medford, Massachusetts 02155.
[2] Preparation of this foreword was supported, in part, by current grants and contracts from The National Center for Responsible Gaming, bwin.com, Massachusetts Family Institute, National Institute on Alcohol Abuse and Alcoholism (NIAAA), National Institute on Mental Health (NIMH), National Institute on Drug Abuse (NIDA), the Massachusetts Council on Compulsive Gambling, and the Nevada Department of Public Health. I extend special thanks to Debi LaPlante, Sarah Nelson, Chris Reilly, and Chrissy Thurmond for their helpful comments on earlier versions of this manuscript.

effects—had quit on their own, so the same pattern might hold for cocaine users. Nicotine dependence is widely accepted as one of the most difficult circumstances to change; this is partly due to how people weave its use into the fabric of their everyday lives. Illegal and more expensive, cocaine use arguably was less integrated into the day-to-day activities of most people who used it. Therefore, we expected that people should be able to stop cocaine use on their own at rates similar to nicotine quitting. We also reasoned, however, that people who used cocaine would not be willing to talk about their natural recovery experience because the community view was that they could not stop on their own and would require treatment—at the time, the treatment most often prescribed was inpatient care. To many people this pathway to recovery was unacceptable. So, they kept their quitting strategy a secret. We opened the floodgates for these people by soliciting their participation with flyers posted in public areas around Boston. When people came to tell us their story, they often began by saying, "I thought I was the only one." Interestingly, though they were unwilling to talk about their self-directed cocaine quitting in general, they were very willing to talk about it with us—perhaps because they knew that we already accepted the idea of natural recovery.

Earlier, as Stephanie and I were preparing to undertake our quitting cocaine project, we received lots of advice from colleagues. Unfortunately, the advice usually was that people could not recover from cocaine dependence without formal treatment, and that we were wasting our time. Norman Zinberg, one of the pioneers in the addiction field who demonstrated that self-control was possible even with the most frightening of illicit drugs (Zinberg, 1984; Zinberg & Harding, 1982; Zinberg, Harding, & Winkeller, 1977; Zinberg & Jacobson, 1976), encouraged us to see the project through. That was all we needed to keep going.

More recently, I have been working to better understand the similarities and differences between substance (e.g., cocaine) and activity (e.g., gambling) addiction. In both cases, treatment seekers are different from people in the community who might have addiction but do not seek treatment (e.g., Berkson's bias; Berkson, 1946); more specifically, very few people seek treatment compared with the number who struggle with either type of problem on their own. Yet, many people recover. With both types of addiction, more people recover on their own, without treatment, than with formal care. What makes it so difficult for people to accept the idea that people struggling with addiction can change their behavior on their own?

In addition to the cynical but unfortunately real concerns about turf and economic issues that treatment providers fear, for example losing treatment opportunities to natural home remedies for addiction, there are other powerful social psychological forces that make it very difficult for people to accept the idea of self-change. When talking about human foibles, Norman Zinberg often quipped, "Consider it projection until proven otherwise." This aphorism is useful when trying to understand the challenges to accepting self-change.

People tend to view the world as they experience it. People tend to think that others experience the world as they do. People think that others require treatment to change because they think their own behavior change is the result of external forces. "I had to stop smoking because my doctor said...." The tendency to project is compounded by the "fundamental attribution error." Ross (1977) first described this error as the tendency for actors to see their own behavior as determined by forces external to them, and for observers to see the very same behavior as determined by the actor's internal dispositions. This "fundamental attribution error" increases the likelihood that observers will think that others who are struggling with addiction are stuck because they "want" to be stuck—that they are not sufficiently motivated to change, for example. Once observers perceive people with addiction to be absent the intrapersonal resources necessary for change, they then deduce that people with addiction need some external force to change. Similarly, they tend to view their own behavior changes as the consequence of external forces.

The dynamics of addiction and the need to attribute causes for both addiction and recovery have important implications for clinicians and public policy makers alike. Sometimes treatment providers and public policy makers intervene with addictive behavior patterns when it is unnecessary, calling too much attention to issues that have limited adverse consequences. These patterns of drug misuse tend to resolve without treatment. Alternatively, if policy makers or treatment providers think that addictive behaviors will resolve without intervention, they might act too slowly. Research must determine the latency of self-change, which problems require policy or treatment interventions to help people change, and which expressions of addiction fall somewhere in between.

To illustrate, while working on the quitting cocaine project, it was common to see public service announcements that touted, "One puff of crack and you will be hooked." This announcement might have kept some people who were ambivalent about whether to try smoking crack from doing it. But, I wonder what effect this message had on the people who already tried smoking crack? This message might have encouraged them to believe that they were doomed to a life of addiction and would not be able to stop. A better, and more scientifically accurate, message would be "one puff of crack and you can stop, just like most of the people who have used it." This public health message and its consequences likely would be very different from the other message and most users would recognize that there were others who understood the nature of drug use and that they were telling the truth.

Understanding natural recovery holds fundamental benefits for treatment providers and treatment protocols. People who have recovered from addiction without formal treatment often have discovered—on their own—some of the essential elements of behavior change. For example, our cocaine quitters often identified loss of health, work, or family to be primary factors that encouraged them to change. Similarly, they identified more healthy substitutes that could take the place of the addiction they wanted to stop. It is very important for treatment providers to learn about the building blocks of natural recovery so that they can integrate or enhance these elements in their treatment. Natural or self-directed changers have learned—on their own—exactly what treatment seekers need to know to help others: how to change behavior for the better and then maintain those changes.

The earlier book of *Promoting Self-Change From Problem Substance Abuse* was a landmark in the field, and this book updates, integrates, and solidifies the best science on this topic. Klingemann and Sobell have provided a fundamental service to the field that is destined to become a watershed event. As more research has become available, they have identified the central perspectives essential to understanding self-change from addictive behaviors and woven them into a coherent explanation of recovery. Yet, despite this vital contribution, the idea of self-change is still likely to face stout challenge: this is because, as I suggested earlier, the idea that people can direct their own escape from addiction is anathema to many observers. In the struggle between (a) what people are disposed to perceive by cultural myth and the dynamics of social perception and (b) what is possible, this volume makes its most important contribution. It shifts from unimaginable to imaginable the process and possibility of self-directed changes from addiction. This shift in perspective holds the potential to revolutionize treatment and recovery. This book can change treatment because it identifies the central elements of human change; it can transform recovery because, in addition to revealing the most fundamental and efficient treatment tactics, it makes clear to people struggling with addiction that they have the capacity for change. If we cannot imagine the possibility of self-directed change, not only will our science be limited unnecessarily to studies of externally directed change, but it also is likely that people will not change without external influence. Just as software lags behind hardware, clinical practice tends to lag behind science. This circumstance suggests that clinicians do not access some of the change options that are available to them. The conventional cultural wisdom lags even further behind clinical protocols, making it difficult for people with addiction to even imagine that they can change without formal treatment or self-help. Yet, some do recover by self-directing their change. Consequently, I suspect that natural recovery is a more powerful force than even self-change proponents now recognize.

In context, the challenges associated with considering self-change inherently limit the full range of change options. This book makes a very special contribution and provides a portal to things yet unimagined and undiscovered about change. Yet, for this book to achieve its full potential, it will be necessary for addiction science to mature. Currently, the field of addiction reflects an underlying belief that change is either not likely or must be coerced. But, Jean Rostand (1962) reminds us, "It is sometimes important for science to know how to forget the things she is surest of.... Nothing leads the scientist so astray as a premature truth" (A Biologist's Thoughts, Chapter 7).

References

Berkson, J. (1946). Limitations of the application of fourfold table analysis to hospital data. *Biometrics, 2*, 47–53.

Ross, L. (1977). The intuitive psychologist and his shortcomings: Distortions in the attribution process. In L. Berkowitz (Ed.), *Advances in experimental social psychology* (Vol. 10, pp. 173–220). New York: Academic Press.

Rostand, J. (1962). *The substance of man.* Garden City, NY: Doubleday.

Shaffer, H. J., & Jones, S. B. (1989). *Quitting cocaine: The struggle against impulse.* Lexington, MA: Lexington Books.

Zinberg, N. E. (1984). *Drug, set, and setting: The basis for controlled intoxicant use.* New Haven: Yale University Press.

Zinberg, N. E., & Harding, W. M. (Eds.). (1982). *Control over intoxicant use.* New York: Free Press.

Zinberg, N. E., Harding, W. M., & Winkeller, M. (1977). A study of social regulatory mechanisms in controlled illicit drug users. *Journal of Drug Issues, 7*, 117–133.

Zinberg, N. E., & Jacobson, R. C. (1976). The natural history of chipping. *American Journal of Psychiatry, 133*, 37–40.

Preface

The literature clearly shows that many individuals with addictive behaviors overcome their problems without professional treatment or self-help groups. Research into the self-change process for many years was impeded by the disease concept that has long dominated the addiction field. However, since the mid-1980s there has been a rapid growth of studies examining the self-change process. Several years ago, the first major review of the literature reported that there were 40 studies of alcohol and drug abusers who changed on their own, with the vast majority published in the last decade (Sobell, Ellingstad, & Sobell, 2000). Chapter 5 of this book reviews the same literature from 1999 through 2005 and found that over this 6-year period 22 studies were published that met the same criteria. In addition, the topic of self-change from substance abuse has gained recognition and acceptance as reflected in the statements from three prominent organizations: (a) "Improvement without formal treatment is not a minor or insignificant phenomenon" (Institute of Medicine, 1990, p.152), (b) "Some individuals (perhaps 20% or more) with Alcohol Dependence achieve long-term sobriety even without active treatment" (American Psychiatric Association, 1994, p. 202), and (c) "The track of this disease is not clear-cut—some people appear to recover from alcoholism without formal treatment" (National Institute on Alcohol Abuse and Alcoholism, 2006).

In the early 1990s, the study of the self-change process started to be approached differently. For example, recent studies have started using qualitative and quantitative methods to describe how individuals change (e.g., life history/life event approach). Two factors have emerged from these newer studies that appear to be strongly associated with the self-change process— motivation for change and a cognitive appraisal process. These findings have important implications for the design of new interventions. In addition, several recent and better designed surveys have provided a basis for more precise estimates of the prevalence of self-change from different addictions. The phenomenon of recoveries from different addictive behaviors (e.g., smoking, alcohol and drug use, gambling) and the macro-societal conditions that may promote recoveries have also been examined. Such research, however, has been scattered around the globe, and the need for a systematic integration of this research and its clinical implications as well as the identification of future research directions has become a priority in the field.

In March 1999, the first international conference on "Natural history of addiction: Recovery from alcohol/tobacco and other drug problems without treatment" was held in Les Diablerets, Switzerland. The conference, which occurred under the umbrella of the Kettil Bruun Society for Social and Epidemiological Research on Alcohol, was sponsored by the Swiss Federal Office of Public Health, and hosted and organized by the Swiss Institute for the Prevention of Alcohol and Other Drug Problems. The conference brought together 29 researchers from more than 10 countries who shared a common interest in self-change/natural recovery. Sociologists, psychologists, health care practitioners, anthropologists, economists, and government policy analysts formed a truly interdisciplinary research group. What made this meeting different from many others was the explicit objective to start a dialogue between researchers, treatment providers, and policymakers and to gain a clearer vision of the treatment implications based on the recent research. The meeting led to several scientific publications including two miniseries in two journals (Klingemann & Sobell, 2001; Sobell et al., 2000). The state-of–the-art scientific review on the study of self-change from the perspective of various disciplines and the rich outcome of the conference's interdisciplinary panel discussions provided the framework for the first book published on self-change from substance abuse (Klingemann et al., 2001). In the subsequent years, the broad positive response to the English book encouraged the Swiss Federal Office of Health to support a German version of the book (Klingemann & Sobell, 2006).

Three years after the Les Diablerets conference in Switzerland, a related conference, "Addiction in the Life Course Perspective," was held in Stockholm in 2002 as part of the thematic meeting of the Kettil Bruun Society for Social and Epidemiological Research on Alcohol and was sponsored by the Nordic Council for Alcohol and Drug Research. The conference attracted 43 participants from 12 countries, representing a diversity of disciplines, and resulted in the book *Addiction and the Life Course* published by the Nordic Council for Alcohol and Drug Research (Rosenqvist, Blomqvist, Koski-Jännes, & Öjesjö, 2004). This entire publication is available at <http://www.nad.fi/index.php?lang=se&id=pub/44>.

We felt that those who have made this book possible, our interview partners, should have a say in the book. Therefore, using original interview transcripts, we had the unique opportunity to mirror our scientific statements with the words, sentiments, and feelings of our respondents about how they recovered on their own. Throughout the book, selected excerpts from such individuals are juxtaposed and matched to various discussions about the self-change process.

Chapter 1 in this volume starts with a historical overview of the phenomenon of self-change. It reviews conceptual and methodological issues, presents a state-of-the-art review of the field of self-change, and discusses barriers to treatment as well as the major models of change. Chapter 2 provides a comprehensive review of the often-cited classic alcohol and drug studies of self-change, many of which were not designed to study self-change explicitly, but nevertheless have provided the early base for documenting the existence of the phenomenon. Chapter 3 looks at what we know about self-change from substance abuse from large-scale population surveys and community studies as well as from smaller samples obtained by advertising and other avenues. The advantages and disadvantages of using various methods are discussed as well as questions that are still unanswered about self-change in large populations. Chapter 4 discusses the more recent natural recovery studies and presents new directions in research in this area. Chapter 5 provides a review of 22 self-change studies with alcohol and drug abusers published over the past 6 years, and compares these findings with an earlier review (Sobell et al., 2000), pointing out methodological shortcomings and priorities for future research.

Because this book has a heavy emphasis on the self-change process with substance abusers, we felt that chapters demonstrating the occurrence and application of the self-change process with other populations would expand the discussion and understanding of the self-change process. Therefore, Chapter 6 presents reviews of the self-change process with five different participant groups: cigarette smokers (6.1), gamblers (6.2), individuals with eating disorders or obesity (6.3), juvenile delinquents (6.4), and stutterers (6.5).

Chapter 7 suggests that although the traditional model would have us believe that there is only one way to resolve an addictive behavior, treatment is, in fact, only "one way to leave your lover" or, put differently, multiple pathways to change exist. This chapter talks about the role of treatment in changing addictive behaviors and concludes with the suggestion that one way of providing services efficiently would be for health care practitioners in the substance abuse field to embrace a stepped-care model of service provision. Based on state-of-the-art research, this chapter offers real and practical suggestions about how health care practitioners can expedite or nurture what might be seen as a time-delayed "natural" process. Chapter 8, in discussing the fact that the majority of substance abusers will never enter treatment, offers alternative nontraditional ways to motivate substance abusers to change (e.g., Internet, self-change materials available other than through traditional avenues).

Chapter 9 expands the discussion of self-change from addiction through an examination of the broader environmental factors that play an important role in substance abusers' recoveries. Too often, decisional processes of self-change are seen as occurring solely within the individual or from interactions between individuals rather than from societal forces. This chapter sets out to show links between the individual clinical view and social factors (e.g., public images of addiction and their changeability, treatment systems, the role of the media and policy measures) as macro-societal aspects. In doing so, it argues that environmental factors are amenable to manipulation to reduce problem use and to promote recovery. An essential request addressed to policymakers is to provide favorable conditions for self-change and to promote maintenance. Chapter 10 presents information about alcohol and drug use from a broad range of cultural settings and then provides a rich discussion of self-change issues across different cultures. This chapter raises questions about specific group needs and cultural variations in the perception of time and ideas on the basic trajectory of life and its goals. For example, the topic of how to assist and treat migrants from various cultural backgrounds has gained increasing importance, particularly in Europe.

Chapter 11, the Self-Change Toolbox, is intended as a reference source for readers by supplying tools, tips, websites, and other informational resources for assessing and promoting self-change. Our hope is that this book and the toolbox will be used as a reference by researchers, health care practitioners, public health specialists, and alcohol and drug policy makers to further understand and promote the self-change process. Although the last decade has witnessed an increased interest in and understanding of the study of self-change, our understanding is by no means complete. Thus, the often-heard phrase that "more research is needed" is relevant. It is hoped that this book will better inform funding agencies and scientists about where the research "Euro" is likely to get its best value.

Lastly, it seems fitting to close with the words of two of the early natural recovery researchers:

The identification of natural recoverers is not anomalous and should not be dismissed casually. These groups have much to teach those who are willing to learn. In order to learn, however, one must first believe that groups such as these exist. (Shaffer & Jones, 1989, p. 5)

Harald Klingemann and Linda Carter Sobell
Zurich and Fort Lauderdale

References

American Psychiatric Association. (1994). *Diagnostic and statistical manual of mental disorders* (4th ed). Washington, DC: Author.

Institute of Medicine. (1990). Broadening the base of treatment for alcohol problems. Washington, DC: National Academy Press.

Klingemann, H.. & Sobell, L. C. (2001). Introduction: Natural recovery research across substance use. *Substance Use & Misuse, 36*, 1409–1416.

Klingemann, H., & Sobell, L. C. (Eds.). (2006). *Selbstheilung von der Sucht [Addiction and self-healing]*. Wiesbaden, Germany: VS Verlag für Sozialwissenschaften.

Klingemann, H., Sobell, L. C., Barker, J., Blomqvist, J., Cloud, W., Ellingstad, T. P., et al. (2001). *Promoting self-change from problem substance use: Practical implications for policy, prevention, and treatment*. Dordrecht: Kluwer Academic Publishers.

National Institute on Alcohol Abuse and Alcoholism. (2006). National epidemiologic survey on alcohol and related conditions. *Alcohol Alert, 70*, 1–5.

Rosenqvist, J., Blomqvist, A., Koski-Jännes, & Öjesjö, L. (2004). *Addiction and the life course* (Vol. 44). Helsinki, Finland: Nordiska Nämnden för Alkohol- OchDrogforskning (Nordic Council for Alcohol and Drug Research).

Shaffer, H. J., & Jones, S. B. (1989). *Quitting cocaine: The struggle against impulse.* Lexington, MA: Lexington Books.

Sobell, L. C., Ellingstad, T. P., & Sobell, M. B. (2000). Natural recovery from alcohol and drug problems: Methodological review of the research with suggestions for future directions. *Addiction, 95*(5), 749–764.

Contents

Contributors

Judith C. Barker
Department of Anthropology, History, & Social Medicine
University of California, San Francisco
San Francisco, CA 94143-0850, USA

Gallus Bischof
Universität zu Lübeck
Klinik für Psychiatrie und Psychotherapie
Ratzeburger Allee 160
23538 Lübeck, Deutschland

Jan Blomqvist
Centrum för Socialvetenskaplig
Alkohol- och Drogforskning (SoRAD)
Stockholms Universitet
S-106 91 Stockholm, Sverige

José Luis Carballo
Facultad de Psicología
Universidad de Oviedo
Oviedo, Asturias, España

Mariam Dum
Center for Psychological Studies
Nova Southeastern University
Ft. Lauderdale, FL 33314-7796, USA

José Ramón Fernández-Hermida
Facultad de Psicología
Universidad de Oviedo
Oviedo, Asturias, España

Patrick Finn
Speech, Language, and Hearing Sciences
University of Arizona
Tucson, AZ 85721-0071, USA

Stephanie Flöter
IFT Institut für Therapieforschung
80804 München, Deutschland

Olaya García-Rodríguez
Facultad de Psicología
Universidad de Oviedo
Oviedo, Asturias, España

Geoffrey Hunt
Institute for Scientific Analysis
Alameda, CA 94501-3685, USA

Ulrich John
Ernst-Moritz-Arndt-Universität Greifswald
Institut für Epidemiologie und Sozialmedizin
17487 Greifswald, Deutschland

Harald Klingemann
University of Zurich
Zurich, Switzerland

Justyna Klingemann
Zaklad Badan nad Alkoholizmem i Toksykomaniami
Instytut Psychiatrii i Neurologii
Sobieskiego 9, 02-957 Warszawa, Polska

Joachim Körkel
University of Applied Sciences
Bärenschanzstrasse 4
D - 90429 Nürnberg, Deutschland

Christoph Kröger
IFT Institut für Therapieforschung
80804 München, Deutschland

Jachen C. Nett
Berner Fachhochschule Fachbereich Soziale Arbeit
CH-3001, Bern, Switzerland

Janet Polivy
Department of Psychology
University of Toronto at Mississauga
Mississauga, ON, L5L 1C6, Canada

Hans-Jürgen Rumpf
Universität zu Lübeck
Klinik für Psychiatrie und Psychotherapie
23538 Lübeck, Deutschland

Roberto Secades-Villa
Facultad de Psicología
Universidad de Oviedo
Oviedo, Asturias, España

Reginald G. Smart
Centre for Addiction and Mental Health
Toronto, ON, M5S 2S1, Canada

Linda Carter Sobell
Center for Psychological Studies
Nova Southeastern University
Ft. Lauderdale, FL 33314-7796, USA

Mark B. Sobell
Center for Psychological Studies
Nova Southeastern University
Ft. Lauderdale, FL 33314-7796, USA

Jukka-Pekka Takala
Helsingin Yliopisto Rikoksentorjuntaneuvosto
PL 25, 00023 Valtioneuvosto, Suomi

Tony Toneatto
Centre for Addiction and Mental Health
Toronto, ON, M5S 2S1, Canada

Andrew Voluse
Center for Psychological Studies
Nova Southeastern University
Ft. Lauderdale, FL 33314-7796, USA

1
The Phenomenon of Self-Change: Overview and Key Issues

Linda Carter Sobell

> The way ahead in alcoholism treatment research should be to embrace more closely the study of 'natural forces' that can then be captured and exploited by planned interventions.
>
> Orford & Edwards, 1977, p. 3

Introduction

In his classic treatise 40 years ago on the study of deviants, Becker (1963) cautioned against studying only extreme cases. Over the years, other researchers have made similar arguments with regard to studying the addictions. For example, Cahalan (1987), based on epidemiological surveys of problem drinkers (Cahalan, 1970, 1987; Cahalan, Cisin, & Crossley, 1969; Cahalan & Room, 1974), used the phrase "tip of the iceberg" to refer to the fact that their survey data demonstrated that clinically defined "alcoholics" constituted only a relatively small proportion of those whose drinking created significant problems for themselves and society. Room (1977) later labeled the distinction between persons with alcohol problems in surveys versus those in clinical studies as the "two worlds of alcoholism." A few years later, based on their well-known longitudinal study, Vaillant and Milofsky (1984) asserted that we cannot understand the natural history of alcoholism by solely looking at clinic samples. Finally, based on a study of Vietnam veterans who used heroin during their tour but stopped on returning to the United States, Robins stated that "[a]ddiction looks very different if you study it in a general population than if you study it in treated cases" (Robins, 1993, p. 1051). Price, Risk, and Spitznagel (2001) conducted a 25-year follow-up of the Vietnam veterans study with the 841 living members of the previously interviewed cohort. It was found that (a) most attempted to quit and the majority succeeded at the time of their last attempt without the aid of traditional drug treatment programs, (b) less than 9% of current drug users had been treated in a formal treatment setting, and (c) "Most drug abusers who had started using drugs by their early 20s appeared to gradually achieve remission. Spontaneous remission was the rule rather than the exception" (p. 1107).

In another large study, the Collaborative Study on the Genetics of Alcoholism, the clinical histories of 3,572 DSM-III-R-defined alcohol dependent individuals who were either (a) never in treatment, (b) in outpatient or Alcoholics Anonymous (AA), or (c) in inpatient treatment were compared. As demonstrated in many other studies, those in inpatient treatment had more serious histories compared to those who had never been in treatment. The authors concluded that "studies using data from inpatient populations may give a skewed picture of the clinical characteristics of alcohol dependence" (Raimo, Daeppen, Smith, Danko, & Schuckit, 1999, p. 1605). With regard to cocaine, Erickson and Alexander (1989) studied naturally recovered cocaine abusers and concluded that the addicts in treatment represented only the tip of the iceberg of all cocaine users. Lastly, today there is no shortage of survey studies supporting the original findings of Cahalan and his colleagues that treated alcohol and drug abusers constitute only a small percentage of all individuals with such problems (Cunningham, 1999b; Cunningham, Lin, Ross, & Walsh, 2000; Dawson, 1996; Dawson et al., 2005; Grant, 1997; Narrow, Regier, Rae, Manderscheid, & Locke, 1993; Roizen, 1977; Room & Greenfield, 1993).

For years, the addiction field has been dominated by an almost exclusive focus on individuals who are severely dependent. The emphasis on severe dependence has resulted in a myopic view of substance abuse problems that has characterized them as progressive, irreversible, and only resolved through treatment. Further support that the traditional view based on treatment populations is myopic comes from studies that show those who recover on their own typically have less serious substance use problems and more intact social resources (e.g., marriages, education, jobs) than those who have sought formal treatment or help (Hodgins & el-Guebaly, 2000; Humphreys, Moos, & Finney, 1995; Sobell, Ellingstad, & Sobell, 2000; Sobell, Sobell, Toneatto, & Leo, 1993; Vaillant & Milofsky, 1984).

If substance use problems are viewed as lying along a continuum ranging from no problems to mild problems to severe problems, rather than as dichotomous (i.e., alcoholic versus not alcoholic, drug addict versus not drug addict) it has profound implications for how one views and treats such individuals. One implication is that there are multiple pathways to recovery, including self-change, a pathway that has largely been ignored by the addiction field. This first chapter has several objectives, most notably to help readers understand where the field is currently and where it is headed. It also provides a historical overview of the phenomenon of self-change, reviews key methodological issues, presents a state-of-the-art review of the field of self-change, and discusses barriers to treatment as well as the major models of change.

The Respondents Speak

Several investigators who have examined the self-change process with substance abusers have reported that such individuals "wanted to tell" their stories (Shaffer & Jones, 1989; Sobell, Sobell, & Toneatto, 1992; Tuchfeld, 1981). In this regard, respondents' stories are used throughout this book to illustrate aspects of the self-change process. Thus, starting with this chapter, quotations from individuals who were interviewed about their successful self-change from an addictive behavior are presented in boxes throughout the book. These short narratives relate to various topics discussed within each chapter. The narratives are not meant to be in-depth descriptions of the entire recovery episode, and details of the respondents are not provided. Rather, the comments are included to give readers a grass-roots flavor of various issues relating to recovery (e.g., reasons for change, barriers to treatment, maintenance factors) discussed in each chapter. The narratives come from several studies of self-change conducted over the years.

Telling My Story

In one of the first studies to comment on respondents' reactions to discussing their self-change from alcohol problem, Tuchfeld (1981) found alcohol abusers to be quite proud of their recovery without formal treatment or help. Some years later Shaffer and Jones (1989), after interviewing cocaine abusers who quit on their own, reported that the "typical cocaine quitter wanted—even felt compelled—to tell us his or her story" (p. 6). Sobell and her colleagues (1992) further noted that many recovered alcohol abusers said they had never talked with others about their recovery. Thus, it appears self-changers from substance use problems find the interview experience helpful and therapeutic.

Is What We Call the Phenomenon Important?

Concepts such as "spontaneous remission," "natural recovery," and "maturing out" are not new. In the medical field, the term *spontaneous* has been used for many years and refers to an improvement in the patient's condition that occurs without treatment (Roizen, Cahalan, & Shanks, 1978). Psychological working definitions of the terms emphasize the individual's own cognitive achievement (i.e., self-initiated recovery or change in behavior; Biernacki, 1986; Marlatt & Gordon, 1985). From a sociological viewpoint, the primary consideration is to exit from a deviant career without formal intervention (Stall, 1983) or to mobilize external resources (i.e., self-organized remission; Happel, Fischer, & Wittfeld, 1993). Lastly, from the perspective of juvenile delinquency the term "maturing out" has been synonymous with no longer engaging in delinquent behaviors (Labouvie, 1996).

In the addictions field over the years, many terms (e.g., *spontaneous remission, auto-remission, untreated remission, self-change, maturing out, burning out, spontaneous recovery, natural recovery, untreated recovery, self-quitters, natural resolution, spontaneous resolution*) have been used to describe individuals who have recovered from an addiction on their own. Although these terms have been used interchangeably, presumably to describe the same phenomenon (i.e., self-change), the notion of spontaneous remission has been challenged as semantically and conceptually imprecise (Institute of Medicine, 1990;

Shaffer & Jones, 1989; Tuchfeld, 1976, 1981). For example, Mulford (1988) has suggested that "'spontaneous remission' is a euphemism for our ignorance of the forces at work" (p. 330). Although some terms used to describe natural recoveries suggest the change has no cause, it is doubtful that any investigator of the phenomenon would view it as "unexplainable," just "unexplained."

Lastly, while there is no currently agreed upon term, the common theme in each phrase is that they presume that an *unwanted* condition is overcome without professional treatment or help. Words such as *natural* and *spontaneous* are increasingly being replaced by more neutral terms like *untreated recovery* or *self-change*. While the various terms noted above have been used interchangeably to refer to a change in a person's substance use in the absence of formal treatment or help, the preferred term that will be used throughout this book will be *self-change*.

Defining Treatment and How Little Is Too Much

Although determining whether treatment has taken place would seem to be a straightforward matter, how treatment episodes are defined in the literature has been very fluid (Sobell et al., 2000). There are also problems with treatment intensity (i.e., number of sessions). For example, do brief physician interventions, often involving a single session and sometimes lasting less than 30 minutes, constitute formal treatment (Fleming & Manwell, 1999; Fleming, Manwell, Barry, Adams, & Stauffacher, 1999; Fleming et al., 2000, 2002; Heather, 1989, 1990, 1994; Law & Tang, 1995)? Further complicating the picture is advice by laypersons such as ministers, rabbis, and friends, or a trip to a detoxification center or emergency room for any reason (e.g., traffic accident, but no psychotherapy provided). In addition, do we consider community or organizational interventions that provide treatment at a broad, social level as formal treatment (e.g., weight loss programs like Weight Watchers or smoking cessation programs such as the American Lung Association; Cunningham & Breslin, 2004; Foulds, 1996; Giffen, 1991; Green et al., 1995; Hughes, Cummings, & Hyland, 1999)? The last two major reviews of this literature show that most studies and surveys provide detailed definitions of what constitutes treatment and self-help (Sobell et al., 2000; Chapter 5), including the most recent National Epidemiologic Survey on Alcohol and Related Conditions (National Institute on Alcohol Abuse and Alcoholism, 2006a).

Recent self-change studies (Bischof, Rumpf, Hapke, Meyer, & John, 2002; Sobell et al., 1993, 2000; Toneatto, Sobell, Sobell, & Rubel, 1999; Tucker, Vuchinich, & Gladsjo, 1991; Tucker, Vuchinich, Gladsjo, Hawkins, & Sherrill, 1989) have addressed the problem of how little treatment is considered treatment by adopting a conservative definition (i.e., any intervention by recognized programs or individuals whose primary goal was to treat individuals with substance use problems). Because brief interventions for substance abusers have been found to be effective, even as little as one session, these must also be considered treatment. In a related regard, recognizing that a great many individuals might attend a few self-help group meetings without seriously adopting a recovery program, some natural recovery studies have now included respondents who had attended one or two self-help group meetings (Sobell et al., 1992, 1993, 2000; Tucker, Vuchinich, & Gladsjo, 1994).

An interesting dilemma occurs when one considers the perspective of treatment from different cultures. For example, one recent self-change study conducted in Germany defined the absence of treatment as no more than five outpatient visits with a physician (Rumpf, Bischof, Hapke, Meyer, & John, 2000). The reason for this is that in Germany, alcohol treatment, until very recently, took the form of psychiatric hospitalization and five outpatient visits, which has been more than enough to be considered a brief intervention in the United States (for these German researchers this did not seem to constitute treatment).

Another issue that has clouded research in this area is that many studies that examine the natural history of change across the life span (i.e., look at the progression of the disorder) include individuals who have used treatment or self-help groups in the past. The most notable among such studies are those by Vaillant (Vaillant, 1995; Vaillant & Milofsky, 1982), and unfortunately, these are often confused and included with natural recovery studies that exclude participants who have used treatment or self-help groups.

Mixing Treated and Untreated Respondents

A serious methodological problem with self-change studies in the addiction field has been combining individuals who had received prior treatment with those who never had prior treatment (Bischof et al., 2002; Cunningham, 1999a; Sobell et al., 1992, 2000; Sobell, Toneatto, & Sobell, 1990). Examples of studies that have combined previously treated with untreated participants are abundant in the literature (Cunningham, 1999a; Ludwig, 1985; Saunders & Kershaw, 1979; Stall, 1983; Tuchfeld, 1976, 1981). Most of these studies are older and did not subscribe to a strict definition of "no treatment." Therefore, substance abusers who were unsuccessfully treated, but later resolved their problem on their own, were included in study samples. For example, 22% of Tuchfeld's (Tuchfeld, 1976, 1981) respondents had, at some time, received treatment for an alcohol problem. In another study (Cunningham, 1999a), the author reported the following:

Of 9,892 adult lifetime drinkers, 2,177 had experienced at least one problem related to their alcohol consumption and, of these, 885 (57.2% male) had experienced no problems in the last year. Estimates of the prevalence of nontreatment recoveries ranged from 87.5% to 53.7% depending on the stringency of the definition of prior alcohol problems employed. (p. 463)

To address this problem, recent self-change studies have not only used stricter definitions of treatment, but have also presented data separately for individuals who had gone to treatment or self-help meetings several years prior to their recovery but said they recovered on their own, from self-changers who had no prior treatment or self-help contact (Klingemann, 1991; Sobell et al., 1993). One important reason for differentiating recovered respondents who have and have not received prior treatment is because several studies have shown that never treated recovered substance abusers and smokers have less severe problem histories, symptoms, and consequences compared to those who were once in treatment but later recovered on their own (Fagerström et al., 1996; Hingson, Scotch, Day, & Culbert, 1980; Raimo & Schuckit, 1998; Sobell, Cunningham, & Sobell, 1996; Sobell et al., 1992; Weisner, 1987).

State-of-the-Art in Self-Change

While methodologically rigorous studies of natural recoveries with substance abusers emerged about a decade ago, published studies and isolated reports of the phenomenon are not new. One of the first reports was in the early nineteenth century by Benjamin Rush (1814), a physician and author of one of the earliest scientific treatises on inebriety. He described several individuals who had recovered from alcohol problems on their own (alcohol treatment as we know it today was nonexistent in the 1800s). Further, some of the recoveries appeared to have become moderate drinkers (i.e., they gave up the evils of "spirituous liquors"). However, serious study of the process of self-change with substance abusers appears to have started in the 1960s (Drew, 1968; Schachter, 1982; Winick, 1962). Given the attention to this area over the last decade (see the Preface to this book), research and published studies on the process of self-change have experienced considerable growth as evidenced by the results from two major systematic reviews of this literature. The first article reported results for 38 studies published over almost four decades (Sobell et al., 2000). The second review (see Chapter 5) found 22 studies that met the same strict inclusion criteria as in the Sobell et al. review, but were published during only a 6-year period (i.e., 1999 through 2005). These two reviews clearly demonstrate that considerable evidence has accumulated showing that natural recovery (i.e., recovery without treatment) or self-change is a major pathway to change for individuals with alcohol and drug problems.

However, the study of self-change has been very uneven across the addiction field. Although self-change has long been a well documented common route to recovery for cigarette smokers (estimates range from 80% to 90% of all those who stop smoking; Carey, Snel, Carey, & Richards, 1989; Fiore et al., 1990; Hughes et al., 1996; Mariezcurrena, 1994; Orleans, Rimer, Cristinzio, Keintz, & Fleisher, 1991; U.S. Department of Health and Human Services, 1988; Chapter 6.1), until the past decade the systematic study of this phenomenon was largely ignored for substance abuse. As reflected by the results of the 22 studies reviewed in Chapter 5, this is now changing. Furthermore, as discussed in other chapters of this book, the process of self-change has been expanded to other addictive behaviors such as gambling (Chapter 6.2) and eating disorders and obesity (Chapter 6.3) and to behaviors outside of the addiction field (Chapter 6.4, crime; Chapter 6.5, stuttering).

Evidence for self-change from addictive behaviors comes from several lines of study: (a) prevalence and longitudinal (i.e., cases identified at two different points in time) studies in the general population (e.g., Cahalan, 1970; Cahalan et al., 1969; Cunningham, 1999a,b; Dawson et al., 2005; Fillmore, Hartka, Johnstone, Speiglman, & Temple, 1988; Sobell, Cunningham, & Sobell, 1996), (b) waiting list control groups (e.g., Alden, 1988; Kissin, Rosenblatt, & Machover, 1968) and follow-ups of clients who left treatment (e.g., Kendell & Staton, 1966), (c) active case finding studies, largely done through media advertisements (e.g., Sobell et al., 1993; Toneatto et al., 1999; Tucker et al., 1989) and snowball techniques (i.e., nomination of someone who respondents know has a problem similar to theirs; Granfield & Cloud, 1996; Schasre, 1966) that specifically recruited and interviewed individuals who have recovered without formal treatment or help (e.g., Biernacki, 1986; Hodgins & el-Guebaly, 2000; Ludwig, 1985; Shaffer & Jones, 1989; Sobell et al., 1993; Tuchfeld, 1976; Tucker et al., 1994), and (d) official registers of addicts (e.g., Snow, 1973; Winick, 1962).

Advantages of Survey and Other Methods for Studying the Process of Self-Change

Surveys have many advantages over other methods for studying self-change, but they also have some disadvantages. Although general population surveys with large samples can provide overall rates of self-change, most contain very few, if any, questions about the actual process of self-change. However, recent convenience samples recruited via media advertisements and snowball samples have typically focused more on recovery issues and how the process of self-change proceeds.

Why Has Self-Change as an Area of Study Been So Long Overlooked or Ignored?

One possible reason why the addiction field has paid little attention to self-change as an area of study (Shaffer & Jones, 1989; Sobell et al., 1992) is that such individuals do not come to the attention of researchers or practitioners, as they do not enter treatment or attend 12-step meetings. Another reason may relate to the fact that individuals who exhibit severe forms of the disorder have occupied most of the public's attention. Thus, many in the field have been blinded to the fact that there are multiple pathways to recovery (i.e., treatment, self-help groups such as AA, self-change). A third reason natural recoveries have long been ignored relates to the disease model of addiction, a model that is wholly inconsistent with self-change (Chiauzzi & Liljegren, 1993; Shaffer & Jones, 1989; Sobell et al., 2000). Advocates of the disease model put forth a tautological argument that "an ability to cease addictive behaviors on one's own suggests that the individual was not addicted in the first place. If one is *not* able to stop independently, then an addiction is present" (Chiauzzi & Liljegren, 1993, p. 306). For some health care professionals (Dupont, 1993; Johnson, 1980; Winick, 1962) as well as the general public (Cunningham, 1999a; Cunningham, Sobell, & Chow, 1993; Cunningham, Sobell, & Sobell, 1999; Ferris, 1994; Rush & Allen, 1997), self-change has been met with disbelief. As reflected by the three quotes in the next box, disease model proponents postulate a progressive, irreversible disorder that can only be resolved through intervention.

Traditionalists Claim Self-Change Is Not Possible

"Addiction is not self-curing. Left alone addiction only gets worse, leading to total degradation, to prison, and, ultimately to death" (Dupont, 1993, p. xi–xii).

"Alcoholism is a fatal disease, 100 percent fatal. Nobody survives alcoholism that remains unchecked.... These people will not be able to stop drinking by themselves. They are forced to seek help; and when they don't, they perish miserably" (Johnson, 1980, p. 1).

"There has been considerable skepticism in both lay and professional circles of the thesis that many addicts never stop using drugs, but continue as addicts until they die"(Winick, 1962, p. 1).

Nonabstinent Outcomes and Natural Recovery

Another issue that runs counter to the disease model of addictions is the claim that individuals can engage in moderate drinking or low-risk drug use (also referred to as *chipping*; see Shaffer & Jones, 1989) as a form of recovery. Studies reporting moderation have, over the years, been met with emotional reactions ranging from a deep-seated disbelief to serious attacks (reviewed in Hunt, 1998; Marlatt, 1983, 1998; Rosenberg & Davis, 1994; Sobell & Sobell, 1995). Reports that some naturally recovered substance abusers successfully returned to low-risk nonproblem drinking or drug use can be viewed as a dual threat to the disease model (i.e., recovering without treatment and reversing the disorder). Both of the recent major reviews of the self-change literature with alcohol and drug abusers have reported low-risk alcohol use to be a very frequent occurrence (Sobell et al., 2000; Chapter 5). Over three quarters (78.6%, 22/28 studies, Sobell et al., 2000; 86.6%, 13/15 studies, Chapter 5) of the studies in these two reviews reported that some alcohol abusers who recovered from an alcohol problem on their own also reported engaging in low-risk nonproblem drinking. These results parallel findings from alcohol treatment outcome studies (Breslin, Sobell, Sobell, & Sobell, 1997; Rosenberg, 1993) and suggest that the way the field views recovery from alcohol problems is not consistent with the empirical literature and is, therefore, in need of change (Sobell & Sobell, 2006). Although fewer studies of natural recoveries from drugs, as opposed to alcohol, have been reported, a similar pattern emerged in the first review (Sobell et al., 2000) where nearly half of the studies reviewed (46.2%, 6/13) reported limited drug use recoveries. This is consistent with reports of controlled opiate use (Blackwell, 1983; Klingemann, 1991; Shewan et al., 1998; Waldorf, 1983; Zinberg, Harding, & Winkeller,1977; Zinberg & Jacobson, 1976) and controlled cocaine use (Cohen & Sas, 1994; Hammersley & Ditton, 1994; Mugford, 1995; Waldorf, Reinarman, & Murphy, 1991). In light of such evidence, an important priority for the addiction field is to develop a conceptualization that accommodates discontinuity over time (i.e., does not declare progressivity to be a required element of substance use disorders), and accommodates multiple pathways to recovery, including moderation and harm reduction (Marlatt, 1998; Witkiewitz & Marlatt, 2006).

What Can Be Gained by Studying the Process of Self-Change?

As reflected by the quotes in the next box, several notable addiction researchers have suggested that much can be gained by studying the self-change process.

- "Addiction looks very different if you study it in general populations compared to treated cases" (Robins, 1993, p. 1051).
- "Clinically defined 'alcoholics' constitute only a relatively small proportion of those whose drinking creates significant problems for themselves and society" (Cahalan, 1987, p. 363).
- "First, we cannot understand the natural history of alcoholism by drawing samples from clinic populations. Alcoholics with the most benign prognoses often never come to clinical attention" (Vaillant & Milofsky, 1984, p. 53).
- "The way ahead in alcoholism treatment research should embrace study of 'natural forces' that can then be captured and exploited by planned interventions" (Oxford & Edwards, 1977, p. 3).
- "If treatment as we currently understand it does not seem more effective than natural healing processes, then we need to understand those healing processes" (Vaillant, 1980, p. 18).

Another compelling reason for studying the process of self-change is that the addiction field has not provided enduring, effective treatments (Emrick, 1982; Miller & Heather, 1986; Sobell et al., 1990). Not one treatment can be pointed to as having demonstrated a high rate of sustained recoveries. In addition, little is known about how to successfully match individuals to treatments (Orford, 1999; Project MATCH Research Group, 1998a,b). An understanding of the self-change process has already been used to design and conduct a more effective intervention program (Sobell et al., 2002). Although few in number, some studies examining the process of self-change have started to shed some light on what triggers and maintains the recovery process (Sobell et al., 2000; Chapter 5).

An additional reason for studying the self-change process is that the vast majority of individuals with addictive behaviors never come to the attention of researchers or clinicians. For example, about three-quarters of ex-smokers and untreated alcohol abusers recover on their own (Dawson et al., 2005; Fiore et al., 1990; Hughes et al., 1996; Orleans, Schoenbach, et al., 1991; Sobell, Cunningham, & Sobell, 1996), and less than 3% of pathological gamblers (i.e., severe cases) have received treatment (National Gambling Impact Study Commission, 1999).

Doing It on My Own: Why I Did Not Seek Formal Treatment or Help

Respondent A: "I just felt that if I couldn't do it on my own a group of people isn't going to help me at all. A very good friend of mine he just got his ten-year pin so... he's very proud of it and he should be but I just couldn't. ... They are friends of mine but I just couldn't. If I can't quit by myself I just didn't see how anyone else was going to help me. I have nothing against AA, don't misunderstand me, it's a good organization but 15 to 20 people aren't going to tell me what to do."

Respondent B: "I felt I had a problem but I didn't figure it was like over the edge sort of thing and I figured it wasn't bad enough that I couldn't cure it myself."

Respondent C: "Well, I think I had the feeling that if I'm gonna beat this thing, it's up to me, and nobody else is going to make me stop drinking. It's my problem and I have to resolve it myself. Why should I go to, and ask somebody else and put my problems on their shoulders, when it's one of my own."

Respondent D: "I guess self pride like I didn't feel ... I wanted to try it without it. I think I may have gone to AA perhaps or some agency if I hadn't been able to beat it myself but initially I just wanted to do it on my own and thought I could."

Respondent E: "Only that I think it's a greater victory because I did it on my own. I didn't need anybody else."

The two recent reviews of the literature (Sobell et al., 2000; Chapter 5) revealed that substance abusers report the following three major reasons for not entering traditional treatment programs: (a) stigma associated with being

---

Stigma and Embarrassment: A Big Barrier

Respondent A: "Yes, because I think people usually look at alcoholics as down-and-outers, you know. And a person that's just a social drinker doesn't want to be associated with those kinds. Like the ones you see down in the lower end of the city, these winos. That's what you class yourself as a true alcoholic."

Respondent B: "I think the strongest one was the embarrassment before my relatives and my friends that I had to go to AA or some other place. If I had gone to those places I was admitting or letting everybody say that I was an alcoholic and to this day I don't think I was an alcoholic. I think I had a heavy drinking problem."

Respondent C: "I don't think anybody wants to be classified as an alcoholic or a drunk rummy. At least I didn't. I was embarrassed, yes."

Respondent D: "I don't feel I'm an alcoholic, period. I have ... I had a drinking problem but the word is terrible."

Respondent E: "Because I'm maybe a private person I wasn't the type that, you know, would go out and seek help and I would be embarrassed if a lot of people were ... heard about the problem."

labeled, (b) beliefs that their problems are not serious enough to require treatment (i.e., traditional programs are often too intense and too demanding for individuals who are not severely dependent), and (c) desire to handle their problem on their own.

Barriers to Treatment or Help-Seeking for Racial/Ethnic Minorities and Women

Several studies have also found significant gender differences in reports of barriers to treatment (Gomberg & Turnbull, 1990; Roman, 1988; Schmidt & Weisner, 1995; Schober & Annis, 1996; Thom, 1986, 1987). One study (Weisner, 1993) that examined differences among problem drinkers in treatment and in the general population found differences in the factors that influence treatment entry for women and men. In another study looking at gender differences, Weisner and Schmidt (1992) found that female problem drinkers were more likely than male problem drinkers to use non-alcohol-specific health care settings, particularly mental health treatment services, and to report greater symptom severity. Others have similarly found that women seek nontraditional avenues of help such as general health and mental health care settings for coping with their alcohol problems (Beckman & Kocel, 1982; Schmidt & Weisner, 1999; Schober & Annis, 1996).

It is likely that the availability and acceptance of professional help and treatment also influences the rates of natural recovery. According to Duckert (1989), the failure of treatment systems to adapt to the specific needs of female addicts and "the lack of more attractive treatment alternatives" (p. 176) are major reasons for the relative unwillingness of women to seek treatment. Therefore, natural recovery would be expected to occur more frequently among women than among men. Given the lower prevalence of problem drinking among women than among men (Blume, 1986) and that among heroin addicts there is a typical male–female ratio of 4:1 (Klingemann, 1994), small absolute numbers of female respondents are to be expected in self-change studies.

In a review of naturally recovered alcohol and drug abusers, the mean percentage of women across all studies was 31.6% (Sobell et al., 2000), a statistic only slightly higher than figures for alcohol treatment facilities,

---

Alcohol Abuse: A Worse Stigma for Women

Respondent A: "I feel that to be labeled an alcoholic, especially as a woman, is degrading and it means you're something kind of like ... you don't have any will power. You make an ass of yourself. It's sort of disgusting to me"

Respondent B: "Yes too embarrassing. Especially ... it's always OK for a man to drink and it's great for a man to seek help but as a woman, you look ... it's not quite the same thing."

Respondent C: "I didn't want to be found out. I didn't ... because I still think, perhaps it's not quite so much now but it is more of a stigma for a woman."

where one-quarter of the clients are female (National Institute on Drug Abuse, 1992). The fact that about one-third of all alcohol and drug abusers who naturally recover are female parallels results from brief treatments where larger than expected samples of females are recruited to treatment through advertisements (e.g., Sanchez-Craig, Neumann, Souzaformigoni, & Rieck, 1991; Sobell & Sobell, 1998).

Only a few studies have looked at gender differences in studies of self-change (Bischof, Rumpf, Hapke, Meyer, & John, 2000; Rounsaville & Kleber, 1985; Tucker & Gladsjo, 1993), and all have found an absence of significant variables as a function of gender between treated and untreated samples of alcohol and opiate abusers. One plausible explanation is that both brief treatments and self-change embody the concept of greater empowerment and thus are more appealing to women compared to entering traditional addiction treatment programs that are viewed as stigmatizing and promoting a sense of powerlessness.

In contrast to the sizable body of literature in the addictions field examining and identifying factors that affect treatment entry by gender, there are "very few studies that inform differences in service use by ethnicity" (Schmidt & Weisner, 1999, p. 79). Despite the fact that access to treatment for minorities has not been widely evaluated, there is evidence that factors such as lack of health insurance and a greater likelihood of living below the poverty level limit access to treatment for Hispanics and African-Americans (Gordis, 1994).

In an excellent review of ethnic and cultural minority groups, Castro, Proescholdbell, Abeita, and Rodriguez (1999) found that (a) past studies have shown that minority clients have questioned seeking mental health and substance abuse services from mainstream agencies, (b) there is a high dropout rate among minority clients who seek counseling, and it has been suggested that one reason for this high dropout rate is because counselors are not culturally empathic (Sue, Fujino, Hu, Takeuchi, & Zane, 1991), and (c) failure to engage clients in treatment either through rapport or raising positive expectations have been factors suggested as likely to affect dropout rates. A further reason for failure to enter treatment and high dropouts is that most substance abuse treatment programs have neither been designed or evaluated for minorities. In another large study of seriously mentally ill adults (Substance Abuse and Mental Health Administration, 2003), less than half received treatment in the past year, with almost half reporting that they either did not feel a need for treatment, could handle problems without treatment (10.4%), feared being committed or having to take medicine (9.25), or because of the stigma associated with seeking treatment (28.2%).

In summary, because of the stigma associated with entering substance abuse treatment in general, coupled with the reluctance of women and minorities to enter mainstream substance abuse programs, self-change studies and interventions for these two groups are critical.

Furthermore, cross-cultural comparisons of self-change within and between countries are needed to determine the generalizability of findings. Lastly, while national surveys have shown treatment utilization to vary by gender and ethnic groups, this may be due to any of several factors (e.g., agency discrimination, lack of interest, failure to recognize a problem, available services are not attractive or do not exist). Thus, one issue for the development of alternative services is to be sensitive to the needs of particular groups and individuals. The old adage of one size fits all is outdated.

Models of Change

Over the past 35 years, several models of change or models of decisional processes with inherent similarities have been posited. Although this chapter is not the forum to review these models in depth, a brief description of the prevailing models will help set the context for the studies and findings reported in subsequent chapters. At the heart of the decisional theories of behavior change is a cognitively based cost–benefit evaluation. Such models look at beliefs and feelings, in addition to their role in how decisions to change behavior occur. According to this view, what drives an addiction is that initially, and perhaps for some time thereafter, the positives of using outweigh the negatives (Orford, 2001, 1986). Over time, individuals weigh the pros and cons of their use and when they perceive that the negatives outweigh the positives, they then are more likely to decide to stop or reduce their use.

In a seminal research article, Eysenck (1952) questioned the effectiveness of psychotherapy for what was then called neurosis. Reviewing treatment studies published up to that time, Eysenck concluded that "roughly two-thirds of a group of neurotic patients will recover or improve to a marked extent within about two years of the onset of their illness" (p. 322). By virtue of his early questioning of the effectiveness of psychotherapy, Eysenck was also one of the first to try to understand the common elements of therapeutic change for behavior and mental health problems. From this time forward, several comprehensive models of change have been proposed that integrate different theoretical models of the change process (e.g., Goldfried, 1982).

Conflict Theory

Janis and Mann's (1968) conflict theory postulates that tension results when there is dissonance between attitudes. To reduce such dissonance, individuals must examine the positive and negative aspects of conflicting viewpoints and make a decision about how to lessen the conflict. Janis and Mann's decision-making model involves five stages of decision-making: (a) appraisal of a challenge, (b) appraisal of alternatives, (c) selection of the best alternative, (d) commitment to the new policy, and (e) adherence to the new policy despite negative feedback (Janis & Mann, 1968, 1977). An individual's effort to resolve tension (i.e., inner conflict) is thought to be a function of the amount of dissonance between beliefs.

Transtheoretical Model of Change

The transtheoretical model of change grew out of efforts to apply a set of common change processes from existing theories of therapy to the process of smoking cessation. In explaining behavior change, Prochaska and DiClemente (1984) used a five-stage model of change (i.e., precontemplation, contemplation, preparation, action, and maintenance) similar to the decision making stages put forth by Janis and Mann (1968). Prochaska and DiClemente's model, however, extends to change outside of therapy (Prochaska, DiClemente, & Norcross, 1992) and asserts that the stage that people are in reflects the likelihood of their changing (Prochaska, 1983). In the stages of change (SC) model, (a) precontemplators are individuals who are not considering changing, (b) contemplators are considering change, (c) preparation occurs when an individual starts to make plans to change, (d) individuals in the action stage are actively engaging in change, (e) individuals in the maintenance stage are sustaining their change, and lastly, (f) if a change attempt fails, the person is viewed as relapsing, and the stage process starts over.

This model has come under increasing scrutiny for not accounting adequately for the complexity of behavior change (Bandura, 1997; Budd & Rollnick, 1996; Carey, Purnine, Maisto, & Carey, 1999; Davidson, 1998; Sutton, 1996). It has been argued that the SC model is a complex way of describing behavior that can better be explained on a continuum, and that actual change from addictive behaviors does not move systematically through discrete stages (Budd & Rollnick, 1996; Carey et al., 1999; Sutton, 1996). In a true stage model, all stages must be passed through and no stage is revisited (Bandura, 1997). Thus, the SC model violates both of these premises because when individuals relapse, the model asserts that they must return to an earlier stage. Furthermore, because many who recover on their own successfully complete the change as soon as they decide to stop, this contradicts a stage development. In this regard, a recent study reported that 42.9% (15/35) of naturally recovered alcohol abusers successfully resolved on their first attempt (King & Tucker, 2000). Finally, it is a force fit to explain cases of true spontaneous remission (e.g., religion conversions) as passing through all stages rapidly, when what seems to occur is a quantum jump from precontemplation to action.

Lastly, although the transtheoretical model (TM) received considerable attention over the past decade and has inspired much of the empirical work on "readiness to change" (RTC), the psychometric literature provides inconsistent support for stages of change (Carey et al., 1999). Several have criticized the TM as being seriously flawed as a true stage model (Bandura, 1997; Brug et al., 2005; Littell & Girvin, 2002; Sutton, 2001; West, 2005, 2006). Carey et al. (1999) suggest that RTC (i.e., the degree to which an individual is motivated to change a problem behavior) may best be thought of as a "multidimensional and continuous construct with complex relationships to behavior, cognition, and environmental content" (p. 245).

Crystallization of Discontent

Baumeister (1996) has conceptualized the change process as related to individuals' personal perception of circumstances surrounding their behavior. He further asserts that people continually reevaluate their beliefs and behaviors in an effort to maintain consistency while also maintaining their beliefs. In this process, individuals make attributions that support their choices. Using examples from marriage and religion, Baumeister explains how people make extreme causal attributions in an effort to support their strongly held commitments or beliefs. Conversely, he posits that people discount disconfirming evidence to retain their commitments or beliefs.

Baumeister (1996) states that if consequences perceived by individuals as negative reach a certain threshold of discomfort, they will begin to see the consequences as related, thereby crystallizing the belief that the consequences are strongly linked with the behavior. He calls this process "crystallization of discontent." Thus, when an individual's perception crystallizes or solidifies negative aspects as related to a belief, affiliation, or behavior, the individual becomes motivated to change the situation. For example, one might end a committed relationship perceived to have become negative because of increased awareness of uncomfortable consequences beyond that which the individual is willing to tolerate. Another example would be a change in political beliefs as one comes to realize that the consequences of such beliefs are unacceptable. In the addiction field, Winick's (1962) maturation hypothesis is a good example of the process of crystallization of discontent. Addicts who quit using drugs talk about the extra "hustle" that is required over time to get drugs, with the strain building such that the negative consequences eventually reach a threshold of discomfort that then motivates behavior change (i.e., drug addicts are no longer willing to do this or they do not have the energy to continue doing drugs). This approach, however, fails to explain the occurrence of relapses (i.e., if discontent has crystallized, why would one again engage in the behavior?).

Becoming an Ex

In a process of change akin to Baumeister's crystallization of discontent, Ebaugh (1988) describes the change process as a role exit that includes developing a perception that a current role is not what individuals desired when they began the role. He refers to this as "Becoming an Ex." A good example of Ebaugh's role exiting involves nuns who, after taking their vows and entering the church, over time start to see things they strongly disagree with about the institution's policies. As their disenfranchisement builds, their commitment in the face of negative consequences (i.e., disagreement with church policy, defrocking) decreases and as the consequences build, dissonance increases between what they personally value and what their role entails. The point where individuals finally decide to exit a role and become motivated to do something different is seen as a focal point where persons have finally crystallized their discontent. Ebaugh (1988) feels "turning points" play an important role in behavior change as they "(a) announce to others and give ultimate reasons for change; (b) reduce cognitive dissonance and conflict; and (c) help mobilize resources" (p. 134).

Major Findings from Self-Change Studies

Although the study of natural recoveries is relatively new, the majority of the more recent studies have several findings in common. The major and notable findings from self-change studies are briefly discussed below.

Self-Change: A Major Pathway to Recovery

Several major surveys have shown that self-change appears to be the dominant pathway to recovery for: (a) *cigarettes* (Fiore et al., 1990; Hughes et al., 1996; Orleans, Rimer, et al., 1991; U.S. Department of Health and Human Services, 1988), (b) *alcohol* (Cunningham, Ansara, Wild, Toneatto, & Koski-Jännes, 1999; Cunningham et al., 2000; Dawson, 1996; Sobell, Cunningham, & Sobell, 1996), (c) *drugs* (Cunningham, 1999b), and (d) *gambling* (Hodgins, Wynne, & Makarchuk, 1999). The majority of the self-change studies of alcohol and drug abusers, included in the two major recent reviews (Sobell et al., 2000; Chapter 5), were conducted in the United States, Europe, and Canada (Sobell et al., 2000). The two recent reviews also found that the majority of self-change studies were conducted with alcohol abusers (75.0%, 30/40, Sobell et al., 2000; 81.8%, 18/22, Chapter 5).

In the first systematic study of natural recovery from marijuana, 25 cannabis abusers who were recovered for at least 1 year described their successful quit attempts, their past substance use, antecedents to recovery, and factors supportive of change through structured interviews and autobiographical narratives (Ellingstad, Sobell, Sobell, Eickleberry, & Golden, 2006). Marijuana cessation appears to have been motivated more by internal rather than external factors, and precipitants of attempts to quit involved more positive cognitive and affective components than social or health factors. The most commonly cited reason for stopping cannabis use was a change in how the participants viewed their cannabis use, followed by negative personal effects. The most commonly reported recovery maintenance factors were avoidance of situations in which cannabis was used, changes in lifestyle, and the development of non-cannabis-related interests. Lastly, over three quarters of respondents reported not seeking treatment because they believed it was not needed or because they wanted to quit on their own.

Can We Believe What They Tell Us?

Corroboration of self-changers' self-reports is important because respondents are being asked to recall events over long time periods. As with treated substance abusers, the primary confirmation of self-reports of self-changers has been by interviewing collaterals and thorough official records (reviewed in Sobell et al., 2000).

In examining the validity of self-reports among naturally recovered substance abusers, four major studies (Blomqvist, 1996; Gladsjo, Tucker, Hawkins, & Vuchinich, 1992; Klingemann, 1991; Sobell, Agrawal, & Sobell, 1997; Sobell et al., 1992, 1993; Tucker, 1995; Tucker et al., 1994) found that such individuals give reasonably accurate accounts of their pre- and post-recovery substance use as compared to reports from collaterals. These results parallel findings from studies of treated substance abusers (Babor, Brown, & Del Boca, 1990; Babor, Steinberg, Anton, & Del Boca, 2000; Maisto & Connors, 1992; Maisto, McKay, & Connors, 1990; Sobell, Toneatto, & Sobell, 1994). Although some studies (King & Tucker, 2000; Sobell et al., 1993; Toneatto et al., 1999) have reported problems in getting respondents to provide the name of someone who knew them when they had their problem (i.e., in the distant past, for example 10–20 years ago), one suggestion has been to incorporate reliability checks (e.g., asking the same questions when first screened into the project and when interviewed at a later date) into the interview process (Sobell et al., 2000). In summary, it can be concluded that naturally recovered substance abusers' reports of their pre- and post-recovery and related experiences generally are consistent with reports from other sources.

Stability of Natural Recoveries

In two recent reviews of self-change studies, it was found that across all studies the average recovery length was about 6 (Sobell et al., 2000) to 8 years (Chapter 5). Because substance use is a highly recurrent disorder (Marlatt & Gordon, 1985) and because several recent studies have suggested that stability of recovery with or without treatment does not seem to occur for at least 5 years (Dawson, 1996; De Soto, O'Donnell, & De Soto, 1989; Jin, Rourke, Patterson, Taylor, & Grant, 1998; Sobell, Sobell, & Kozlowski, 1995), it is suggested that studies of the self-change process use a minimum recovery period of 5 years or more. Such a recovery period parallels findings from the medical field showing that a survival rate of 5 or more years is associated with very stable outcomes from serious diseases (e.g., Bonadonna & Robustelli, 1988; Devita, Hellman, & Rosenberg, 1985).

Longitudinal studies of self-changers can also be used to examine how a change in the use of one substance relates to changes in other behaviors. There have been a few reports of respondents stopping one drug but increasing the use of another (Biernacki, 1986; Sobell et al., 1994), and one longitudinal study found that close to one-half of naturally recovered alcohol abusers reported increases in the use of nonalcoholic beverages within the first 6 months of stopping drinking alcohol; one-quarter also reported that they ate more sweet things, and about one-fifth reported smoking more cigarettes as well as eating more food (Sobell et al., 1995). However, some studies have contradicted the above findings by reporting that cessation of alcohol problems was associated with an increase in the likelihood of subsequent smoking cessation (Breslau et al., 1996).

A final issue concerns evaluating the use and abuse of all drugs, and not just the substance from which the person recovered. For example, the onset of heavy drinking has been reported by some naturally recovered cocaine abusers (Toneatto et al., 1999). In another study, for some naturally recovered heroin addicts who were totally abstinent, "the use of other drugs, especially alcohol, continued for longer periods and eventually became a problem in themselves" (Biernacki, 1986, p. 126).

What Triggers Self-Change? Thinking about Changing

One of the most common ways that self-change has been reported to occur is by a process described as a "cognitive appraisal" or a "cognitive evaluation" (i.e., individuals report that their initiation of change was preceded by a process of weighing the pros and cons of changing their substance use and eventually becoming committed to change). With the exception of gambling (Hodgins & el-Guebaly, 2000), cognitive appraisals have been reported across a variety of substances: (a) cigarettes (Carey et al., 1989), (b) drugs such as cocaine and heroin (Biernacki, 1986; Klingemann, 1992; Toneatto et al., 1999; Waldorf et al., 1991), and (c) alcohol (Granfield & Cloud, 1996; Klingemann, 1992; Ludwig, 1985; Sobell et al., 1993; Tucker et al., 1991). Further support for a cognitive appraisal process comes from the two major reviews of the literature. In the first review (Sobell et al., 2000), 27.5% of the studies reported such reasons for recovery, and 42.5% reported health-related reasons. In the second review (Chapter 5), three reasons (family-, health-, and finance-related) were endorsed by over one-half of the respondents. Cognitive appraisal was endorsed as a reason by 36.4% of respondents. Cognitive processes also have been reported for treated alcohol abusers with long-term recoveries (Amodeo

---

Recoveries Described as Cognitive Appraisals

Respondent A: "You know, I had thought about it for awhile and I had made up my mind that I wanted to do it. To me, I had a problem. It was a big problem. It was a bigger problem than I certainly thought that I had. And once I came to grips with it and realized that there was something wrong there ... that once I started thinking along those lines, it wasn't too long before I discovered what the problem was and why it was there. So if it's staring you in the face, I mean you got to do something about it ... so I just made up my mind to stop drinking. But this ... didn't happen Tuesday, Thursday, or Wednesday ... there's a lot more to it than that. I mean it's hard for me to sit here and tell you how I was thinking Tuesday, 1978. Or how I was thinking Wednesday, but the overall picture ... that's about as plain as I can make it ... how it came about. It was a process of ... over a period of time. It was a gradual thing ... it was probably over a year, maybe 18 months time."

Respondent B: "I looked at myself as being dirt, that I had not achieved more than that; when you are 36 years old, you begin to draw kind of a balance sheet, you realize you are you are down on the ground and you have spent everything on alcohol."

& Kurtz, 1990). Collectively, the results from several studies suggest that ongoing cognitive evaluations are central to the change process for many substance abusers who had problems but recovered on their own.

Recoveries associated with cognitive evaluations as opposed to recoveries precipitated by discrete events are of particular interest, as such recoveries have implications for clients in treatment as well as for individuals who want to change on their own but do not want to enter treatment. If a cognitive appraisal process (e.g., a balance sheet evaluating the pros and cons of continuing to use or not use) facilitates the resolution of substance abuse problems, then outcomes for clients might be improved by having them engage in an appraisal of their substance use. A decisional balance process has been used with smokers and for weight loss (Mann, 1972; Velicer, DiClemente, Prochaska, & Brandenberg, 1995), with college students to reduce alcohol use (Carey, Carey, Maisto, & Henson, 2006), and with problem drinkers in a large community intervention (Sobell, Cunningham, Sobell et al., 1996; Sobell, et al., 2002).

Maintaining Recoveries

In terms of coping strategies for maintaining recovery, the literature is scant but consistent. The single biggest factor associated with maintaining recoveries has been social support or a positive milieu, particularly from friends and family (reviewed in Carey et al., 1989; Klingemann, 1991; Sobell et al., 1993, 2000; Tuchfeld, 1981; Chapter 5). These findings are consistent with the literature showing that a positive family milieu or social support is the single most notable factor associated with positive outcomes in treatment studies (Billings & Moos, 1983; Moos, Finney, & Chan, 1982). For drug abusers, a common strategy for avoiding relapse has been to leave the environment where drugs are used and to break off social relationships with friends who use drugs (Sobell et al., 2000; Waldorf et al., 1991)

> **Resolved Alcohol Abuser**
>
> "[I stayed] away from old playmates and the old playground with people who drink and use ... [and stayed] connected with positive people in positive environments."

Conclusions and Future Directions

Multiple and converging lines of evidence have led to the recognition of self-change as an important pathway to recovery from alcohol and drug problems (American Psychiatric Association, 1994; Institute of Medicine, 1990; National Institute on Alcohol Abuse and Alcoholism, 2006b; Sobell et al., 2000). Research on the process of self-change has also led to the development of alternative interventions for problem drinkers (Chapter 8).

As reviewed earlier, research on the self-change process is important for several reasons, including the fact that the addiction field does not have enduring, effective treatments and has failed to reach large numbers of individuals with less severe problems. In this regard, Humphreys and Tucker (2002) persuasively argue that addiction intervention systems need to be responsive to the full range of problems, resources, treatment preferences, goals, motivations, and behavior-change pathways, including self-change. In conclusion, it is time for the addiction field to respond to the entire continuum of addictive behaviors by offering multiple and varied behavior-change pathways, including self-change.

As noted in two recent reviews (Sobell et al., 2000; Chapter 5), future studies of self-change need to be methodologically sound, including uniformly reporting demographic and substance use history information. If not, it will be impossible to draw conclusions across studies. In addition, a minimum recovery interval of 5 or more years has been suggested in order to draw valid conclusions that are based on stable recoveries. It will also be important to identify substance related differences (e.g., environmental change such as moving may be an important factor in natural recoveries from heroin, but less important for alcohol) and commonalities (e.g., social support may be a helpful maintenance factor for all substance abusers). Finally, since one of the goals of studying natural recoveries is to understand what factors might be associated with successful recoveries and to test those factors in clinical interventions, an in-depth qualitative understanding of what drives and maintains recovery in the absence of treatment or self-help is critical.

In summary, the proliferation of self-change studies in the addiction field and the findings of low-risk alcohol and drug use provide empirical support for a conceptualization of multiple pathways for recovery from addictive behaviors, including moderation and harm reduction. As well, the evidence clearly demonstrates that substance abuse problems should be viewed as lying along a continuum from no problems to mild problems to severe problems, rather than as a dichotomy. Such a view, of course, has implications for the types and intensities of services that can be offered. Lastly, with one exception (Sobell et al., 2001), there have been no investigations of the self-change processes across different cultural or social contexts (Klingemann, 2001). As discussed in Chapters 5 and 10, to substantiate that the phenomenon of self-change and what triggers it is not culture specific, cross-cultural evaluations are needed. Although the concept of self-change runs counter to the disease model of addictions and has been met with disbelief, there has been a significant increase in research in this area in the past decade.

References

Alden, L. (1988). Behavioral self-management controlled drinking strategies in a context of secondary prevention. *Journal of Consulting and Clinical Psychology, 56,* 280–286.

American Psychiatric Association. (1994). *Diagnostic and statistical manual of mental disorders* (4th ed.). Washington, DC: Author.

Amodeo, M., & Kurtz, N. (1990). Cognitive processes and abstinence in a treated alcoholic population. *International Journal of the Addictions, 25*, 983–1009.

Babor, T. F., Brown, J., & Del Boca, F. K. (1990). Validity of self-reports in applied research on addictive behaviors: Fact or fiction? *Addictive Behaviors, 12*, 5–32.

Babor, T. F., Steinberg, K., Anton, R., & Del Boca, F. (2000). Talk is cheap: Measuring drinking outcomes in clinical trials. *Journal of Studies on Alcohol, 61*(1), 55–63.

Bandura, A. (1997). The anatomy of stages of change. *American Journal of Health Promotion, 12*(1), 8–10.

Baumeister, R. F. (1996). The crystallization of discontent in the process of major life change. In T. F. Heatherton & J. L. Weinberger (Eds.), *Can personality change?* (pp. 281–297). Washington, DC: American Psychological Association.

Becker, H. S. (1963). *Outsiders.* New York: Free Press.

Beckman, L. J., & Kocel, K. M. (1982). Treatment-delivery system and alcohol abuse in women: Social policy and implications. *Journal of Social Issues, 38*, 139–151.

Biernacki, P. (1986). *Pathways from heroin addiction recovery without treatment.* Philadelphia: Temple University Press.

Billings, A. G., & Moos, R. H. (1983). Psychosocial processes of recovery among alcoholics and their families: Implications for clinicians and program evaluators. *Addictive Behaviors, 8*, 205–218.

Bischof, G., Rumpf, H. J., Hapke, U., Meyer, C., & John, U. (2000). Gender differences in natural recovery from alcohol dependence. *Journal of Studies on Alcohol, 61*(6), 783–786.

Bischof, G., Rumpf, H. J., Hapke, U., Meyer, C., & John, U. (2002). Remission from alcohol dependence without help: How restrictive should our definition of treatment be? *Journal of Studies on Alcohol, 63*(2), 229–236.

Blackwell, J. S. (1983). Drifting, controlling and overcoming: Opiate users who avoid becoming chronically dependent. *Journal of Drug Issues, 13*, 219–235.

Blomqvist, J. (1996). Paths to recovery from substance misuse: Change of lifestyle and the role of treatment. *Substance Use and Misuse, 31*, 1807–1852.

Blume, S. B. (1986). Women and alcohol: A review. *Journal of the American Medical Association, 256*, 1467–1470.

Bonadonna, G., & Robustelli, G. (1988). *Handbook of medical oncology.* Milano, Italy: Masson.

Breslau, N., Peterson, E., Schultz, L., Andreski, P., & Chilcoat, H. (1996). Are smokers with alcohol disorders less likely to quit? *American Journal of Public Health, 86*(7), 985–990.

Breslin, F. C., Sobell, S. L., Sobell, L. C., & Sobell, M. B. (1997). Alcohol treatment outcome methodology: State of the art 1989–1993. *Addictive Behaviors, 22*(2), 145–155.

Brug, J., Kremers, S., Conner, M., Harre, N., McKellar, S., & Whitelaw, S. (2005). The transtheoretical model and stages of change: A critique. Observations by five commentators on the paper by Adams, J. and White, M. (2004) Why don't stage-based activity promotion interventions work? *Health Education Research, 20*(2), 244–258.

Budd, R. J., & Rollnick, S. (1996). The structure of the Readiness to Change Questionnaire: A test of Prochaska & DiClemente's transtheoretical model. *British Journal of Health Psychology, 1*, 365–376.

Cahalan, D. (1970). *Problem drinkers: A national survey.* San Francisco: Jossey-Bass.

Cahalan, D. (1987). Studying drinking problems rather than alcoholism. In M. Galanter (Ed.), *Recent developments in alcoholism* (Vol. 5, pp. 363–372). New York: Plenum Press.

Cahalan, D., Cisin, I. H., & Crossley, H. M. (1969). *American drinking practices*. New Brunswick, NJ: Rutgers Center of Alcohol Studies.

Cahalan, D., & Room, R. (1974). *Problem drinking among American men*. New Brunswick, NJ: Rutgers Center of Alcohol Studies.

Carey, K., Carey, M., Maisto, S., & Henson, J. (2006). Brief motivational interventions for heavy college drinkers: A randomized controlled trial. *Journal of Consulting and Clinical Psychology, 74*(5), 943–954.

Carey, K. B., Purnine, D. M., Maisto, S. A., & Carey, M. P. (1999). Assessing readiness to change substance abuse: A critical review of instruments. *Clinical Psychology-Science and Practice, 6*(3), 245–266.

Carey, M. P., Snel, D. L., Carey, K. B., & Richards, C. S. (1989). Self-initiated smoking cessation: A review of the empirical literature from a stress and coping perspective. *Cognitive Therapy and Research, 13*, 323–341.

Castro, F. G., Proescholdbell, P. J., Abeita, L., & Rodriquez, D. (1999). Ethnic and cultural minority groups. In B. S. McCrady & E. E. Epstein (Eds.), *Addictions: A comprehensive guidebook* (pp. 499–526). New York: Oxford University Press.

Chiauzzi, E. J., & Liljegren, S. (1993). Taboo topics in addiction treatment: An empirical review of clinical folklore. *Journal of Substance Abuse Treatment, 10*, 303–316.

Cohen, P., & Sas, A. (1994). Cocaine use in Amsterdam in non deviant subcultures. *Addiction Research, 2*, 71–94.

Cunningham, J. A. (1999a). Resolving alcohol-related problems with and without treatment: The effects of different problem criteria. *Journal of Studies on Alcohol, 60*(4), 463–466.

Cunningham, J. A. (1999b). Untreated remissions from drug use: The predominant pathway. *Addictive Behaviors, 24*(2), 267–270.

Cunningham, J. A., Ansara, D., Wild, T. C., Toneatto, T., & Koski-Jännes, A. (1999). What is the price of perfection? The hidden costs of using detailed assessment instruments to measure alcohol consumption. *Journal of Studies on Alcohol, 60*(6), 756–758.

Cunningham, J. A., & Breslin, F. C. (2004). Only one in three people with alcohol abuse or dependence ever seek treatment. *Addictive Behaviors, 29*(1), 221–223.

Cunningham, J. A., Lin, E., Ross, H. E., & Walsh, G. W. (2000). Factors associated with untreated remissions from alcohol abuse or dependence. *Addictive Behaviors, 25*(2), 317–321.

Cunningham, J. A., Sobell, L. C., & Chow, V. M. C. (1993). What's in a label? The effects of substance types and labels on treatment considerations and stigma. *Journal of Studies on Alcohol, 54*, 693–699.

Cunningham, J. A., Sobell, L. C., & Sobell, M. B. (1999). Changing perceptions about self-change and moderate-drinking recoveries from alcohol problems: What can and should be done? *Journal of Applied Social Psychology, 29*(2), 291–299.

Davidson, R. (1998). The transtheoretical model: A critical overview. In W. R. Miller & N. Heather (Eds.), *Treating addictive behaviors* (2nd ed., pp. 25–38). New York: Plenum Press.

Dawson, D. A. (1996). Correlates of past-year status among treated and untreated persons with former alcohol dependence: United States, 1992. *Alcoholism: Clinical and Experimental Research, 20*, 771–779.

Dawson, D. A., Grant, B. F., Stinson, F. S., Chou, P. S., Huang, B., & Ruan, W. J. (2005). Recovery from DSM-IV alcohol dependence: United States, 2001–2002. *Addiction, 100*(3), 281–292.

De Soto, C. B., O'Donnell, W. E., & De Soto, J. L. (1989). Long-term recovery in alcoholics. *Alcoholism: Clinical and Experimental Research, 13*, 693–697.

Devita, V. T. J., Hellman, S., & Rosenberg, S. A. (1985). *Cancer: Principles and practice of oncology* (2nd ed.). New York: J. P. Lippincott.

Drew, L. R. (1968). Alcoholism as a self-limiting disease. *Quarterly Journal of Studies on Alcohol, 29*, 956–967.

Duckert, F. (Cartographer). (1989). "Controlled drinking": A complicated and contradictory field. In F. Duckert, A. Koski-Jännes, & S. Rönnberg (Eds.), *Perspectives on controlled drinking* (pp. 39–54). Helsinki: Nordic Council for Alcohol and Drug Research, NAD Publication No. 17.

Dupont, R. L. (1993). Foreword, in G. R. Ross *Treating adolescent substance abuse.* Boston: Allyn & Bacon.

Ebaugh, H. R. F. (1988). *Becoming an ex: The process of role exit.* Chicago: University of Chicago Press.

Ellingstad, T. P., Sobell, L. C., Sobell, M. B., Eickleberry, L., & Golden, C. J. (2006). Self-change: A pathway to cannabis abuse resolution. *Additive Behaviors, 31*(3), 519–530.

Emrick, C. D. (Ed.). (1982). *Evaluation of alcoholism psychotherapy methods.* New York: Gardner Press.

Erickson, P. G., & Alexander, B. K. (1989). Cocaine and addictive liability. *Social Pharmacology, 3*, 249–270.

Eysenck, H. J. (1952). The effects of psychotherapy: An evaluation. *Journal of Consulting Psychology, 16*, 319–324.

Fagerström, K. O., Kunze, M., Schoberberger, R., Breslau, N., Hughes, J. R., Hurt, R. D., et al. (1996). Nicotine dependence versus smoking prevalence: Comparisons among countries and categories of smokers. *Tobacco Control, 5*, 52–56.

Ferris, J. (1994, June). *Comparison of public perceptions of alcohol, drug and other tobacco addictions—moral vs. disease models.* Paper presented at the 20th annual Alcohol Epidemiology Symposium, Ruschlikon, Switzerland.

Fillmore, K. M., Hartka, E., Johnstone, B. M., Speiglman, R., & Temple, M. T. (1988, June). *Spontaneous remission of alcohol problems: A critical review.* Paper commissioned and supported by the Institute of Medicine, Washington, DC.

Fiore, M. C., Novotny, T. E., Pierce, J. P., Giovino, G. A., Hatziandreu, E. J., Newcomb, P. A., et al. (1990). Methods used to quit smoking in the United States. *Journal of the American Medical Association, 263*, 2760–2765.

Fleming, M., & Manwell, L. B. (1999). Brief intervention in primary care settings: A primary treatment method for at-risk, problem, and dependent drinkers. *Alcohol Health & Research World, 23*(2), 128–137.

Fleming, M. F., Manwell, L. B., Barry, K. L., Adams, W., & Stauffacher, E. A. (1999). Brief physician advice for alcohol problems in older adults: A randomized community-based trial. *Journal of Family Practice, 48*, 378–384.

Fleming, M. F., Mundt, M. P., French, M. T., Manwell, L. B., Stauffacher, E. A., & Barry, K. L. (2000). Benefit-cost analysis of brief physician advice with problem drinkers in primary care settings. *Medical Care, 38*(1), 7–18.

Fleming, M. F., Mundt, M. P., French, M. T., Manwell, L. B., Stauffacher, E. A., & Barry, K. L. (2002). Brief physician advice for problem alcohol drinkers: Long-term efficacy and benefit-cost analysis. *Alcoholism: Clinical and Experimental Research, 26*(1), 36–43.

Foulds, J. (1996). Strategies for smoking cessation. *British Medical Bulletin, 52*, 157–173.

Giffen, C. A. (1991). Community intervention trial for smoking cessation (COMMIT): Summary of design and intervention. *Journal of the National Cancer Institute, 83*, 1620–1628.

Gladsjo, J. A., Tucker, J. A., Hawkins, J. L., & Vuchinich, R. E. (1992). Adequacy of recall of drinking patterns and event occurrences associated with natural recovery from alcohol problems. *Addictive Behaviors, 17*, 347–358.

Goldfried, M. R. (1982). *Converging themes in psychotherapy.* New York: Springer.

Gomberg, E. S. L., & Turnbull, J. E. (1990, June). *Alcoholism in women: Pathways to treatment.* Paper presented at the Research Society on Alcoholism Annual Meeting, Toronto, Ontario, Canada.

Gordis, E. (1994). Alcohol and minorities. *Alcohol Alert* (NIAAA), No. 23 PH 347, 1–5.

Granfield, R., & Cloud, W. (1996). The elephant that no one sees: Natural recovery among middle-class addicts. *Journal of Drug Issues, 26*(1), 45–61.

Grant, B. F. (1997). Barriers to alcoholism treatment: Reasons for not seeking treatment in a general population sample. *Journal of Studies on Alcohol, 58*(4), 365–371.

Green, S. B., Corle, D. K., Gail, M. H., Mark, S. D., Pee, D., Freedman, L. S., et al. (1995). Interplay between design and analysis for behavioral intervention trials with community as the unit of randomization. *American Journal of Epidemiology, 142*(6), 587–593.

Hammersley, R., & Ditton, J. (1994). Cocaine careers in a sample of Scottish users. *Addiction Research, 2*, 51–70.

Happel, H.-V., Fischer, R., & Wittfeld, I. (1993). *Selbstorganisierter Ausstieg. Überwindung der Drogenabhängigkeit ohne professionelle Hilfe (Endbericht).* Frankfurt: Integrative Drogenhilfe an der Fachhochschule Ffm L.V.

Heather, N. (1989). Psychology and brief interventions. *British Journal of Addiction, 84*, 357–370.

Heather, N. (1990). *Brief intervention strategies.* New York: Pergamon.

Heather, N. (1994). Brief interventions on the world map. *Addiction, 89*, 665–667.

Hingson, R., Scotch, N., Day, N., & Culbert, A. (1980). Recognizing and seeking help for drinking problems. *Journal of Studies on Alcohol, 11*, 1102–1117.

Hodgins, D. C., & el-Guebaly, N. (2000). Natural and treatment-assisted recovery from gambling problems: A comparison of resolved and active gamblers. *Addiction, 95*(5), 777–789.

Hodgins, D. C., Wynne, H., & Makarchuk, K. (1999). Pathways to recovery from gambling problems: Follow-up from a general population survey. *Journal of Gambling Studies, 15*, 93–104.

Hughes, J. R., Cummings, K. M., & Hyland, A. (1999). Ability of smokers to reduce their smoking and its association with future smoking cessation. *Addiction, 94*(1), 109–114.

Hughes, J. R., Fiester, S., Goldstein, M., Resnick, M., Rock, N., Ziedonis, D., et al. (1996). Practice guidelines for the treatment of patients with nicotine dependence. *American Journal of Psychiatry, 153*(10 Suppl.), 1–31.

Humphreys, K., Moos, R. H., & Finney, J. W. (1995). Two pathways out of drinking problems without professional treatment. *Addictive Behaviors, 20*(4), 427–441.

Humphreys, K., & Tucker, J. A. (2002). Toward more responsive and effective intervention systems for alcohol-related problems: Introduction. *Addiction, 97*(2), 126–132.

Hunt, M. (1998). *The new know-nothings: The political foes of the scientific study of human nature.* Piscataway, NJ: Transaction Publishers.

Institute of Medicine. (1990). *Broadening the base of treatment for alcohol problems.* Washington, DC: National Academy Press.

Janis, I. L., & Mann, L. (Eds.). (1968). *A conflict-theory approach to attitude change and decision making.* New York: Academic Press.

Janis, I. L., & Mann, L. (1977). *Decision-making: A psychological analysis of conflict, choice, and commitment.* New York: Free Press.

Jin, H., Rourke, S. B., Patterson, T. L., Taylor, M. J., & Grant, I. (1998). Predictors of relapse in long-term abstinent alcoholics. *Journal of Studies on Alcohol, 59*(6), 640–646.

Johnson, V. E. (1980). *I'll quit tomorrow* (rev. ed.). San Francisco: Harper & Row.

Kendell, R. E., & Staton, M. C. (1966). The fate of untreated alcoholics. *Quarterly Journal of Studies on Alcohol, 27*, 30–41.

King, M. P., & Tucker, J. A. (2000). Behavior change patterns and strategies distinguishing moderation drinking and abstinence during the natural resolution of alcohol problems without treatment. *Psychology of Addictive Behaviors, 14*(1), 48–55.

Kissin, B., Rosenblatt, S. M., & Machover, K. (1968). Prognostic factors in alcoholism. *Psychiatric Research Reports, 24*, 22–43.

Klingemann, H. K. H. (1991). The motivation for change from problem alcohol and heroin use. *British Journal of Addiction, 86*, 727–744.

Klingemann, H. K. H. (1992). Coping and maintenance strategies of spontaneous remitters from problem use of alcohol and heroin in Switzerland. *International Journal of the Addictions, 27*, 1359–1388.

Klingemann, H. K. H. (1994). Environmental influences which promote or impede change in substance behaviour. In G. Edwards & M. M. Laer (Eds.), *Addiction: Process of change* (Vol. 34, pp. 131–161). New York: Oxford University Press.

Klingemann, H. K. H. (2001). Natural recovery from alcohol problems. In N. Heather, T. J. Peters, & T. Stockwell (Eds.), *International handbook of alcohol dependence and problems* (pp. 649–662). New York: John Wiley & Sons.

Labouvie, E. (1996). Maturing out of substance abuse: Selection and self-correction. *Journal of Drug Issues, 26*, 457–476.

Law, M., & Tang, J. L. (1995). An analysis of the effectiveness of interventions intended to help people stop smoking. *Archives of Internal Medicine, 155*(18), 1933–1941.

Littell, J. H., & Girvin, H. (2002). Stages of change: A critique. *Behavior Modification, 26*(2), 223–273.

Ludwig, A. M. (1985). Cognitive processes associated with "spontaneous" recovery from alcoholism. *Journal of Studies on Alcohol, 46*, 53–58.

Maisto, S. A., & Connors, G. J. (1992). Using subject and collateral reports to measure alcohol consumption. In R. Z. Litten & J. Allen (Eds.), *Measuring alcohol consumption: Psychosocial and biological methods* (pp. 73–96). Totowa, NJ: Humana Press.

Maisto, S. A., McKay, J. R., & Connors, G. J. (1990). Self-report issues in substance abuse: State of the art and future directions. *Behavioral Assessment, 12*, 117–134.

Mann, L. (1972). Use of a "balance sheet" procedure to improve the quality of personal decision making: A field experiment with college applicants. *Journal of Vocational Behavior, 2*, 291–300.

Mariezcurrena, R. (1994). Recovery from addictions without treatment: Literature review. *Scandinavian Journal of Behaviour Therapy, 23*, 131–154.

Marlatt, G. A. (1983). The controlled drinking controversy: A commentary. *American Psychologist, 38*, 1097–1110.

Marlatt, G. A. (Ed.). (1998). *Harm reduction: Pragmatic strategies for managing high-risk behaviors.* New York: Guilford.

Marlatt, G. A., & Gordon, J. R. (1985). *Relapse prevention.* New York: Guilford Press.

Miller, W. R., & Heather, N. (1986). *Treating addictive behaviors: Processes of change.* New York: Plenum.

Moos, R. H., Finney, J. W., & Chan, D. (1982). The process of recovery from alcoholism. II. Comparing spouses of alcoholic patients and matched community controls. *Journal of Studies on Alcohol, 43,* 888–909.

Mugford, S. K. (1995). Recreational cocaine use in three Australian cities. *Addiction Research, 3,* 95–108.

Mulford, H. (1988). Enhancing the natural control of drinking behavior: Catching up with common sense. *Contemporary Drug Problems, 17,* 321–334.

Narrow, W. E., Regier, D. A., Rae, D. S., Manderscheid, R. W., & Locke, B. Z. (1993). Use of services by persons with mental and addictive disorders: Findings from the National Institute of Mental Health epidemiologic catchment area program. *Archives of General Psychiatry, 50,* 95–107.

National Gambling Impact Study Commission. (1999). *Final Report.* Washington, DC: U.S. Government Printing Office.

National Institute on Alcohol Abuse and Alcoholism. (2006a). *Alcohol use and alcohol use disorders in the United States: Main findings from the 2001–2002 National Epidemiologic Survey on Alcohol and Related Conditions (NESARC).* Bethesda, MD: National Institutes of Health.

National Institute on Alcohol Abuse and Alcoholism. (2006b). National epidemiologic survey on alcohol and related conditions. *Alcohol Alert, 70,* 1–5.

National Institute on Drug Abuse. (1992). *Highlights from the 1989 National Drug and Alcoholism Treatment Unit Survey (NDATUS).* Rockville, MD: National Institute on Drug Abuse.

Orford, J. (Ed.). (1986). *Critical conditions for change in the addictive behaviors.* New York: Plenum Press.

Orford, J. (1999). Future research directions: A commentary on Project MATCH. *Addiction, 94*(1), 62–66.

Orford, J. (2001). Addiction as excessive appetite. *Addiction, 96*(1), 15–31.

Orford, J., & Edwards, G. (1977). *Alcoholism: A comparison of treatment and advice with a study of the influence of marriage.* New York: Oxford University Press.

Orleans, C. T., Rimer, B. K., Cristinzio, S., Keintz, M. K., & Fleisher, L. (1991). A national survey of older smokers: A treatment needs of a growing population. *Health Psychology, 10,* 343–351.

Orleans, C. T., Schoenbach, V. J., Wagner, E. H., Quade, D., Salmon, M. A., Pearson, D. C., et al. (1991). Self-help quit smoking interventions: Effects of self-help materials, social support instructions, and telephone counseling. *Journal of Consulting and Clinical Psychology, 59,* 439–448.

Price, R. K., Risk, N. K., & Spitznagel, E. L. (2001). Remission from drug abuse over a 25-year period: Patterns of remission and treatment use. *American Journal of Public Health, 91*(7), 1107–1113.

Prochaska, J. O. (1983). Self-changers versus therapy versus Schachter [Letter to the editor]. *American Psychologist, 38,* 853–854.

Prochaska, J. O., & DiClemente, C. C. (1984). *The transtheoretical approach: Crossing traditional boundaries of therapy.* Homewood, IL: Dow Jones-Irwin.

Prochaska, J. O., DiClemente, C. C., & Norcross, J. C. (1992). In search of how people change. *American Psychologist, 47,* 1102–1114.

Project MATCH Research Group. (1998a). Matching alcoholism treatments to client heterogeneity: Project MATCH three-year drinking outcomes. *Alcoholism: Clinical and Experimental Research, 22,* 1300–1311.

Project MATCH Research Group. (1998b). Matching alcoholism treatments to client heterogeneity: Treatment main effects and matching effects on drinking during treatment. *Journal of Studies on Alcohol, 59*(6), 631–639.

Raimo, E. B., Daeppen, J. B., Smith, T. L., Danko, G. P., & Schuckit, M. A. (1999). Clinical characteristics of alcoholism in alcohol-dependent subjects with and without a history of alcohol treatment [comment]. *Alcoholism: Clinical & Experimental Research, 23*(10), 1605–1613.

Raimo, E. B., & Schuckit, M. A. (1998). Alcohol dependence and mood disorders. *Addictive Behaviors, 23*(6), 933–946.

Robins, L. N. (1993). Vietnam veterans' rapid recovery from heroin addiction: A fluke or normal expectation? *Addiction, 88*, 1041–1054.

Roizen, R. (1977). *Barriers to alcoholism treatment.* Berkeley, CA: Alcohol Research Group.

Roizen, R., Cahalan, D., & Shanks, P. (1978). Spontaneous remission among untreated problem drinkers. In D. B. Kandel (Ed.), *Longitudinal research on drug use: Empirical findings and methodological issues* (pp. 197–221). Washington, DC: Hemisphere.

Roman, P. M. (1988). Treatment issues. In National Institute on Alcohol Abuse and Alcoholism (Ed.), *Women and alcohol use: A review of the research literature* (ADM 88-1574, pp. 38–45). Washington, DC: U. S. Government Printing Office.

Room, R. (Ed.). (1977). *Measurement and distribution of drinking patterns and problems in general populations.* Geneva: World Health Organization.

Room, R., & Greenfield, T. (1993). Alcoholics Anonymous, other 12 step movements and psychotherapy in the United States population, 1990. *Addiction, 88*, 555–562.

Rosenberg, H. (1993). Prediction of controlled drinking by alcoholics and problem drinkers. *Psychological Bulletin, 113*, 129–139.

Rosenberg, H., & Davis, L. A. (1994). Acceptance of moderate drinking by alcohol treatment services in the United States. *Journal of Studies on Alcohol, 55*, 167–172.

Rounsaville, B. J., & Kleber, H. D. (1985). Untreated opiates addicts: How do they differ from those seeking treatment? *Archives of General Psychiatry, 42*, 1072–1077.

Rumpf, H. J., Bischof, G., Hapke, U., Meyer, C., & John, U. (2000). Studies on natural recovery from alcohol dependence: Sample selection bias by media solicitation? *Addiction, 95*(5), 765–775.

Rush, B. (1814). *An inquiry into the effects of ardent spirits upon the human body and mind* (8th ed.). Brookfield: E. Merriam & Company.

Rush, B., & Allen, B. A. (1997). Attitudes and beliefs of the general public about treatment for alcohol problems. *Canadian Journal of Public Health, 88*, 41–43.

Sanchez-Craig, M., Neumann, B., Souzaformigoni, M., & Rieck, L. (1991). Brief treatment for alcohol dependence: Level of dependence and treatment outcome. *Alcohol and Alcoholism, S1*, 515–518.

Saunders, W. M., & Kershaw, P. W. (1979). Spontaneous remission from alcoholism: A community study. *British Journal of Addiction, 74*, 251–265.

Schachter, S. (1982). Recidivism and self-cure of smoking and obesity. *American Psychologist, 37*, 436–444.

Schasre, R. (1966). Cessation patterns among neophyte heroin users. *International Journal of the Addictions, 1*, 23–32.

Schmidt, L., & Weisner, C. (1995). The emergence of problem-drinking women as a special population in need of treatment. In M. Galanter (Ed.), *Recent developments in alcoholism* (Vol. 12, pp. 309–334). New York: Plenum Press.

Schmidt, L. A., & Weisner, C. M. (1999). Public health perspectives on access and need for substance abuse treatment. In J. A. Tucker, D. A. Donovan, & G. A. Marlatt

(Eds.), *Changing addictive behavior: Bridging clinical and public health strategies* (pp. 67–96). New York: Guilford Press.

Schober, R., & Annis, H. M. (1996). Barriers to help-seeking for change in drinking: A gender-focused review of the literature. *Addictive Behaviors, 21*(1), 81–92.

Shaffer, H. J., & Jones, S. B. (1989). *Quitting cocaine: The struggle against impulse.* Lexington, MA: Lexington Books.

Shewan, D., Dalgarno, P., Marshall, A., Lowe, E., Campbell, M., Nicholson, S., et al. (1998). Patterns of heroin use among a non-treatment sample in Glasgow (Scotland). *Addiction Research, 6*(3), 215–234.

Snow, M. (1973). Maturing out of narcotic addiction in New York City. *International Journal of the Addictions, 8*, 921–938.

Sobell, L. C., Agrawal, S., Annis, H., Ayala-Velazquez, H., Echeverria, L., Leo, G. I., et al. (2001). Cross-cultural evaluation of two drinking assessment instruments: Alcohol Timeline Followback and Inventory of Drinking Situations. *Substance Use and Misuse, 36*(3), 313–331.

Sobell, L. C., Agrawal, S., & Sobell, M. B. (1997). Factors affecting agreement between alcohol abusers' and their collaterals' reports. *Journal of Studies on Alcohol, 58*(4), 405–413.

Sobell, L. C., Cunningham, J. A., & Sobell, M. B. (1996). Recovery from alcohol problems with and without treatment: Prevalence in two population surveys. *American Journal of Public Health, 86*(7), 966–972.

Sobell, L. C., Cunningham, J. A., Sobell, M. B., Agrawal, S., Gavin, D. R., Leo, G. I., et al. (1996). Fostering self-change among problem drinkers: A proactive community intervention. *Addictive Behaviors, 21*(6), 817–833.

Sobell, L. C., Ellingstad, T. P., & Sobell, M. B. (2000). Natural recovery from alcohol and drug problems: Methodological review of the research with suggestions for future directions. *Addiction, 95*(5), 749–764.

Sobell, L. C., & Sobell, M. B. (1995). Alcohol consumption measures. In J. P. Allen & M. Columbus (Eds.), *Assessing alcohol problems: A guide for clinicians and researchers* (pp. 55–73). Rockville, MD: National Institute on Alcohol Abuse and Alcoholism.

Sobell, L. C., Sobell, M. B., Leo, G. I., Agrawal, S., Johnson-Young, L., & Cunningham, J. A. (2002). Promoting self-change with alcohol abusers: A community-level mail intervention based on natural recovery studies. *Alcoholism: Clinical and Experimental Research, 26*, 936–948.

Sobell, L. C., Sobell, M. B., & Toneatto, T. (1992). Recovery from alcohol problems without treatment. In N. Heather, W. R. Miller, & J. Greeley (Eds.), *Self-control and the addictive behaviours* (pp. 198–242). New York: Maxwell MacMillan.

Sobell, L. C., Sobell, M. B., Toneatto, T., & Leo, G. I. (1993). What triggers the resolution of alcohol problems without treatment? *Alcoholism: Clinical and Experimental Research, 17*, 217–224.

Sobell, L. C., Toneatto, A., & Sobell, M. B. (1990). Behavior therapy (Alcoholism and substance abuse). In A. S. Bellack & M. Hersen (Eds.), *Handbook of comparative treatments for adult disorders* (pp. 479–505). New York: John Wiley.

Sobell, L. C., Toneatto, T., & Sobell, M. B. (1994). Behavioral assessment and treatment planning for alcohol, tobacco, and other drug problems: Current status with an emphasis on clinical applications. *Behavior Therapy, 25*, 533–580.

Sobell, M. B., & Sobell, L. C. (1995). Controlled drinking after 25 years: How important was the great debate? *Addiction, 90*, 1149–1153.

Sobell, M. B., & Sobell, L. C. (1998). Guiding self-change. In W. R. Miller & N. Heather (Eds.), *Treating addictive behaviors* (2nd ed., pp. 189–202). New York: Plenum Press.

Sobell, M. B., & Sobell, L. C. (2006). Obstacles to the adoption of low risk drinking goals in the treatment of alcohol problems in the United States: A commentary. *Addiction Research & Theory, 14*(1), 19–24.

Sobell, M. B., Sobell, L. C., & Kozlowski, L. T. (1995). Dual recoveries from alcohol and smoking problems. In J. B. Fertig & J. A. Allen (Eds.), *Alcohol and tobacco: From basic science to clinical practice* (NIAAA Research Monograph No. 30, pp. 207–224). Rockville, MD: National Institute on Alcohol Abuse and Alcoholism.

Stall, R. (1983). An examination of spontaneous remission from problem drinking in the bluegrass region of Kentucky. *Journal of Drug Issues, 13*, 191–206.

Substance Abuse and Mental Health Administration. (2003). *Reasons for not receiving treatment among adults with serious mental illness* (Vol. 2003). Rockville, MD: U.S. Department of Health and Human Services.

Sue, S., Fujino, D. C., Hu, L., Takeuchi, T., & Zane, N. W. S. (1991). Community mental health services for ethnic minority groups: A test of the cultural responsiveness hypothesis. *Journal of Consulting and Clinical Psychology, 59*, 533–540.

Sutton, S. (1996). Can stages of change provide guidelines in the treatment of addictions? In G. Edwards & C. Dare (Eds.), *Psychotherapy, psychological treatments and the addictions* (pp. 189–205). London: Cambridge University Press.

Sutton, S. (2001). Back to the drawing board? A review of applications of the transtheoretical model to substance use. *Addiction, 96*(1), 175–186.

Thom, B. (1986). Sex differences in help-seeking for alcohol problems—1. The barriers to help-seeking. *British Journal of Addiction, 81*, 777–788.

Thom, B. (1987). Sex differences in help-seeking for alcohol problems—2. Entry into treatment. *British Journal of Addiction, 82*, 989–997.

Toneatto, T., Sobell, L. C., Sobell, M. B., & Rubel, E. (1999). Natural recovery from cocaine dependence. *Psychology of Addictive Behaviors, 13*(4), 259–268.

Tuchfeld, B. S. (1976). *Changes in patterns of alcohol use without the aid of formal treatment: An exploratory study of former problem drinkers.* Research Triangle Park, NC: Research Triangle Institute.

Tuchfeld, B. S. (1981). Spontaneous remission in alcoholics: Empirical observations and theoretical implications. *Journal of Studies on Alcohol, 42*, 626–641.

Tucker, J. A. (1995). Predictors of help-seeking and the temporal relationship of help to recovery among treated and untreated recovered problem drinkers. *Addiction, 90*(6), 805–809.

Tucker, J. A., & Gladsjo, J. A. (1993). Help seeking and recovery by problem drinkers: Characteristics of drinkers who attend Alcoholics Anonymous or formal treatment or who recovered without assistance. *Addictive Behaviors, 18*, 529–542.

Tucker, J. A., Vuchinich, R. E., & Gladsjo, J. A. (1991). Environmental influences on relapse in substance use disorders. *International Journal of the Addictions, 25*, 1017–1050.

Tucker, J. A., Vuchinich, R. E., & Gladsjo, J. A. (1994). Environmental events surrounding natural recovery from alcohol-related problems. *Journal of Studies on Alcohol, 55*, 401–411.

Tucker, J. A., Vuchinich, R. E., Gladsjo, J. A., Hawkins, J. L., & Sherrill, J. T. (1989, November). *Environmental influences on the natural resolution of alcohol problems without treatment.* Paper presented at a poster session at the annual meeting of the Association for the Advancement of Behavior Therapy, Washington, DC.

U.S. Department of Health and Human Services. (1988). *The health consequences of smoking: Nicotine addiction. A report of the Surgeon General.* Washington, DC: U.S. Government Printing Office.

Vaillant, G. E. (Ed.). (1980). *The doctor's dilemma* (27A, CD ed.). London: Croom Helm.

Vaillant, G. E. (1995). *The natural history of alcoholism revisited.* Cambridge, MA: Harvard University Press.

Vaillant, G. E., & Milofsky, E. S. (1982). Natural history of male alcoholism. IV. Paths to recovery. *Archives of General Psychiatry, 39,* 127–133.

Vaillant, G. E., & Milofsky, E. S. (1984). Natural history of male alcoholism: Paths to recovery. In D. W. Goodwin, K. T. V. Dusen, & S. A. Mednick (Eds.), *Longitudinal research in alcoholism* (pp. 53–71). Kluwer-Nijhoff Publishing.

Velicer, W. F., DiClemente, C. C., Prochaska, J. O., & Brandenberg, N. (1995). Decisional balance measure for assessing and predicting smoking status. *Journal of Personality and Social Psychology, 48,* 1279–1289.

Waldorf, D. (1983). Natural recovery from opiate addiction: Some social-psychological processes of untreated recovery. *Journal of Drug Issues, 13,* 237–280.

Waldorf, D., Reinarman, C., & Murphy, S. (1991). *Cocaine changes: The experience of using and quitting.* Philadelphia, PA: Temple University.

Weisner, C. (1987). The social ecology of alcohol treatment in the U. S. In M. Galanter (Ed.), *Recent developments in alcoholism* (Vol. 5, pp. 203–243). New York: Plenum Press.

Weisner, C. (1993). Toward an alcohol treatment entry model: A comparison of problem drinkers in the general population and in treatment. *Alcoholism: Clinical and Experimental Research, 17,* 746–752.

Weisner, C., & Schmidt, L. (1992). Gender disparities in treatment for alcohol problems. *Journal of the American Medical Association, 268,* 1872–1876.

West, R. (2005). Time for a change: Putting the Transtheoretical (Stages of Change) Model to rest. *Addiction, 100*(8), 1036–1039.

West, R. (2006). The transtheoretical model of behaviour change and the scientific method. *Addiction, 101*(6), 774–778.

Winick, C. (1962). Maturing out of narcotic addiction. *Bulletin on Narcotics, 14,* 1–7.

Witkiewitz, K., & Marlatt, G. A. (2006). Overview of harm reduction treatments for alcohol problems. *International Journal of Drug Policy, 17*(4), 285–294.

Zinberg, N. E., Harding, W. M., & Winkeller, M. (1977). A study of social regulatory mechanism in controlled illicit drug users. *Journal of Drug Issues, 7,* 117–133.

Zinberg, N. E., & Jacobson, R. C. (1976). The natural history of "chipping." *American Journal of Psychiatry, 133,* 37–40.

2
Self-Change from Alcohol and Drug Abuse: Often-Cited Classics

Jan Blomqvist

The Setting

As maintained by Toulmin (1961), a certain event or condition can appear as a phenomenon—something that is problematic and needs explaining—only against the background of some inferred "state of natural order." This proposition is worth bearing in mind when revisiting and trying to summarize the key findings and major implications of some of the studies that have historically been most often cited in the debate over the existence, incidence, and character of self-change in addictive behaviors. Admittedly, the selection of studies for the following brief review has been, by necessity, somewhat arbitrary. Nonetheless, it is evident that the vast majority of what may be termed the "classics" in this field originated in the United States in the 1960s and 1970s. To some extent, this may be explained by the dominance, in a global perspective, of U.S. alcohol and drug research at the time. However, the attention paid to these studies and the controversy raised by the issue of self-change may also be reflective of a cultural setting particularly conducive for making this topic stand out. Through the influence of the alcohol movement, the popular "disease model" of drinking problems had, by the early 1960s, become an almost uncontested foundation in alcohol research as well as policy in the United States (Mulford, 1984). According to this model, alcoholism is an irreversible and inexorably progressive process due to some inborn characteristics in certain people. Similarly, but for different reasons, narcotic drugs (i.e., at the time opium and its derivatives) were assumed to have chemical properties that made them capable of enslaving users, more or less instantly and for life. Consequently, increasing resources were spent on the creation of treatment facilities for people with drinking problems and in preventing any use of narcotic drugs.

While terms like *natural recovery* or *spontaneous remission* may initially seem compatible with a medical or biochemical notion of addiction, the suggestion that problem drinking or heroin use might be transient conditions struck at the heart of widespread and firmly rooted beliefs, and challenged strong vested interests in the prevention and treatment fields. Had social-psychological or "natural processes" models been generally accepted to account for addictive problems, the idea that many people may grow out of their problematic drinking or drug use with time would, in all probability, simply have stood out as "the natural thing" (Mulford, 1984; Peele, 1985).

Before proceeding to a review of the "classics," it should be pointed out that many of the studies that, at the time, were most frequently quoted as evidence for the existence of self-change were designed to address other research questions. Therefore, potential failures in providing a conclusive basis for judgment on this specific issue should not necessarily be attributed to flaws and weaknesses in the methodology of these studies. In effect, to the extent that self-change or some semantic equivalent was used in these studies, the term was typically adopted as a provisional metaphor for putative and still little understood psychological and/or social processes.

The "Pioneering Studies"

Charles Winick (1962), often referred to as the researcher who first drew attention to the phenomenon of self-change, conjectured that a "maturing out" process might be partly responsible for the fact that approximately two-thirds of the 16,725 addicts (defined as regular users of opiates) originally reported to the Federal Bureau of Narcotics between 1953 and 1954 were not reported again at the end of 1959. Based on the experience that only a slight minority of regular narcotic users could avoid coming to the attention of the authorities during a 2-year period, he argued that inactive status, with consideration for an uncertain number who had died, indicated the cessation of drug use. Winick also found that almost three-quarters of the 7,234 addicts who had become inactive during the period 1955–1960 had ceased their drug use before the age of 38. In addition, a comparison of the age distribution of the inactive sample with that of the total population of registered addicts up to 1955 showed that persons between 30 and 40 years old were clearly overrepresented in the former group. Finally, the mean length of the addiction period among the inactive cases was found to have been 8.6 years and more than 80% were reported to have stopped their use before the tenth year of their addiction.

These findings led Winick to speculate about a natural "life cycle" of heroin addiction. Essentially, the hypothesis was that opiate addicts begin their habit as a way of coping with the emotional challenges and strains of early adulthood and cease with their habit when they belatedly, as the result of some homeostatic process, were able to confront and cope with adult responsibilities without using drugs. As a designation of this putative process, he chose the street term *maturing out*. In a later analysis, Winick (1964) plotted the length of the addiction in inactive cases against age at onset. This analysis corroborated that the vast majority of the inactive cases had started their use in their late teens or early 20s and had stopped using in their late 20s or 30s. However, a small subgroup of persons with a very early onset proved to have been addicted for a considerably longer time than the average of the group, meaning that there was an inverse correlation between age of onset and length of addiction. Winick's conclusion was that these data essentially supported his "maturing out" notion regarding the majority of "intermediate users," but that long-term addicts as well as a small group of short-term users may require other designations. In retrospect, the major merit of Winick's study is that it drew attention to the fact, unrecognized or even denied at the time, that a substantial number of addicted heroin users achieve enduring abstinence with time. At the same time, his calculations contain a good deal of uncertainty, lacking data for certain critical variables (e.g., mortality rates, potential treatment effects, exact dates of cessation of drug use). Moreover, the proposed explanation did not rely on empirical data for the emotional experiences of the respondents.

A few years later, the Australian psychiatrist Les Drew (1968) called attention to the fact that a large number of clinical studies unanimously showed that the quotient of identified alcoholics, in relation to the population in a specific age-group, tended to peak prior to the age of 50 years and then decrease substantially. Drawing on the results of other studies, Drew acknowledged that one reason for the reduction of alcohol problems in older age groups might be related to increased mortality among alcohol abusers and, to a lesser degree, the beneficial effects of treatment. However, viewing these explanations as insufficient, he also found reason to conclude that a process of self-change probably accounts for a significant proportion of alcohol abusers who cease to appear in alcohol statistics as their age increases. As potential forces involved in such a process, Drew suggested a number of factors accompanying aging (e.g., increasing maturity and responsibility, decreasing drive, increasing social withdrawal, changing social pressures, declining financial resources). Among factors that may hamper self-change processes included social isolation and the early onset of severe complications of alcohol abuse. As in Winick's case, what makes Drew's paper somewhat of a milestone is not its empirical data, which were less than perfect, but rather it presented a strong and not easily ignored case against the notion of alcohol abuse as an inexorably progressive and irreversible condition, widely accepted at the time, although it largely lacked an empirical basis (Pattison, Sobell, & Sobell, 1977).

Subsequent Research on Self-Change

The literature pertaining to self-change published in the decades following the "pioneering studies" presents a rather disparate mix of treatment and population studies, cross-sectional and longitudinal studies, and other addiction studies. This chapter will present a selection of such studies that were published before what may be called the "second wave" of self-change research commenced in the early 1990s. Although varying with regard to sample size, type, overall research questions, and methods, the studies to be discussed were selected because they were seminal reports that produced new insights and/or raised controversy and public debate at the time of publication. As will soon be obvious, the studies selected all address either drug or alcohol problems. Research concerning self-change for gambling, smoking, and a number of other problems is discussed in later chapters in this volume. It should be pointed out, however, that there were some early forerunners of today's research on self-change from other addictions as well. Schachter (1982), in a seminal article, presented data on the self-cure of smoking and obesity in two different nontherapeutic populations. In short, this study showed that about two thirds of those who had, in a lifetime perspective, tried to stop smoking or reduce their weight, had in fact succeeded. The success rates of self-change in the Schachter study were higher than those usually reported for people who were treated for smoking or obesity. Schachter argues that this discrepancy may partly be due to self-selection into treatment of the severest cases, but that the main explanation is likely to be the fact that treatment studies typically report the outcome of a single attempt to quit smoking or to lose weight, whereas self-change studies reflect the cumulative effects of multiple efforts. Emphasizing that treatment studies may give rise to flawed conclusions about the intractability of addiction problems, the author implicitly points to the need for longitudinal research on self-change as well as on the role of treatment in life-change (Blomqvist, 1996).

The following pages will first examine a limited number of studies in the drug research field that can be deemed "classic" works pertaining to the issue of self-change. This will be followed by a somewhat larger number of similar studies in the alcohol research field. To enhance comprehension, each section contains a summary table of the aims, results, and main implications of the reviewed studies.

Studies of Drug Use and Drug Addiction

Table 2.1 shows a variety of information from four classic self-change drug studies that are discussed below.

Treatment Studies

Winick's study, based on official records of known drug users, may be seen as prototypical of many of the early self-change studies in the drug field. Unfortunately, studies of drug use and drug addiction in the general population are still rare (Sobell, Ellingstad, & Sobell, 2000). As for treatment research in the drug field, a limited number of studies during the 1960s and 1970s indicated that only a rather small percentage, seldom more than 1 in 10, remained continuously abstinent for 5–10 years after hospital treatment (Maddux & Desmond, 1980). However, with one exception, these studies did not include a control group that would have allowed for analyses exploring rates of and

TABLE 2.1. Characteristics of classic studies on self-change in drug use.

Author (year)	Winick (1962, 1964)	Snow (1973)	Burt Associates (1977)	Robins (1974a,b, 1993); Robins, Davis, & Goodwin (1974); Robins, Davis, & Nurco (1974); Robins, Helzer, & Davis (1975); Robins, Helzer, Hesselbrock, & Wish (1980)
Data sources; respondents	Official records of regular opiate users (Federal Bureau of Narcotics)	Records of drug addicts in New York (New York City Narcotics Register)	360 heroin addicts followed up 1–3 years after treatment	Enlisted men, returning from Vietnam in September 1971
Principal aims	To assess the long-term outcome of registered drug users	To replicate Winick's studies, taking into account factors such as mortality and institutionalization	To evaluate the National Treatment Association's Program by comparing treated and minimally treated subjects	To estimate drug use and problems among servicemen in Vietnam and the need for drug addiction treatment after returning home
Main results	About 2/3 became inactive in a 5-year period. The majority stopped after < 10 years use, in their late 20s or 30s	About 1/4 stopped using in a 4-year period	Almost 1/3 had recovered (no use and social stability during 2 months before interview) and 1/3 had improved. Subjects who stayed ≤ 5 days did not differ from those who stayed longer	Almost 1/2 of all men had used opiates in Vietnam, and 20% had been addicted. The great majority did not resume use on return. Of those who did, less than 10% got readdicted, mostly for only a brief period. Less than 20% of those who were addicted in Vietnam had shown any signs of readdiction 3 years after return

(Continued)

TABLE 2.1. Characteristics of classic studies on self-change in drug use—Cont'd.

Conclusions bearing on self-change	There may be a natural life cycle of drug addiction, and most addicts seem to "mature out" of their addiction	"Maturing out" may be less common than suggested in Winick's studies	Many heroin addicts positively change in a relatively short time frame. Treatment does not seem to add to the recovery rate	Drug addiction is not a unitary and intractable disorder, but a complex and often transitory phenomenon. Transitions between use, addiction, and recovery are probably driven by different sets of factors
Comments	The number who actually stopped may have been exaggerated. The putative "maturing out" process was not supported by empirical data	The lower rate of recoveries may partly be explained by the unique situation in New York and/or by changes in the drug scene since Winick's studies	The study and control groups may not have been fully comparable. The "recovery" criterion may have captured temporary changes	The "Vietnam experience" may have been a facsimile of drug use and addiction in the population, demonstrating much more flux and "natural recovery" than in treatment-seeking groups

forces behind untreated recovery (Sobell, Sobell, Toneatto, & Leo, 1993). The one exception was Burt Associates's (1977) evaluation of the National Treatment Association programs, based on interviews 1 to 3 years later with 81% of the 360 initially treated heroin addicts. Here, one-third of these individuals had stayed in treatment 5 days or less and were used as a comparison group. Almost one third (29%) were found to be "fully recovered" (i.e., no use of illicit drugs and no arrests plus social stability during the 2 months prior to the interview) and an additional 37% were judged as "partly recovered." The crucial findings pertaining to self-change were that there were no significant differences between the treated and control groups and time in treatment was not associatied with outcome. However, the study does not give evidence that the treatment and control groups were comparable in relevant aspects. Moreover, the 2-month criterion for assessing recovery may be cited as evidence for confounding a temporary hiatus in one's drug use with stable recovery.

The Vietnam Experience

The most frequently cited and hotly debated self-change study in the drug field is Lee Robins's follow-up of returning Vietnam veterans, published in a series of reports and articles during the period 1973–1980. This study was originally set up by the Nixon administration through the Special Action Office on Drug Abuse Prevention to estimate the size of the drug use problem among servicemen in Vietnam and after their return, and to provide a basis for planning proper treatment facilities. The study employed two samples of all enlisted men who left Vietnam to return home in September 1971. The first was a simple random sample of all eligible respondents. The other was a random sample of all men who had screened "drug positive" by urine tests before departure. Since all men were warned they would be screened, not having managed to stop using before leaving was seen as a sign of stronger addiction. After correcting for a small overlap between the samples and deducting a minority who could not be reached for an interview, the two samples were comprised of 451 and 469 men, respectively. The first reported analyses concerned respondents' drug use in Vietnam and during the first 8–12 months after their return to the United States (Robins, 1974a,b; Robins, Davis, & Goodwin, 1974; Robins, Davis, & Nurco, 1974). A later analysis was based on data from a 3-year follow-up of the same samples (Robins, Helzer, Hesselbrock, & Wish, 1980). As for drug use in Vietnam, the study found that almost half of Army enlisted men had used narcotics; 34% had tried heroin and 38% had tried opium. Further, approximately 80% had used marijuana (not classified as a narcotic in this study). Almost half of those who had used narcotics had done so more than weekly for greater than 6 months. Overall, one out of five (20%) of all returning men admitted to having been "addicted" to narcotics while in Vietnam (i.e., had felt "strung out" and experienced repeated and prolonged withdrawal symptoms). The predominant route of administration was smoking and less than 10% had ever injected. Compared with soldiers who used no drugs or only marijuana, drug users tended to be younger, more often single, less well-educated, reared in broken homes, and from larger cities. However, most of the men who used narcotic drugs in Vietnam had not used before service and showed no signs of pre-Vietnam social deviance.

Regarding drug use during the first year after return, only about 10% of the general sample and one third of those who had tested "drug positive" at departure proved to have used any narcotics. More interestingly, less than one in ten of all men who had used since returning had experienced any signs of addiction. In the drug positive sample the corresponding proportion was one in five. That is, only 7% in the drug positive sample and 12% of all men who had been addicted in Vietnam were found to still have been addicted after returning stateside (Robins, Davis, & Goodwin, 1974; Robins, Davis, & Nurco, 1974). When the veterans were followed for an additional 2-year period, these figures rose somewhat. Nonetheless, fewer than 20% of those who were addicted in Vietnam and had resumed narcotic use in the United States were found to have been addicted at any time, and mostly for only a brief period in the 3 years since returning. Collectively, these results were clearly at odds with conventional beliefs at the time. They were counter to reported outcomes of treated cases that generally had shown high rates of readdiction after as short a time period as 6 months. Analyses of the addicted veterans' reception toward treatment further showed that the intervention was at best responsible for only a tiny fraction of the remarkable recovery rates. In effect, less than 2% of those who had used narcotics in Vietnam and only 6% in the "drug-positive" sample went to drug abuse treatment after returning to the United States (Robins, Helzer, & Davis, 1975). Moreover, those who sought treatment showed the same readdiction rates as clients in other treatment outcome studies. Lastly, the results indicated that recovery from drug addiction did not require abstention. In effect, even among those who were addicted in Vietnam and had used heroin regularly after return, half of the cases were not re-addicted.

The results presented by Robins and her colleagues were met with considerable skepticism by the press as well as large parts of the research community (Robins, 1993). In fact, attempts to dispute or explain away their findings still continue, even in the scientific literature. Apart from raising suspicions that the results were tailored to satisfy military authorities' interests in demonstrating that soldiers serving in Vietnam had not been consigned to a life-enduring dependence on drugs, critics have concentrated on attempts to show that the results lack generalizability. One line of reasoning has been that the Vietnam veterans never were "real addicts." The argument put forth is that the strains and misery of war made addiction a "normal reaction" and that the relatively benign outcome after return was thus irrelevant to addiction in the United States. Another line of thinking states that the veterans' circumstances after return made them different from addicts who started their heroin use in the United States (i.e., returning meant living in a new setting where one would not know where to access heroin and where factors that could serve as stimuli to relapse were essentially absent). In her "look back" article two decades after the initial study, Robins (1993) finds reasons to repudiate these objections and defends most of the original conclusions. Concerning the explanation of addiction in Vietnam, she highlights that addiction had generally begun before the soldiers were exposed to combat and that the dose–response curve, strongly indicative of a causal link, did not apply to the relation between combat exposure and addiction. Moreover, the respondents themselves did not explain their heroin use as a reaction to fear or stress, but rather as a way of making the boring life in the Army more endurable and enjoyable, factors that may explain casual use in the United States as well. Since, like under "normal" conditions, earlier antisocial behavior was indeed an important pre-dictor for drug addiction in Vietnam, the author is inclined to see high avail-ability and lack of alternative recreational activities as the main explanations for the remarkable rate of use; this was also seen among young men without earlier signs of personal or social problems. The argument that the impressive recovery rates after return could be explained by very limited availability and lack of stimuli to use in the new environment, is clearly contradicted by the fact that only a small fraction of those who continued using in the United States actually became readdicted.

According to Robins herself (1993), looking back over the past two decades the most important implications of the study, although still not entirely incor-porated in public and scientific views of heroin use, are as follows: (a) "Few of the Vietnam addicts would have become addicted if they had remained in the US. However, their history of brief addiction followed by spontaneous recov-ery, both in Vietnam and afterwards, was not out of line with the American experience; only with American beliefs" (p. 1051), (b) addiction looks very different if one studies it in a general population rather than in treated cases, and (c) addiction is a complex and multifaceted phenomenon and further understanding would be facilitated if the focus was shifted from attempts to grasp the entity of addiction to the transitions between use, addiction, and recovery; the latter are probably driven by different sets of interacting forces.

What Did the "Classics" Teach Us about Drug Addiction?

At the surface, the studies just reviewed seem to indicate that recovery rates are very high among "situational" heroin addicts, such as most of Robins's enlisted men, moderately high to high among narcotic addicts in official registers, and remarkably low among treatment-seeking addicts. Certainly, all of the studies may have claimed to have contributed knowledge in demonstrating that the prevailing notion of heroin as an instantly and interminably addictive drug was a myth, related to its legal status and official rhetoric rather than to empirical facts. The most probable explanation of these widely varying estimates of self-change is—besides methodological divergences—that these different types of studies covered rather different points on the heroin use and abuse continuum. Without reliable data allowing for a comparison between studies of different drug problem severity, it may be conjectured that heroin use and addiction among enlisted men in Vietnam may, except for the high overall prevalence, have been a fairly good facsimile of heroin use and addiction in the general population. Although a small proportion became readdicted after returning, for most of these users addiction turned out to be a transient condition, strongly influenced by environmental and developmental factors. The veterans who did become readdicted may be more representative of a much smaller group whose problematic heroin use is intertwined with a number of other social and psychological problems, and who eventually seek treatment. In this group, possibly with an earlier onset of heroin use than the average user and often with a relatively long history of problematic use before the first admission, addiction often seems to have developed into a truly self-defeating process that may be difficult to break with or without professional help. Indeed, prevailing notions of heroin addiction as a generally progressive and irreversible condition may even function as a self-fulfilling prophecy in accelerating such a process.

As for studies of "heroin addicts" in official registers, these may have covered a continuum ranging from users registered only for minor drug offenses to severely addicted and recurrently treated persons, which would explain the middle-range rates of self-change found in these studies. However, due to methodological flaws in Winick's nonetheless pioneering study, the author's conclusion that about two thirds of all registered addicts eventually "mature out" of their addiction may have been somewhat exaggerated. Snow (1973), in a replication based on data in the New York City Narcotics Register, tried to account for respondents who had died, been admitted to treatment, or were institutionalized and found that about one-fourth of the registered addicts had "matured out" of their addiction over a 4-year period. On the other hand, the lower rate found by Snow may also, at least partly, be explained by the unique situation in New York City and/or overall changes in the drug scene between the 1950s and the 1960s.

In their review of the incidence literature on self-change from heroin addiction, Waldorf and Biernacki (1979) concluded that studies over the past two decades had amply demonstrated that a significant number of heroin addicts naturally recover from their addiction without treatment intervention. At the same time they deplored the virtual absence of studies providing information concerning the psychological, social, and environmental mechanisms and processes that may be used to bring about such changes. In addition, they pointed to the need to explore the characteristics and resources of people who recover naturally and to compare these with their treated counterparts and with the larger population. With this review, and the same authors' subsequent attempt to put their proposed research program into practice (1981; Biernacki, 1986; Waldorf, 1983), the "second wave" of research on self-change, which provides the main focus for this book, may be said to have commenced, at least regarding the area of drugs.

Studies of Alcoholism, Drinking Patterns, and Drinking Problems

Table 2.2 shows a variety of information from nine classic self-change alcohol studies that are discussed below.

TABLE 2.2. Characteristics of classic studies on self-change in alcohol use.

Author (year)	Drew (1968)	Kendell & Staton (1966)	Kissin, Rosenblatt, & Machover (1968)
Data sources; respondents	Literature review of studies reporting prevalence rates for alcoholism by age groups	Subjects who declined or were refused treatment for their alcoholism at the Maudsley Hospital (London) and a comparison group of clients who were treated at the same clinic	Clients treated in three different programs and an untreated wait-list control group
Principal aims	To assess changes in alcoholism rates over the life span	To assess treatment effects and "spontaneous recovery" in alcoholics	To compare the outcome of different treatments and of an untreated control group
Main results	Studies from different countries display a common pattern in that the quotient of alcoholics in relation to the population in a specific age group peaks before the age of 50 and decreases substantially thereafter	Half of the untreated subjects had recovered (no serious disruption due to drinking) at the follow-up, 2–13 years after initial assessment. The improvement rate in treated subjects was similar, except for more abstinent cases	Improvement (largely abstinent and socially/vocationally stable for 6+ months at a 1-year follow-up) ranged between 17% and 20% in the treated groups, but was only 4% in the untreated group
Conclusions bearing on self-change	The decrease of alcoholism in older age groups is not sufficiently explained by increased mortality and potential treatment effects. There may be a process of "spontaneous recovery" driven by factors normally accompanying aging	"Spontaneous recovery" seems to be relatively common. Treatment promotes abstinence, but does not seem to add to overall improvement	"Spontaneous recovery" in alcoholism is relatively rare and treated clients fare much better
Comments	The data used did not allow for an exact estimation of the impact of factors such as increased mortality or potential treatment effects. The study presented a strong case against the notion of alcoholism as an inexorably progressive and irreversible "disease"	Previous treatment experiences in the study groups were not reported. Treated and untreated samples may not have been comparable in all significant aspects	Using a wait-list group as control may have biased results. Study attrition was almost 50% and may have seriously jeopardized valid conclusions

(Continued)

TABLE 2.2. Characteristics of classic studies on self-change in alcohol use—Cont'd.

Author (year)	Cahalan (1970); Cahalan, Cisin, & Crossley (1969); Knupfer (1972)	Cahalan & Room (1974)	Clark (1976); Clark & Cahalan (1976)
Data sources; respondents	National and regional probability samples of adult U.S. citizens	National ($n = 1561$) and regional ($n = 780$) probability samples of adult American men	Cahalan's and Room's regional (San Francisco) sample followed up 4 years after the initial interview
Principal aims	To give a detailed and representative account of American drinking practices and drinking problems	To analyze drinking problems, their intercorrelations, and their associations with drinking and with demographic and contextual factors	To assess the development over time of problem drinking and drinking problems
Main results	Drinking patterns and various drinking problems were found to be strongly associated with such factors as ethnicity, social class, sex, and age. Heavy drinking and drinking problems were found to be much less prevalent in women and in the older age group. More than 3/4 of all recoveries from problematic drinking occurred without treatment (Knupfer, 1972)	Strong ethnic and socioeconomic determinants were found for both drinking and problem drinking. Specific drinking problems were found to be only modestly intercorrelated and to vary with contextual and ecological factors. Heavy drinking and drinking problems were found to be more prevalent among men than women, and much more prevalent in younger than in older age groups	"Loss of control" as a problem-drinking symptom was found to come and go over rather brief periods (Clark, 1976). Specific symptoms showed low persistence over time, even if continued involvement with some problems was relatively common. A great proportion of all respondents with some drinking problems at Time 1 reported a complete absence of problems at Time 2
Conclusions bearing on self-change	The traditional alcoholism notion is ill fitted to capture the general population's drinking experiences. Drinking problems tend to be transitory, generally passing with age without treatment	Problem drinking is a heterogeneous condition and problem drinkers constitute a heterogeneous group. People may shift in and out of problem categories, depending on age and changing contextual factors	There is a great deal of flux in problem drinking. The "key symptoms" of the alcoholism paradigm are not a one-way gate to worse problems
Comments	The studies relied on cross-sectional data and did not directly address change over time. "Problem drinking" was predominantly assessed by a simple summary score	Analyses were mainly based on cross-sectional data, and did not directly address change over time	The follow-up period may be claimed to have been too brief to capture the prolonged course of problem drinking

(Continued)

Author (year)	Roizen, Cahalan, & Shanks (1978)	Fillmore (1975, 1987a,b); Fillmore & Midanik (1984); Temple & Fillmore (1985)	Valliant (1983, 1995)
Data sources; respondents	A subsample of 521 men in the San Francisco sample with some drinking problem at Time 1 and no treatment experience at Time 2	Probability samples followed up over extended periods, sometimes (Fillmore, 1987b) complemented by cross-sectional analyses of various birth cohorts	Men in a community ("Core City") sample, followed up from adolescence until their old age. Additional data from a college sample and a follow-up of a clinical sample
Principal aims	To explore variations in the rate of "spontaneous remission" related to initial problem severity and different outcome standards	To explore variations in drinking and drinking problems over the life span among men and women	To explore the long-term course of alcoholism and alcohol abuse
Main results	Improvement rates varied between 11% and 71%, depending on criteria used for defining problem drinking at Time 1 and improvement at Time 2. The proportion with no problems at all at Time 2 varied between 12% (Ss scoring the highest at Time 1) and 30% (Ss scoring the lowest at Time 1)	Among men, the incidence of heavy drinking and drinking problems was found to be highest in early adulthood, decreasing with age; the chronicity of problem drinking was found to be highest in middle age. In women, heavy drinking and drinking problems were much less common in younger years, increasing slightly in the middle years, and decreasing thereafter. Chances of remission were found to vary greatly with sex and age with the lowest rates in middle-aged women	At the age of 47, more than 1/2 of all men ever classified as alcohol abusers but never subjected to formal treatment were abstinent or drinking without symptoms. Among abusers who did receive treatment, almost 1/2 were symptom-free, of whom the majority were abstinent. Of all previous abusers drinking without symptoms at the age of 47, 1/3 later relapsed into alcohol abuse as compared with < 1/5 of those who were abstinent. Of all dependent subjects later to have achieved abstinence for 2+ years, 4/10 later relapsed, sometimes after as long as 10 years
Conclusions bearing on self-change	Since there is no natural boundary between alcoholics and nonalcoholics in the population, "natural recovery" can be equated with a number of arbitrary standards. Dealing with remission as a prognostic and diagnostic issue requires different research designs and will yield different results	Drinking patterns and drinking problems vary with sex and age, are susceptible to cultural norms, and are often transitory. Only certain combinations of early problem drinking signs seem to predict chronicity of problems	Alcoholism has its own dynamics and is best envisaged as a disease, in the same vein as hypertension or coronary disorders. Abstinence is the only viable alternative to addictive drinking and principles of AA may be said to comprise the fundamental elements of effective remedy
Comments	The study may be claimed to have had crucial implications for further research on "natural recovery"	Controlling for potential bias due to specific historical conditions or unique aspects of particular birth cohorts did not alter overall conclusions	An alternative interpretation of the data is that up to 1/2 of all alcohol abusers, depending on the definition used, recover naturally and that the "natural course" of alcohol problems is better captured by a "natural process" than by a disease model

Studies of Identified Alcohol Abusers

Drew's (1968) seminal article, building on secondary cross-sectional data, included no attempts at estimating the incidence of self-change among indivduals with alcohol problems. However, Smart (1975), in the first extensive literature review in this area, reports a number of studies that followed untreated identified alcohol abusers or problem drinkers at two time points. Except for a few early investigations of mostly anecdotal interest, the studies conducted between 1965 and 1975 yielded overall recovery rates varying between 4% and 40% and annual recovery rates between 1% and 33%. A closer examination reveals that these varying results are most likely due to differences regarding study groups (e.g., registered abusers, self-identified alcohol abusers in health surveys, convicted felons identified as alcohol abusers, etc.), recovery criteria (e.g., not found in treatment records, abstinent, drinking without problems, etc.), and follow-up periods (ranging from 6 months to 13 years).

As maintained by Smart, another problem with many of these studies is that untreated alcohol abusers may differ from those who seek and receive treatment in important respects influencing prognosis. Thus, studies of self-change should do as treatment studies and use control groups. However, the only two studies of self-change among treatment-seeking alcohol abusers that had been reported at that time also showed clearly different results. Kendell and Staton (1966) found that one-half of a group of diagnosed alcohol abusers, who were either refused or declined treatment (at Maudsley Hospital in London) and who received no treatment during the follow-up period, had improved at the follow-up 2 to 13 years later; that is, they had not experienced serious disruption due to drinking. In contrast, Kissin, Rosenblatt, and Machover (1968), in a comparative study of three different treatments, found that no more than 4% of an untreated control group had improved in a 1-year period after the assessment. Improvement, in this case, was defined as total abstinence or near-total abstinence and social and vocational stability during the previous 6 months. Further, Kendell and Staton found that the improvement rates in their untreated sample differed little from those in a treated sample from the same hospital (except for a higher proportion of abstinent cases in the latter group), while Kissin and colleagues found the treated respondents to have faired much better (recovery rates ranging between about 17% and 20%) than their untreated counterparts. However, it should be noted that the total attrition in the latter study was almost 50%, although the rates within different samples were not reported; in addition, all dropouts were classified as not improved. Thus, the reported data may well have underrated remission in the total sample and overrated the difference between treated and untreated samples. Moreover, it is unclear whether the treated and untreated groups in any of the studies were really comparable. That is, Kendell and Staton actually borrowed their treated comparison group from another study. Kissin and colleagues, for their part, tried to assign clients randomly to a wait-list, but had to drop from their control group respondents whose request for treatment persisted beyond the 6 months they had been advised to wait, and who then had to be assigned to a treatment group.

In summary, as pointed out by Blomqvist (1996), making inferences about self-change from control or wait-list groups in treatment studies may, in fact, be a rather unreliable endeavor. On the one hand, because treatment effects may be cumulative, such groups should ideally include only previously untreated respondents. On the other hand, this may make them truly incomparable to treatment groups in which readmitted clients, probably representing the severest cases, are likely to be clearly overrepresented. Further, this type of study design presupposes clients voluntarily seeking treatment. However, reluctance to enter treatment may be a typical characteristic of "self-change" and even part of the motivation to change (Blomqvist, 1996).

The "Problem Drinking" Paradigm

Whereas studies of treatment-seeking respondents, identified as alcohol abusers, may give a rather circumscribed picture of self-change, a quite different type of evidence, at least indirectly bearing on the same issue, comes from emerging survey research on drinking and drinking problems in the general population, mainly by Don Cahalan and his colleagues in the Social Research Group (later called the Alcohol Research Group) at Berkeley. In a forerunner to the Berkeley group's publications, Cahalan, Cisin, and Crossley (1969) described the detailed drinking patterns of adult Americans, based on personal interviews with 2,756 persons, representative of the total population and conducted in late 1964 and early 1965. In summary, this study showed that drinking patterns, as well as a variety of "drinking problems" with different prevalence rates, were strongly associated with factors such as ethnic origin, social class, sex, and age. The finding most relevant to the discussion of self-change was that both drinking and "heavy drinking" were much less common among both men and women aged 50 and older than in younger age groups. Following up a subsample of the same respondents approximately 3 to 4 years later, Cahalan (1970) more directly addressed the issue of problem drinking. Based on the heterogeneity and variability of drinking-related problems (even over rather short periods of time) found in the study, Cahalan argued that "problem drinking," at least as a provisional concept, might better capture the realities of the general population's troubles with alcohol than the traditional alcoholism notion. Concerning self-change, this study showed that problem drinking (defined as 7 or greater on an 11-item problem scale) was much more common in the younger than the older age groups. Whereas one-quarter of all men aged 21–29 scored as problem drinkers, this was true for only 13% of the men aged 51–60 and only 1% of those over 70 years old. The prevalence of problem drinking increased with lower socioeconomic status, and women showed a much lower prevalence than did men. Nonetheless, the decline of problems with age was observable in all groups. Using a similar additive problem-drinking score, Knupfer (1972) examined drinking problems in two adult San Francisco probability samples (one male, and one of both sexes). Among her findings, about one-third of those who ever scored "high" on the drinking score were stably recovered, and less than one-quarter of all recoveries had included any kind of treatment.

While these early surveys, favoring summary problems scores as the dependent variable in their analyses, came close to substituting "drinking problems" for "alcoholism" as a new unitary concept (Room, 1983), Cahalan and Room's (1974) "Problem Drinking Among American Men" adopted a disaggregated approach, a concept entirely different from the old alcoholism paradigm. This study utilized data from the samples previously investigated by Cahalan and colleagues, supplemented by an additional, national probability sample of adult men interviewed in 1969. The pooled data from the first two surveys yielded a total of 1,561 men aged 21 to 59, and the supplementary sample included 978 men in the same age range. In addition, the book presented some initial analyses of a probability sample of 786 San Francisco men interviewed in late 1967 and early 1968. The core finding of this study was that problem designations seem to be arbitrary and transitory, and that people moved readily into and out of problem categories. Regarding prevalence of problems, the study showed that between 6% and 24% of all men exhibited at least some signs of 1 of 13 types of actual or potential drinking problems during the last 3 years. The prevalence rates of problems of "high severity" of each type were considerably lower (often only one-half of that of "minimal severity" of the same problem). Although about three-quarters of those with one problem of high severity also had at least one other problem, the overall picture was that of a very heterogeneous collection of drinking problems and people with drinking problems. Thus, even if pairwise comparisons of the problem measures showed moderately high intercorrelations, these were predominantly attributable to the large proportion of men with no problems at all. One interesting finding, for example, was that symptomatic drinking (signs of physical dependence) was more strongly associated with psychological dependence than with heavy intake. The study also confirmed earlier findings, indicating strong ethnic and socioeconomic determinants of drinking and drinking problems. For instance, problem drinking patterns and tangible consequences of drinking were both associated with a disadvantaged status with regard to socioeconomy, ethnicity, family history, and work history. Further, this study showed the great influence of contextual or ecological factors on drinking patterns and drinking problems. For example, whereas living in an abstaining neighborhood was negatively correlated with both drinking and heavy drinking, those who did drink in this environment were more likely than others to be very heavy drinkers. At the same time, while heavy drinkers in dry neighborhoods did not appear to be more personally maladjusted than other heavy drinkers, the proportion experiencing tangible consequences was markedly higher. Finally, the researchers once again found heavy intake as well as problem drinking patterns to be most common in the younger age groups, declining with age.

Studies Directly Addressing Change over Time

In summary, the results of the referenced studies indicated that there may be a great deal of flux in problem drinking, and that the pattern of progressive worsening of problems, suggested by the "alcoholism" paradigm, was in many respects ill fitted to account for problem drinking in the general population. However, the analyses were mainly based on cross-sectional data and did not provide direct evidence about change over time in drinking patterns and problems. Thus, for example, they may have left room for other explanations regarding the decline in drinking problems with age other than simply self-change (e.g., generational differences in drinking habits, increased mortality among problem drinkers, potential treatment effects). It is true that Cahalan provided some longitudinal analyses in his 1970 book; that is, using a summary index of problem drinking (based on psychological dependence and frequent intoxication), he showed that 22% of the men and 9% of the women had changed their problem drinking status materially, in either direction, since the original interview 3–4 years earlier. In addition, both this study and the subsequent study by Cahalan and Room included some retrospective data, indicating a substantial "maturing out" of potentially severe drinking problems.

However, it was not until Clark's (1976) and Clark and Cahalan's (1976) reporting of data obtained by a second wave of interviews, from the San Francisco sample about 4 years later, that the Berkeley group more directly addressed the issue of change, based on repeated observations of the same respondents. In the first of these articles, Clark related "loss of control," the core concept of the alcoholism paradigm, to other measures of heavy drinking and drinking problems. To summarize his findings, this variable was only one among many in predicting drinking problems, and loss of control over drinking, instead of being a one-way gate to worse problems, appeared to come and go over even as brief a period as 4 years. Clark and Cahalan presented further data challenging the alleged progressiveness of alcoholism by failing to demonstrate either the persistence of "early symptoms" of alcoholism over longer periods or the accumulation of further drinking problems over time among respondents with such symptoms. Rather, these analyses showed that even if continued involvement in *some* alcohol problems was common, continuity of any *particular* problem over time was low. Moreover, one quarter to one-half (depending on the particular problem) of all respondents with drinking problems at the time of the first interview reported a complete absence of problems 4 years later.

Finally, in a seminal study based on a subsample of the same panel, Roizen, Cahalan, and Shanks (1978) directly addressed the question of self-change among untreated problem drinkers. The sample consisted of the 521 men who reported some drinking problems at the time of the first interview, who never had any contact with a treatment agency or group, and who could be reached at the follow-up, about 4 years after the first interview. By using a variety of criteria for problem drinking at Time 1 as well as for improvement at Time 2,

Roizen and colleagues found improvement rates varying from 11% to 71%. The highest rate was obtained when problem drinking was defined as 11 points on an 11-item overall problem scale, and improvement was measured as a drop of 1 or more points at Time 2. When the criterion was shifted to "no problems at all" at Time 2 (virtually no one was totally abstinent), the recovery rate dropped to 12% in the group with the highest problem score at Time 1 and to 30% among those with the lowest score at Time 1. In a subsample of 57 men defined to match a clinical population in problem severity, the improvement rates, depending on criteria, ranged from 14% to 59%. These findings, showing that remission can be equated with a variety of more or less arbitrary standards, falling between abstinence and any improvement, were described by the authors as a corollary of the fact that there is no natural boundary between alcohol abusers and non-alcohol abusers in the general population. In addition, they highlighted that the question of remission from alcohol problems does not constitute a single research problem, but rather a number of problems requiring different approaches. For example, they pointed out that dealing with remission as a "prognostic" problem (i.e., following diagnosed or "known" cases to explore factors associated with improvement and persistence) presumes the validity of the diagnostic measures that placed the respondents in the problem category in the first place. However, longitudinal studies of individuals' drinking problems can also be viewed as a way of testing various diagnostic categories; at least, in essence, they are assumed to capture a lifelong condition. Indeed, the tautological claim that self-change simply represents a diagnostic failure in the first place can still be heard. By a number of analyses, the authors demonstrated that designing one's study to address, for example, prognostic versus diagnostic research questions may yield different results, even when the same data are utilized.

Longitudinal Research

Although the Berkeley group's panel studies demonstrated great variability in drinking and drinking problems over time, the study periods were relatively short, not allowing for definite conclusions about the long-term course of problem drinking. This limitation was partly overcome by a series of studies by Kaye Fillmore who adopted a much longer time frame. In the first study in this series, Fillmore (1975) followed 206 respondents from a large study of drinking patterns and problems among 17,000 U.S. college students, initially interviewed 20 years earlier. Even if the sample size was small—the study was designed to explore the feasibility of a larger study which was subsequently not funded—the results replicated the findings of earlier cross-sectional studies by showing a substantial decrease in most types of drinking problems from early adulthood to middle age. For example, according to a summary score, 42% of the men were "problem drinkers" during their college years, but only 17% in middle age.

However, the type of problem characteristic of early problem drinking did not prove to be a particularly good predictor of later problems. Rather, as the author concluded, unique combinations of early problems tended to predict unique combinations of later problems. For example, among men, early drinking-related problems such as accidents, arrests, belligerence, or interference with schoolwork did not predict later problems unless associated with recurrent intoxication and symptomatic drinking. Further, binge drinking tended to precede other early problems and to predict later problems only if associated with symptomatic drinking. A noteworthy finding was that "psychological dependence" was the measure yielding the highest prevalence rates at both time points, but had a relatively low overlap with other measures and was a poor predictor of future problem drinking. The author concludes that psychological dependence might, to a certain degree, be an American drinking norm rather than a symptom of problem drinking. Another important finding, emphasized by Fillmore, was the tangible difference between men and women with regard to the prevalence of problem drinking as well as specific drinking problems and changes over time. For example, the decline in problem drinking with age was characteristic of men only. Actually, women, with a much lower prevalence of any drinking problems during their college years, had slightly more problems in their middle age. Based on a closer analysis of these divergences, the author found them to indicate the influence of norms and social expectations in men's and women's drinking.

During the following years, Fillmore provided further evidence of the variability over time of drinking patterns and problems in both men (Fillmore & Midanik, 1984; Temple & Fillmore, 1985) and women (Fillmore, 1987a). In a methodologically important article (Fillmore, 1987b), she supplemented longitudinal data with cross-sectional analyses of different birth cohorts. In this way the study was able to control for potential bias in the longitudinal analyses, due to specific historical conditions (e.g., prohibition or wartime) and other unique aspects of specific birth cohorts. Even with these controls, the study reiterated the findings that the incidence of heavy drinking, among men, was relatively high in early adulthood, decreasing with age, and that chronicity of alcohol problems (persistence over the study periods, 5–7 years) was highest in the middle years, decreasing thereafter. Reviewing evidence of self-change from alcohol problems for a committee of the Institute of Medicine, Fillmore, Hartka, Johnstone, Speiglman, and Temple (1988) made the following summary statement:

[There is] a higher prevalence of problems in youth, but erratic and non-chronic with a 50–60 percent chance of remission both in the long and short term among men and more than 70 percent chance of remission among women; in middle age, a much lower prevalence, but chronic with a 30–40 percent chance of remission among men and about a 30 percent chance among women; in older age, a great deal lower prevalence of problems, which were more likely chronic, with a 60–80 percent chance of remission among men and a 50–60 percent chance of remission among women. (p. 29)

Is Self-Change Part of the "Natural History" of Alcoholism?

Notwithstanding that remission levels were shown to be highly responsive to measurement criteria, the Berkeley group's population studies demonstrated a substantial amount of self-change in drinking problems, even among people with high problem drinking scores. However, even if these studies may be claimed to have disproved the conventional picture of such problems as long-lasting, inexorably worsening with time, and even interminable, most of them obtained their data at only two time points, often with a relatively short time period elapsing between them. Thus, they may still be criticized for not being able to fully refute the possibility that alcohol abusers or severe problem drinkers are strongly susceptible to relapse even after a rather long period of abstinence or problem-free drinking. This question is one of the main themes in George Vaillant's (1983, 1995) now 50-year-long study of the long-term course of alcohol problems. Although in many respects it is the most impressive research endeavor to date in this field, it has yielded the most varying interpretations and has caused the most heated debates. Vaillant's study is based on data from Harvard Medical School's Study of Adult Development, following a community sample of 660 men from adolescence into late middle life and further into old age. The respondents fell into the following two groups: an upper-middle-class College sample of 204 persons and a less privileged Core City sample of 456 persons. In his major report from 1983, Vaillant follows the 110 surviving persons in the Core City sample ever classified as alcohol abusers (defined as greater than 4 points on the Problem Drinking Scale for at least 1 year) until the age of 47. In addition, he occasionally reports on the outcome of the 26 abusers in the College sample, and some data from an 8-year follow-up of 106 persons in a clinical sample, treated in a program combining individual counseling, psychoeducation, and regular Alcohol Anonymous (AA) meetings.

Regarding the origin and nature of addiction to alcohol, Vaillant (1983), not totally unlike the referenced population studies, finds developing alcohol abuse to be associated with ethnic background, early social problems, and parents' alcohol problems, but not with, for example, childhood emotional problems or environmental weaknesses. Nonetheless, based on the alleged persistence of addictive drinking and the high intercorrelations between a number of measures of alcohol abuse and dependence, he maintains that alcoholism is a unitary phenomenon and is best envisaged as a disease, in the same vein as it makes sense to regard hypertension or coronary arterial disorders as diseases. In both versions of his book, Vaillant further asserts that total abstinence is the only viable alternative to addictive drinking and that the principles of AA can be said to comprise all that is necessary to achieve such a solution. However, as pointed out by Peele (1983), these conclusions are not unambiguously supported by the empirical findings of Vaillant's own study. For example, more than one-quarter of the untreated alcohol abusers in the Core City sample were stably abstinent at the age of 47, and almost as many were drinking without symptoms (Vaillant, 1983). Among abusers in the same sample who had hospital or clinic visits during the follow-up period (and whose alcohol abuse was often more clearly "progressive"), slightly less than one-half had ceased with their abuse, predominantly by becoming abstinent. In contrast, less than one-third of the clinical sample (who had been referred to AA as part of their treatment) were judged to be in stable remission at the 8-year follow-up, and only 5% had not relapsed at any time during the follow-up period (Vaillant, 1983).

To support his conclusions in the face of the above-cited findings, Vaillant, in the original edition of his book, takes the view that a return to social drinking, which was a common outcome among the untreated abusers in the Core City sample, should not, by necessity, be equated with stable recovery. Rather, he maintains, giving a number of case histories as examples, that a return to "a symptomatic drinking" pattern constitutes a rather ambiguous outcome, often representing borderline cases between moderate drinking and alcohol abuse. In the updated version, based on an additional 12-year follow-up (Vaillant, 1995), he presents evidence claimed to demonstrate that ex-abusers may drink for extended periods without symptoms and still relapse, and that the period of continuous abstinence required to be able to predict stable remission may in fact be much longer than the 6-month criterion adopted in many treatment studies. The empirical findings cited to support these claims are, for instance, that almost one-third of the Core City abusers, judged to be drinking socially at the age of 47, later relapsed into alcohol abuse as compared with less than one-fifth of the abstainers. Further, following up all 56 men in the combined Core City and College samples who were ever judged to have been dependent on alcohol (DSM-III; APA, 1980) and later to have achieved abstinence for greater than 2 years, Vaillant finds that 4 out of 10 relapsed at some later time point, in some cases after as long as 10 years or more. In regards to predictors of stable abstinence, he finds that neither childhood antecedents, risk factors for alcohol abuse, nor most indicators of problem severity can single out future abstainers from future chronic cases. However, becoming abstinent was moderately associated with being of Irish (as opposed to French-Mediterranean) ancestry, having ever been a binge drinker, and being extensively involved in AA.

In summary, and largely in accordance with other studies, Vaillant's longitudinal endeavor may be said to have shown that many alcohol abusers—perhaps as many as one-half, depending on how broadly "abuse" is defined—eventually do recover naturally, at least sometimes, without quitting their drinking altogether. At the same time, his data indicate that for a smaller group the problem may develop into a more or less "chronic" stage, from which sustained abstinence indeed seems to be the safest route. Although admitting that alcoholism can be defined by a sociological model just as well as by a medical model (Vaillant, 1983), the author insists that its course in these latter cases seems to be driven by its own dynamic, legitimizing the use of the disease notion.

The "Classics" in the Alcohol Field: A Summary Appraisal

Perhaps the best way of resolving the apparent contradictions in some of Vaillant's conclusions, and of reconciling the seemingly diverging images of self-change given by studies of identified alcohol abusers and epidemiological research, is to paraphrase Room (1977), who talks about "the two worlds of alcohol problems." Thus, from the clinical perspective, addiction to alcohol may well be viewed as an inexorably progressive "disease," manifested by increasing and increasingly stereotypic drinking, accompanied by a continuous alienation from conventional life and normal social networks, and with relatively few examples of stable remission, either "spontaneously" or with the help of treatment. In population probability samples, on the other hand, alcohol problems will typically stand out as relatively common, heterogeneous and poorly intercorrelated, and largely transient, with self-change as the typical outcome. However, this does not necessarily mean that these two types of studies deal with groups of people who are initially and vitally different. Rather, they may be seen as focusing on different parts of a continuum, the field of vision in clinical studies typically restricted to the one end, or even as using different paradigms and language to account for representations of basically the same phenomena. In fact, the seemingly progressive and predictable course of alcoholism, as it appears in clinical studies, is likely to be a "retrospective illusion," created by a number of overlapping factors (e.g., that it is indeed the severest cases that tend to turn up in treatment and often do so repeatedly, that they generally come to treatment when they are at the bottom of a cycle, and/or that people may adapt the stories they tell clinicians to what they believe to be viable in this context; Peele, 1999). As amply illustrated by examples from Mulford (1984), the empirical facts that some individuals' drinking tends to evolve into a vicious circle, and that the option of stable remission decreases—and is likely to require more strain—the deeper into this circle a person has come, do not prove that there are vital inborn differences between future alcohol abusers and future non-alcohol abusers.

As evidenced by this review, research and debate on self-change in the addiction field, possibly due to the perceived controversial nature of the topic, has long focused on incidence and prevalence rates. Only a few of the early studies (e.g., Ludwig, 1985; Saunders & Kershaw, 1979; Tuchfeld, 1981) addressed reasons for quitting or cutting down drinking among untreated respondents. However, due to differences in scope and methods and levels of analysis, the findings of these studies are difficult to compare and can scarcely claim to have given a consistent picture of the forces behind self-change. What has contributed to later theorizing in the field, however, is Tuchfeld's (1981) suggestion that treated and untreated recoveries may be similar in form but different in content, and Vaillant's (1983) attempt to discern the common "healing forces" behind enduring solutions. At the methodological level, the study first reported by Sobell, Sobell, and Toneatto in 1992 introduced several important improvements (e.g., a thorough assessment of respondents' drinking histories to ensure that there were recoveries from severe alcohol problems, structured inventories to record environmental changes, comparisons with a nonrecovered control group to avoid attributing recovery to events and experiences common to all problem drinkers). Thus, setting a standard for investigations to come, this study can be seen as the first in the "second wave" of self-change research in the alcohol field.

Summing Up: Conclusions and Implications

What can safely be deduced about self-change from these "early classics"? In order to give a valid answer to this question, it might be helpful to return to the opening remarks of this chapter. The notion of self-change first attracted attention and became the subject of dispute and controversy at a time and place where the intended phenomenon was perceived as a challenge and threat to widely cherished notions of drug and alcohol problems and to strongly vested interests in the expanding prevention and treatment fields. During the same period, much of the empirical data that furnished the, at times, heated debate emerged as the side products of research essentially focusing on other issues. Consequently, the "classics" cannot be claimed to have given conclusive answers to simplistic questions such as "How common is self-change?" or "Who is the typical self-changer?". Rather, and perhaps more importantly, they may be claimed to have settled a number of widespread, but poorly substantiated, beliefs about drug and alcohol use related problems which, at the time, permeated both the popular mind and society's ways of trying to deal with these issues. In summary, they showed such problems to be multifaceted and heterogeneous, and more strongly associated with ethnic, sociocultural, and contextual factors than with, for example, heredity or childhood experiences. Contrary to what had been commonly believed regarding the long-term course of drug use or problem drinking, the research demonstrated a great deal of variability and flux over often rather short periods and a general decline of most types of problems with age. It needs to be emphasized, however, that this general picture does not refute the existence of a continuum of individual "problem careers," ranging from temporary and relatively mild to long-lasting and increasingly severe problems, showing great resistance to any change effort, with or without treatment.

Overall, these findings fit rather poorly with traditional disease or dependence paradigms and demonstrate the need for more complex explanatory models, taking into account psychological and sociodemographic factors as well as culturally and subculturally induced values, options, and alternatives (Blomqvist, 1998; Mulford, 1984; Peele, 1985). Concerning the incidence of self-change, the early studies have amply demonstrated that people rather often change drug use and drinking habits, perceived by themselves or others to be a problem, for the better. At the same time, they have clearly indicated that recovery rates are highly sensitive to measurement (i.e., criteria used to define "addiction" and "improvement," length of study periods). Certainly, the incidence rates may also depend on how the boundary between treatment interventions and naturally occurring events and processes is drawn (Blomqvist, 1996; Moos, 1994).

By demonstrating that "'spontaneous recovery' is no more a unitary phenomenon than is addiction itself" (Blomqvist, 1996, p. 1819), the studies discussed in this chapter may be viewed as helpful in pointing toward future research in this area regarding more complex and possibly more fruitful questions than incidence rates or allegedly stable predictors of self-change. At least indirectly, they revealed that there may not be a single route out of one uniform condition defined as addiction, but rather multiple paths out of a wide range of more or less severe substance use-related predicaments. Moreover, the options for stable recovery as well as the specific course of the change process may vary with problem severity in addition to personal and sociocultural circumstances. This, of course, does not make continued research any less urgent, but rather calls for more sophisticated attempts to uncover the complex web of interacting biological, psychological, social, and cultural forces that may assist people in overcoming self-defeating engagements in drug or alcohol use, irrespective of whether this process partly occurs within the context of formal treatment (Blomqvist & Cameron, 2002). Viewed in this light, the vast implications of the studies reviewed in this chapter may be claimed to be far from having been fully acknowledged by all, either in the general public or in the research and treatment fields. Indeed, as will become evident from other chapters in this book, many of the issues raised by these early publications are still strikingly topical.

References

American Psychiatric Association. (1980). *Diagnostic and statistical manual of mental disorders* (3rd ed.). Washington, DC: Author.

Biernacki, P. (1986). *Pathways from heroin addiction. Recovery without treatment.* Philadelphia: Temple University Press.

Blomqvist, J. (1996). Paths to recovery from substance misuse: Change of lifestyle and the role of treatment. *Substance Use and Misuse, 31*(13), 1807–1852.

Blomqvist, J. (1998). *Beyond treatment? Widening the approach to alcohol problems and solutions.* Doctoral dissertation, Stockholm University: Department of Social Work.

Blomqvist, J., & Cameron, D. (2002). Editorial: Moving away from addiction: Forces, processes and context. *Addiction Research and Theory, 10*(2), 115–118.

Burt Associates. (1977). *Drug treatment in New York City and Washington, DC: Follow-up studies.* NIDA.

Cahalan, D. (1970). *Problem drinkers: A national survey.* San Francisco: Jossey-Bass.

Cahalan, D., Cisin, I. H., & Crossley, H. M. (1969). *American drinking practices: A national survey of behaviour and attitudes* (Monograph No. 6). New Brunswick, NJ: Rutgers Center of Alcohol Studies.

Cahalan, D., & Room, R. (1974). *Problem drinking among American men.* New Brunswick, NJ: Rutgers University Press.

Clark, W. B. (1976). Loss of control, heavy drinking and drinking problems in a longitudinal study. *Journal of Studies in Alcohol, 37*, 1256–1290.

Clark, W. B., & Cahalan, D. (1976). Changes in problem drinking over a four-year span. *Addictive Behaviors, 1*, 251–260.

Drew, L. R. H. (1968). Alcoholism as a self-limiting disease. *Quarterly Journal of Studies on Alcohol, 29,* 956–967.

Fillmore, K. M. (1975). Relationships between specific drinking problems in early adulthood and middle age: An exploratory 20-year follow-up study. *Journal of Studies on Alcohol, 36,* 882–907.

Fillmore, K. M. (1987a). Women's drinking across the life course as compared to men's. *British Journal of Addiction, 82,* 801–811.

Fillmore, K. M. (1987b). Prevalence, incidence, and chronicity of drinking patterns and problems among men as a function of age: A longitudinal and cohort analysis. *British Journal of Addiction, 82,* 77–83.

Fillmore, K. M., Hartka, E., Johnstone, B. M., Speiglman, R., & Temple, M. T. (1988). *Spontaneous remission from alcohol problems: A critical review.* Prepared for the Institute of Medicine Committee for the Study of Treatment and Rehabilitation Services for Alcoholism and Alcohol Misuse.

Fillmore, K. M., & Midanik, L. (1984). The chronicity of alcohol problems by age among men: A longitudinal study. *Journal of Studies on Alcohol, 45,* 228–236.

Kendell, R. E., & Staton, M. C. (1966). The fate of untreated alcoholics. *Quarterly Journal of Studies on Alcohol, 27,* 30–41.

Kissin, B., Rosenblatt, S. M., & Machover, S. (1968). Prognostic factors in alcoholism. *Psychiatric Research Reports, 24,* 22–43.

Knupfer, G. (1972). Ex-problem drinkers. In M. Roof, L. N. Robins, & M. Pollack (Eds.), *Life history research in psychopathology* (Vol. 2, pp. 256–280). Minneapolis: The University of Minnesota Press.

Ludwig, A. M. (1985). Cognitive processes associated with 'spontaneous' recovery from alcoholism. *Journal of Studies on Alcohol, 46,* 53–58.

Maddux, J. F., & Desmond, D. P. (1980). New light on the maturing out hypothesis in opioid dependence. *Bulletin of Narcotics, 32*(1), 15–25.

Moos, R. (1994). Treated or untreated, an addiction is not an island unto itself. *Addiction, 89,* 507–509.

Mulford, H. (1984). Rethinking the alcohol problem: A natural processes model. *Journal of Drug Issues, 14,* 31–43.

Pattison, E. M., Sobell, M. B., & Sobell, L. C. (1977). *Emerging concepts of alcohol dependence.* New York: Springer.

Peele, S. (1983, June 26). Disease or defense? Review of the 'Natural history of alcoholism' by George E. Vaillant. *New York Times Book Review,* p. 10.

Peele, S. (1985). *The meaning of addiction. Compulsive experience and its interpretation.* Toronto: Lexington Books.

Peele, S. (1999, March). *Natural remission as a natural process. Models of addiction/ remission and their consequences.* Paper presented at the International Conference on Natural History of the Addictions, Les Diablerets, Switzerland.

Robins, L. N. (1974a). *The Vietnam drug user returns* (Special Action Office Monograph, Series A, No. 2). Washington, DC: U.S. Government Printing Office.

Robins, L. N. (1974b). A follow-up study of Vietnam veterans' drug use. *Journal of Drug Issues, 4,* 61–63.

Robins, L. N. (1993). Vietnam veterans' rapid recovery from heroin addiction: A fluke or normal expectation? (The Sixth Thomas James Okey Memorial Lecture). *Addiction, 88,* 1041–1054.

Robins, L. N., Davis, D. H., & Goodwin, D. W. (1974). Drug use by Army enlisted men in Vietnam: A follow-up on their return home. *American Journal of Epidemiology, 99,* 235–249.

Robins, L. N., Davis, D. H., & Nurco, D. N. (1974). How permanent was Vietnam drug addiction? *American Journal of Public Health, Suppl. 64*, 38–43.

Robins, L. N., Helzer, J. E., & Davis, D. H. (1975). Narcotic use in Southeast Asia and afterwards: An interview study of 898 Vietnam returnees. *Archives of General Psychiatry, 32*, 955–961.

Robins, L. N., Helzer, J. E., Hesselbrock, M., & Wish, E. (1980). Vietnam veterans three years after Vietnam: How our study changed our view of heroin. In L. Brill & C. Winick (Eds.), *Yearbook of substance use and abuse* (pp. 213–230). New York: Human Science Press.

Roizen, R., Cahalan, D., & Shanks, P. (1978). Spontaneous remission among untreated problem drinkers. In D. B. Kandel (Ed.), *Longitudinal research on drug use: Empirical findings and methodological issues* (pp. 197–221). Washington, DC: Hemisphere Publishing.

Room, R. (1977). Measurement and distribution of drinking patterns and problems in general populations. In G. Edwards et al. (Eds.), *Alcohol related disabilities* (pp. 62–87). Geneva: World Health Organization.

Room, R. (1983). Sociological aspects of the disease concept of alcoholism. In R. G. Smart, E. B. Glaser, Y. Israel, H. Kalant, R. E. Popham, & W. Schmidt (Eds.), *Research advances in alcohol and drug problems* (Vol. 7, pp. 47–91). New York: Plenum Press.

Saunders, W. M., & Kershaw, P. W. (1979). Spontaneous remission from alcoholism: A community study. *British Journal of Addiction, 74*, 251–265.

Schachter, S. (1982). Recidivism and self-cure of smoking and obesity. *American Psychologist, 37*(4), 436–444.

Smart, R. G. (1975). Spontaneous recovery in alcoholics: A review and analysis of the available research. *Drug and Alcohol Dependence, 1*, 277–285.

Snow, M. (1973). Maturing out of narcotic addiction in New York City. *International Journal of the Addictions, 8*(6), 921–938.

Sobell, L. C., Ellingstad, T. P., & Sobell, M. B. (2000). Natural recovery from alcohol and drug problems: Methodological review of the research with suggestions for future directions. *Addiction, 95*(5), 749–764.

Sobell, L. C., Sobell, M. B., & Toneatto, T. (1992). Recovery from alcohol problems without treatment. In N. Heather, W. R. Miller, & J. Greeley (Eds.), *Self-control and addictive behaviors* (pp. 198–241). New York: Pergamon Press.

Sobell, L. C., Sobell, M. B., Toneatto, T., & Leo, G. I. (1993). What triggers the resolution of alcohol problems without treatment? *Alcoholism: Clinical and Experimental Research, 17*, 217–224.

Temple, M. T., & Fillmore, K. M. (1985). The variability of drinking patterns among young men, age 16–31: A longitudinal study. *International Journal of the Addictions, 20*, 1595–1620.

Toulmin, S. (1961). *Foresight and understanding*. London: Hutchinson.

Tuchfeld, B. S. (1981). Spontaneous remissions in alcoholics: Empirical observations and theoretical implications. *Journal of Studies on Alcohol, 42*, 626–641.

Vaillant, G. E. (1983). *The natural history of alcoholism*. Cambridge, MA: Harvard University Press.

Vaillant, G. E. (1995). *The natural history of alcoholism revisited*. Cambridge, MA: Harvard University Press.

Waldorf, D. (1983). Natural recovery from opiate addiction. Some social-psychological processes of untreated recovery. *Journal of Drug Issues, 13*(2), 237–280.

Waldorf, D., & Biernacki, P. (1979). Natural recovery from heroin addiction: A review of the incidence literature. *Journal of Drug Issues, 9*(2), 282–289.

Waldorf, D., & Biernacki, P. (1981). The natural recovery from opiate addiction: Some preliminary findings. *Journal of Drug Issues, 9*(1), 61–76.

Winick, C. (1962). Maturing out of narcotic addiction. *Bulletin on Narcotics, 14*(1), 1–7.

Winick, C. (1964). The life cycle of the narcotic addict and of addiction. *Bulletin on Narcotics, 16*(1), 1–11.

3
Natural Recovery or Recovery without Treatment from Alcohol and Drug Problems as Seen from Survey Data

Reginald G. Smart

Much of what is known about self-change or recovery without treatment from alcohol and drug problems comes from general population studies or special samples from sources other than treatment centers. In this chapter, reports from large-scale population surveys and community studies as well as those from smaller samples obtained by advertising or other means will be reviewed. Such studies provide good estimates of how many people in the larger society have alcohol and drug problems that resolved without formal treatment. These studies also help in understanding the characteristics of those who recover without treatment. The advantages and disadvantages of using various interview methods and what questions are still unanswered about natural recovery in large populations will be examined. Finally, practical suggestions based on this research will be discussed.

Early Drinking Survey Results

Some of the earliest interest in natural recovery occurred because of drinking surveys that showed declines in drinking with age. Cahalan and Room (1974) found in their American Drinking Practices Survey that 25% of males aged 21–29 had high scores on a drinking problem scale. However, only 13% of those aged 50–59 and 19% over 70 years old had high problem scores. These results were obtained for both males and females and were stronger among the higher social classes than the lower ones. Because the Cahalan and Room study was a cross-sectional survey and not a longitudinal one, no estimate was made regarding how many individuals stopped drinking on their own as opposed to with active treatment. Later studies using longitudinal data have generally shown that drinking practices remain stable rather than decrease (Glynn, Bouchard, LoCastro, & Laird, 1985; Temple & Leino, 1989). Some have argued that the difference between the cross-sectional and longitudinal studies is accounted for largely by the higher mortality of heavy drinkers, allowing only light and moderate drinkers to reach the older years (Stall, 1987; Temple & Leino, 1989). However, others have noted that mortality rates are an insufficient cause, and natural recovery is an important factor (Drew, 1968; Harford & Samorajski, 1987).

Specialized Survey Studies of Natural Recovery

Several efforts have been made to determine rates of natural recovery or recovery without treatment in surveys of general populations. There is considerable variability in the survey methods used, the definitions of natural recovery, and how alcohol problems are defined.

The earliest survey of natural recovery used a health questionnaire at three time points in the early 1960s. Bailey and Stewart (1967) found that at their first survey, 91 people had a current or previous drinking problem. By the second and third follow-ups, only 13 and 6 participants, respectively, were drinking within normal limits. None had psychotherapy but half had medical care related to drinking and could therefore be considered naturally recovered. This study showed a very low rate of natural recovery compared with that found in later investigations. As this report has a very small sample size, less confidence can be placed in the results of these findings.

In the early 1990s, surveys of natural recovery became larger and more numerous and sophisticated. For example, Hasin and Grant (1995) carried out the first large-scale survey of natural recovery. They used data from the National Health Interview Study conducted in 1988 which had used a well-designed sample of 43,809 people aged 18 and over in the 50 U.S. states and the District of Columbia. They identified former drinkers, who comprised about 19% of the total sample; of this group, 21% were alcohol dependent and 42% were alcohol abusers according to DSM-IV criteria. However, only 33% of those who were alcohol dependent and 17% of those who were alcohol abusers had attended Alcoholics Anonymous (AA) or sought any other kind of treatment, thus indicating that the majority had solved their alcohol problems without help. Moreover, many reported social pressure to cut down their drinking, which may have been sufficient to make them stop drinking.

Several important surveys of recovery without treatment have also been conducted in Canada. Sobell, Cunningham, and Sobell (1996) used data from a national survey ($n = 11,634$) and an Ontario survey ($n = 1,034$). They defined problem drinkers as those who usually drank seven or more drinks per occasion. Most of those who resolved their alcohol problems ($n = 322$ and $n = 70$, respectively) did so without using any formal treatment. The proportion of recovery without treatment was remarkably similar in the two surveys (77.5% and 77.7%, respectively). However, there was a large difference in how many problem drinkers returned to moderate drinking rather than abstinence (38% versus 63%, respectively). One reason suggested for the likelihood of returning to social drinking was that socioeconomic and income levels are higher in Ontario than in the country as a whole.

Cunningham, Lin, Ross, and Walsh (2000) found several groups of heavy drinkers in a natural recovery study. One group had significant alcohol problems over a long time and resolved them through abstinence or treatment while another group experienced fewer problems but "matured out" of them as they aged. Another group recovered from problems and were able to drink moderately and have fewer problems than the abstinent groups. It was found that nontreatment recoveries among those with alcohol problems varied between 53.7% and 87.5%, depending on how many alcohol-related problems the drinker had experienced. The greater the number of problems, the lower was the percentage of participants who were self-remitters. Recoveries without treatment were less frequent among those with more serious alcohol problems. However, even among those who had six or more problems, 53.7% recovered without formal treatment.

Similar to the Canadian studies cited above, Weisner, Matzger, and Kaskutas (2003) found that alcohol dependent people who received treatment were more likely to become abstinent than those who were untreated in a California survey with a 1-year follow-up. Having more heavy drinkers in one's social network, higher psychiatric morbidity, and more social consequences of alcoholism were inversely related to recovery in both treated and untreated groups.

Bischof, Rumpf, Hapke, Meyer, and John (2001) studied natural recovery among those in a German general population survey. They recruited 32 individuals with alcohol dependence who were "fully remitted" without treatment for alcohol problems and compared them with 26 participants who were currently alcohol dependent. Unlike results from other studies, those who recovered without treatment had higher levels of dependency, less social pressure to quit drinking, and more driving while intoxicated. However, they had more work satisfaction, better finances, and more stable relationships. Compared with male alcohol dependents, females who remitted had less social pressure to change, less satisfaction with life, more health problems, and drove less when impaired (Bischof, Rumpf, Hapke, Meyer, & John, 2000a). This is the only known study which explores sex differences in self-change in detail. Further studies with larger samples are needed to explore such differences in greater depth. The above surveys demonstrate that the majority of individuals who report having solved alcohol problems did so without treatment or AA involvement. It should also be noted that there is little variation across studies, and natural survey rates are usually 75% or greater.

While less work has focused on natural recovery from drug use, several studies have been conducted by Cunningham and colleagues. The first study used the Canadian Alcohol and Drugs Survey conducted on a national sample (n = 12,155) in 1994 (Cunningham, Koski-Jännes, & Tonneato, 1996). Former drug users who had not used in the past year were identified. Very few had ever had any drug related treatment, especially among regular marijuana users (16.0%), LSD users (14.1%), and cocaine/crack users (16.0%). However, treatment rates were higher for speed (20.4%) and heroin users (34.5%). Overall, this study did not relate treatment to drug use or serious drug problems and some of the sample sizes were small, especially for individuals treated for speed and heroin use.

A later study done with an Ontario sample examined the reasons why drug users quit (Cunningham, 1999). This study identified 109 former cannabis users who had used 50 times or more and 26 former cocaine users who had used 10 times or more. Only 1.8% of the cannabis users and none of the cocaine users reported that they quit because of treatment or doctors' advice. Most mentioned factors such as growing up, personal changes, changes in responsibilities, health concerns, or disappointments with drug effects as the main reasons for stopping their drug use.

Community Studies of Self-Change

Several community-based studies of self-change from drinking problems have been conducted using a variety of approaches. In the first, Newman (1965) used the records of police, treatment, social agencies, and clergy to identify alcoholics in 1951. A total of 688 were found in an Ontario county and in 1961, a follow-up was conducted to examine how many participants had recovered. In this study, individuals were defined as "recovered" if they did not reappear in any records at follow-up. Overall, only 29.4% of the problem drinkers, 14.2% of the alcohol addicts, and 10% of the chronic alcoholics recovered without treatment. These findings are far lower than would be expected from survey results. However, the criteria used were quite different; that is, people with drinking problems were not self-identified as in other surveys, but were classified through records. Thus, these cases may have been more serious than those typically seen in surveys.

A community-based study of people in the Clydeside area of Scotland by Saunders and Kershaw (1979) also found a lower rate of self-change than did most surveys. This investigation covered 228 people who said that they "drank too much in the past." Some were still drinking too much, while others were episodic drinkers or misclassified based on surveys that are more intensive. However, there were 41 past problem drinkers, none of whom had been treated for alcoholism. Most reduced their drinking because of marriage, job changes, physical illness, or family advice. Moreover, three stated that advice from their general practitioner was important in reducing their drinking. Of the 19 respondents classified as alcoholics, 7 had received alcoholism treatment or had attended AA. The remaining 63% (12 cases) had recovered without treatment, but some of those appeared to have had medical advice or treatment for other ailments. As with the problem drinkers, marriage, job changes, and physical illness were the most important factors in recovery for the people who are "definitely alcoholics."

Leung, Kinzie, Boehnlein, and Shore (1993) conducted a 19-year follow-up of 100 people in a small Indian community. Only 46 could be reinterviewed but others ($n = 25$) were followed through medical charts or death certificates. Alcohol abuse and dependence diagnoses were made using DSM-III criteria. In total, 46 had stopped drinking and of those only 8 (17%) had specific alcohol treatment. Most mentioned family pressures and social and financial problems as the most important factors in recovery, although many could give no reasons.

Cameron, Manik, Bird, and Sinorwalia (2002) compared two small groups of whites and people from the Indian subcontinent who had "grown out of alcohol problems" without treatment. For both groups, physical health, self-esteem, and ability to cope and work were factors in promoting self-change. Social networks and family status and honor were more important factors for the Indians compared with the group of whites.

In another small study, male Navajos who "aged out" of alcohol problems without treatment were interviewed (Quintero, 2000). It was found that important factors in success included health and religious concerns, having a traditional Navajo way of life, and increased child-rearing responsibilities.

Russell et al. (2002) investigated samples of alcoholics identified in previous community studies and found 83 "naturally recovered" individuals. Those who recovered were more often married and had better coping mechanisms, higher self-esteem, social networks with fewer heavy drinkers, and less drug use and intoxication histories.

Overall, it is striking that so few studies involve high-risk groups such as individuals from alcoholic families, American Indians, or other aboriginal peoples. Current knowledge of natural recovery in these groups is, therefore, sparse and needs to be investigated further.

The community studies reviewed above give a wide range of recovery rates without treatment. It is notable, however, that the sample sizes and characteristics vary greatly as do the criteria for alcohol problems and dependency. In addition, only a few communities have been studied and they may not be representative of large populations.

Drug Users and Natural Recovery

Several studies of natural recovery among abusers of drugs such as opiates, cocaine, and cannabis are now available, many with large samples. The largest of these involved recoveries among 841 American Vietnam veterans who had positive urines for drugs on leaving Vietnam in 1971 (Price, Risk, & Spitznagel, 2001). A follow-up 25 years later showed that most drug abusers achieved recovery without treatment. Only about 20% were treated for their drug problems, however, most achieved recovery with a "cold turkey" approach. There was a lower rate of natural recovery for opiates. Not only does this study have interesting results, but it is also one of the very few with a long-term follow-up.

However, it supplies no psychosocial reasons for the natural recoveries or any assessment of why some drug abusers did not recover without treatment.

Several smaller studies have explored the psychosocial reasons for natural recoveries among drug abusers. For example, Toneatto, Sobell, Sobell, and Rubel (1999) studied 50 abstinent, untreated former cocaine users and 21 active, untreated cocaine users. The two groups did not differ in demographics, drug history, or psychiatric problems. However, recovery was related to a cognitive appraisal of the pros and cons of further cocaine use, with recovered individuals assessing the problem of cocaine abuse as not being worth the consequences.

Similar findings were reported by Blomqvist (2002) who studied 25 treated former drug users and 25 self-remitters gathered from advertisements and other sources in Sweden. Among the most often perceived reasons for natural recoveries were intrapsychic factors (i.e., wanting to quit), frightening or humiliating experiences, situational changes in life, legal problems, and positive influences from others. This report showed that both alcohol and drug abusers remitted because of rational decisions and some negative consequences.

Latkin, Knowlton, Hoover, and Mandell (1999) studied 335 former drug addicts and abusers in an HIV prevention program who ceased drug use. The main factor in natural recoveries was that remitters had fewer members of their social network who used drugs; other variables did not seem to be as important. Although this report demonstrates the possible influence of social factors in natural recovery, it does not allow for easy comparisons to other studies of the same type.

Only one known paper makes any cross-national comparisons of natural recovery among alcohol and drug abusers. Sobell et al. (2001) compared alcohol and cocaine abusers in Canada with heroin abusers in Switzerland. Cognitive factors were the most important reasons for cessation followed by emotional and behavioral monitoring. Many drug abusers go through a cognitive appraisal in trying to remit without treatment. This process seems to be similar across cultural setting and type of substance involved.

Advantages of Survey and Other Methods for Studying Natural Recovery

Although survey sampling methods have some disadvantages, they also have many advantages over other designs for studying natural recovery. Surveys usually involve large samples of the general population and hence can give overall estimates for rates of natural recovery. Due to their size, they normally identify large numbers of problem drinkers or alcohol abusers and can break them down into several subgroups. However, most surveys contain very few questions about recovery without treatment. Studies not using surveys but snowball methods or special samples of recovered problem drinkers are typically focused on recovery issues and how recovery proceeds. They usually contain many more questions on how recovery was achieved and go in depth about the motivation for recovery. This study design is more likely to answer questions about how and why recovery occurs, but not about the number of alcoholics or problem drinkers who recover without treatment.

Snowball, Media-Derived, and Convenience Samples in Self-Change Studies

Numerous efforts have been made to study self-change with snowball, samples derived from media advertisements, and other nonrepresentative methods. Various follow-up studies such as those by Vaillant (1983), Fillmore (1987), and others established that the natural history of alcohol problems involves fluctuations over time and that some people recover with increasing age while others do not. Regarding wait-list control groups, several studies have found that some participants in these groups got better without treatment (Kendall and Staton, 1966; Kissin, Rosenblatt, & Machover, 1968).

Reasons for recovery and details of how it happens are best understood from the various studies of recovered alcohol abusers. Numerous investigations have used individuals who responded to media contacts. These are not true population studies, but rather surveys of people who have come forward because of advertisements in newspapers, radio, or television. The early studies of Tuchfeld (1981) and Ludwig (1985) used newspaper advertisements to attract people who had recovered from alcohol problems without treatment. Tuchfeld's 51 alcohol abusers reported that they recovered mainly because of personal illness or accidents, better education about alcohol problems, religious experiences, direct interventions by friends or relatives, and financial or other problems created by alcohol. In addition, most responders gave more than one reason. Ludwig's questions were different and he found that his 29 participants had recovered because they had hit a personal bottom, had a physical illness, a change in lifestyle, or a religious experience; a few simply lost interest in alcohol. These reasons have been repeated in later studies as well.

Klingemann (1991) used newspapers and radio to assemble samples of recovered alcohol abusers and heroin users in Switzerland. About half of the naturally recovered alcohol cases returned to social drinking, although all but a few of the heroin users stopped altogether. In general, the problems of both groups were the same before and after recovery. Both groups were self-conscious remitters who decided that, after hitting bottom or having health, financial, and other problems, their addiction career should end. Klingemann showed that there are several major stages in recovery, such as the motivation for change, implementing this decision, and developing and maintaining a new identity.

One of the largest and most comprehensive studies of alcohol problems derived from media interviews was conducted by Sobell, Sobell, Toneatto, and Leo (1993). They recruited and interviewed 182 respondents and classified them into the following groups: (a) resolved abstinent without treatment, (b) resolved nonabstinent, (c) resolved abstinent with treatment, and (d) non-resolved (i.e., control group). To corroborate respondents' self-report, they also interviewed relatives or friends. The largest group was resolved abstinent without treatment ($n = 71$), followed by nonresolved ($n = 62$). In the overall sample, only 28 participants were abstinent and had ever sought treatment. There were no differences within the various resolved groups or in comparisons with the nonresolved group. Most recoveries involved cognitive appraisals of drinking (i.e., pros and cons of continuing to drink) and the support of spouses. Similar results were also found by Tucker, Vuchinich, and Gladsjo (1994) in their study that examined participants 2 years before and 1 year after their abstinence.

Granfield and Cloud (1996) also studied both alcohol and drug users but employed a snowball sample of 46 middle-class individuals with stable lives, jobs, and families. Although these people had much to lose by continuing their addictive careers, they were reluctant to enter treatment. Most participants in this study never adopted addictive lifestyles or identities, which probably helped in their recovery. Many of these findings were repeated in Burman's (1997) study of 38 alcohol abusers in New Jersey obtained through the media. Individuals who recovered eventually felt that they had too much to lose by continuing their addictive careers.

Only one study (Copeland, 1998) focused on women in recovery. Copeland assembled 32 cases of women who recovered on their own by advertisement in Sydney, Australia. Most changed because of concerns for current and future psychological and physical health and existential crises. A conflict developed between their impoverished lives and their self-concept as intelligent, middle-class women. Compared with men, these women seemed to change residences, social activities, and sexual partners more frequently. However, this study had no direct comparisons with male self-changers.

Among the largest and most comprehensive recent studies using convenience or media samples are those by Bischof and colleagues. In one study, Bischof, Rumpf, Hapke, Meyer, and John (2003) entered 178 media-recruited natural remitters into a cluster analysis. They found one group with high levels of dependence, low alcohol-related problems and low social support and dependence, high social support, and late onset of alcohol problems. They concluded that natural remitters are a heterogeneous group and that understanding natural recovery must take this into account. Further investigation is needed into the various subgroups among natural remitters looking at age, sex, extent of drinking problems, and other factors.

Bischof, Rumpf, Hapke, Meyer, and John (2000b) have also explored the triggering mechanisms in natural recovery. They studied 93 remitters and 42 self-help group participants. There were more similarities than differences in the successful recoveries of the two groups. However, self-help attendees talked to more people about their recovery and sought more social support in dealing with craving than did natural remitters.

Rumpf, Bischof, Hapke, and John (1999) and Rumpf, Bischof, Hapke, Meyer, and John (2000) have also shown that individuals solicited through the media, compared with those in a representative survey, are more likely to be abstinent in the last months, more dependent, less satisfied with life prior to natural recovery, and possess better coping skills. This is an interesting and important finding because it reinforces the idea that there are likely to be different results when different sampling methods are used. Therefore, comparisons of other sampling methods (e.g., word of mouth, convenience, snowball-derived) could be of value.

Several studies have focused on age as an important sample selection variable. For example, a study using a very small sample size of 5 younger males and 7 females was reported by Finfgeld and Lewis (2002), but the results are difficult to interpret. However, Vik, Cellucci, and Ivers (2003) studied 91 college students and found that 22% reduced their heavy drinking without treatment. In these analyses, marital status and church attendance were both important predictors.

Only one known study of older problem drinkers has been published (Walton, Mudd, Blow, Chermack, & Gomberg, 2000). Through advertising, 78 older adults with drinking problems were recruited. At a 3-year follow-up, 48 participants were reinterviewed and only 11.4% were resolved. Health problems were the main reason for decreased drinking. Overall, this study seems to show a low rate of natural recovery for older adults. It would be worth repeating this study with a larger sample and a broader list of maintenance factors. It would also be useful to conduct studies comparing natural recovery rates among different age groups, especially if the design controlled for the extent of alcohol problems.

Do Those Who Recover Naturally Have Fewer Problems Than Those Who Seek Treatment?

Questions have been raised about whether people who recover from alcohol problems are able to do so because they have fewer problems or alcoholic symptoms than those who need treatment to recover. Saunders and Kershaw (1979) were among the first to note that natural recovery appeared to occur most readily in less severe cases. However, they did not show detailed analyses that supported this claim, although a few others have been able to supply such data.

Several survey studies have shown that those who recover with treatment may have fewer problems than those who seek treatment. For example, a national study by Hasin and Grant (1995) found that only 27% of those who were former drinkers experienced a compulsion to drink, 21% had a DSM-IV diagnosis of alcohol dependence, and 42% had a diagnosis of alcohol abuse. These rates would be substantially less than those found in individuals being treated in alcoholism treatment centers. The two surveys reported by Sobell et al. (1996) showed that persons who were resolved abstinent with treatment were much more likely to have more alcohol problems than those abstinent or nonabstinent without treatment. Also, those who were abstinent with treatment in media-derived studies had higher scores on the MAST, drank more drinks per day, and had more alcohol-related consequences than those who were abstinent without treatment (Sobell et al., 1993). It appears from surveys that natural recovery is most likely with problem drinkers at an early stage in their career, before alcohol-related problems become too overwhelming. However, Klingemann's (1991) study showed that samples from the media were similar to those in surveys and clinic populations. This finding is not surprising considering that Rumpf, Bischof, Hapke, and John (1999) have demonstrated that media-derived natural remitters were more dependent and less often abstinent than were the same groups from population surveys. We should not forget, however, that those who recover on their own do typically have substantial alcohol problems.

What Can We Conclude about Self-Change?

When all the survey and special studies are considered together, the following conclusions emerge:

- Most population surveys show that the large majority of people with alcohol problems can and do resolve them without formal treatment or self-help groups.
- While there are fewer relevant studies, it appears that most former illicit drug abusers stop using drugs without formal treatment. Information about whether prescription drug users can do the same, however, is not yet available.
- Community studies of self-change are few in number. Using different methods than survey designs, some community studies find the same results as surveys while others find lower levels of self-change.
- Survey studies of self-change are larger and more useful in estimating the frequency of problems and recovery rates. However, special studies of self-selected groups are more often used to investigate the paths to recovery and the motivation for change.
- Reasons for self-change are many and varied. Health and cognitive appraisals of the pros and cons of continuing to use versus stopping are two of the more salient reasons for changing.
- There is some evidence from surveys that people who recover without treatment may have fewer alcohol problems (i.e., less dependent) than those who recover through treatment.

Clearly, studies of self-changers show that there are multiple pathways to recovery. However, self-change is the predominant pathway to recovery for many alcohol and drug abusers.

Important areas of research which deserve future investigation are the following:

- Ethnic subgroups and how their natural recovery rates may vary from the general population.
- Individual differences between groups of those who recover on their own, depending on their characteristics before their recovery.

- Gender differences in natural recoveries and factors explaining them.
- High-risk groups for alcohol and drug problems such as aboriginal groups and those from families of alcohol and drug abusers. They may have additional problems with natural recovery compared with groups at lower risk.
- Effects of different recruiting methods on the selection of natural recoveries among different respondent groups.

References

Bailey, M. B., & Stewart, J. (1967). Normal drinking by persons reporting previous problem drinking. *Quarterly Journal of Studies on Alcohol, 28*, 305–315.

Bischof, G., Rumpf, H.-J., Hapke, U., Meyer, C., & John, U. (2000a). Gender differences in normal recovery from alcohol dependence. *Journal of Studies on Alcohol, 61*, 783–786.

Bischof, G., Rumpf, H.-J., Hapke, U., Meyer, C., & John, U. (2000b). Maintenance factors of recovery from alcohol-dependence in treated and untreated individuals. *Alcoholism: Clinical and Experimental Research, 14*, 1773–1777.

Bischof, G., Rumpf, H.-J., Hapke, U., Meyer, C., & John, U. (2001). Factors influencing remission from alcohol dependence without formal help in a representative population. *Addiction, 96*, 1327–1336.

Bischof, G., Rumpf, H.-J., Hapke, U., Meyer, C., & John, U. (2003). Types of natural recovery from alcohol dependence: A cluster analytic approach. *Addiction, 98*, 1737–1746.

Blomqvist, J. (2002). Recovery with and without treatment: A comparison of resolutions of alcohol and drug problems. *Addiction Research and Theory, 10*, 119–158.

Burman, S. (1997). The challenge of sobriety, natural recovery without treatment, and self-help groups. *Journal of Substance Abuse, 9*, 41–61.

Cahalan, D., & Room, R. (1974). *Problem drinking among American men*. New Brunswick, NJ: Rutgers Center of Alcohol Studies.

Cameron, D., Manik, G., Bird, R., & Sinorwalia, A. (2002). What may we be learning from so-called spontaneous remission in ethnic minorities? *Addiction Research and Theory, 10*, 175–182.

Copeland, J. (1998). A qualitative study of self-managed change in substance dependence among women. *Contemporary Drug Problems, 25*, 321–347.

Cunningham, J. A. (1999). Untreated remissions from drug use, the predominant pathway. *Addictive Behaviors, 24*, 267–270.

Cunningham, J. A., Koski-Jännes, A., & Tonneato, T. (1996). *Why do people stop their drug use? Results from a general population*. Unpublished manuscript. Toronto: Centre for Addiction and Mental Health.

Cunningham, J. A., Lin, E., Ross, H. E., & Walsh, G. W. (2000). Factors associated with untreated remission from alcohol abuse or dependence. *Addictive Behaviors, 25*, 317–321.

Drew, L. R. (1968). Alcoholism as a self-limiting disease. *Quarterly Journal of Studies on Alcohol, 29*, 956–967.

Fillmore, K. M. (1987). Prevalence, incidence, and chronicity of drinking patterns and problems among men as a function of age: A longitudinal and cohort analysis. *British Journal of Addiction, 82*, 77–83.

Finfgeld, D. L., & Lewis, I. M. (2002). Self-resolution of alcohol problems in young adulthood: A process of recurring solid ground. *Quantitative Health Research, 12*, 581–592.

Glynn, R. J., Bouchard, G., LoCastro, J., & Laird, N. (1985). Aging and generational effects on drinking behavior in men: Results from the Normative Aging Study. *American Journal of Public Health, 15*, 1413–1419.

Granfield, R., & Cloud, W. (1996). The elephant that no one sees: Natural recovery among middle-class addicts. *Journal of Drug Issues, 26*, 45–61.

Harford, J. T., & Samorajski, T. (1987). Alcohol in the geriatric populations. *Journal of American Geriatric Society, 30*, 18–24.

Hasin, D. S., & Grant, B. F. (1995). AA and other help seeking for alcohol problems: Former drinkers in the US general population. *Journal of Substance Abuse, 7*, 281–292.

Kendell, R. E., & Staton, M. C. (1966). The fate of untreated alcoholics. *Quarterly Journal of Studies on Alcohol, 27*, 30–41.

Kissin, B., Rosenblatt, S. M., & Machover, S. (1968). Prognostic factors in alcoholism. *Psychiatric Research Reports, 24*, 22–43.

Klingemann, H. K. (1991). The motivation for change from problematic alcohol and heroin use. *British Journal of Addiction, 86*, 727–744.

Latkin, C. A., Knowlton, A., Hoover, D., & Mandell, W. (1999). Drug network characteristics as a predictor of cessation of drug use among adult injection drug users: A perspective study. *American Journal of Drug and Alcohol Abuse, 25*, 463–473.

Leung, P. K., Kinzie, J. D., Boehnlein, J. K., & Shore, J. H. (1993). A prospective study of the natural course of alcoholism in a Native American village. *Journal of Studies on Alcohol, 54*, 733–738.

Ludwig, A. M. (1985). Cognitive processes associated with "spontaneous" recovery from alcoholism. *Journal of Studies on Alcohol, 46*, 53–58.

Newman, A. R. (1965). *Alcoholism in Frontenac County*. Doctoral dissertation, Queens University, Kingston.

Price, R. K., Risk, N. K., & Spitznagel, E. L. (2001). Remission from drug abuse over a 25-year period: Pattern of remission and treatment use. *American Journal of Public Health, 7*, 1107–1113.

Quintero, G. (2000). The lizard in the green bottle: "Aging out" of problem drinking among Navajo men. *Social Science and Medicine, 51*, 1031–1045.

Rumpf, H.-J., Bischof, G., Hapke, U., & John, U. (1999). *Studies on natural recovery from alcohol dependence: Sample selection bias by media solicitation?* Unpublished manuscript. Lubeck: Medical University of Lubeck.

Rumpf, H.-J., Bischof, G., Hapke, U., Meyer, C., & John U. (2000). Studies on natural recovery from alcohol dependence: Sample selection bias by media solicitation? *Addiction, 95*, 765–775.

Russell, M., Peirce, R. S., Chan, A. W., Wieczorek, W. F., Moscato, B. S., & Nochajski, T. H. (2002). Natural recovery in a community based sample of alcoholics: Study design and descriptive data. *Substance Use and Misuse, 36*, 1417–1441.

Saunders, W. M., & Kershaw, P. W. (1979). Spontaneous remission from alcoholism: A community study. *British Journal of Addictions, 74*, 251–265.

Sobell, L. C., Cunningham, J. A., & Sobell, M. B. (1996). Recovery from alcohol problems with and without treatment: Prevalence in two population surveys. *American Journal of Public Health, 7*, 966–972.

Sobell, L. C., Klingemann, H., Toneatto, T., Sobell, M. B., Agrawal, S., & Leo, G. (2001). Alcohol and drug abusers' perceived reasons for self change in Canada and

Switzerland: Computer-assisted content analysis. *Substance Use and Abuse, 36,* 1467–1500.

Sobell, L. C., Sobell, M. B., Toneatto, T., & Leo, G. (1993). What triggers the resolution of alcohol problems without treatment? *Alcoholism: Clinical and Experimental Research, 17,* 217–224.

Stall, R. (1987). Research issues concerning alcohol consumption among aging populations. *Drug and Alcohol Dependence, 19,* 195–213.

Temple, M. T., & Leino, V. (1989). Long term outcomes of drinking: A 20 year longitudinal study of men. *British Journal of Addiction, 84,* 889–899.

Toneatto, T., Sobell, L. C., Sobell, M. B., & Rubel, E. (1999). Natural recovery from cocaine dependence. *Psychology of Addictive Behaviors, 13,* 259–268.

Tuchfeld, B. S. (1981). Spontaneous remission in alcoholics: Empirical observations and theoretical implications. *Journal of Studies on Alcohol, 42,* 626–641.

Tucker, J. A., Vuchinich, R. E., & Gladsjo, J. A. (1994). Environmental events surrounding natural recovery from alcohol-related problems. *Journal of Studies on Alcohol, 56,* 401–411.

Vaillant, G. E. (1983). *The natural history of alcoholism.* Cambridge, MA: Harvard University Press.

Vik, P., Cellucci, T., & Ivers, H. (2003). Natural reduction of binge drinking among college students. *Addictive Behaviors, 28,* 643–655.

Walton, M. A., Mudd, S. A., Blow, F. C., Chermack, S. T., & Gomberg, E. S. (2000). Stability in the drinking habits of older problem drinkers recruited from non-treatment settings. *Journal of Substance Abuse Treatment, 18,* 169–177.

Weisner, C., Matzger, H., & Kaskutas, L. A. (2003). How important is treatment? One year outcomes of treated and untreated alcohol-dependent individuals. *Addiction, 98,* 901–911.

4
Remission without Formal Help: New Directions in Studies Using Survey Data

Hans-Jürgen Rumpf, Gallus Bischof, and Ulrich John

This chapter reviews natural recovery research over the past years and focuses on new methodological approaches such as sampling methods, definitions of untreated remission, and longitudinal study designs. It will also address neglected areas in the field such as gender and cross-cultural differences. The current studies partly overcome shortcomings of their earlier predecessors. This chapter mainly focuses on alcohol problems.

In general, studies can be divided into investigations that give frequency estimates of natural remission and those that aim to examine triggering and maintaining factors affecting the remission process. These latter studies are characteristically more in-depth and initially start with descriptive investigations (first generation studies), followed by research using control groups (second generation studies). Both types of studies predominantly used snowball sampling or media solicitation for subject recruitment and were based on qualitative as well as quantitative research methods. Due to methodological shortcomings (see below), the third generation studies started to use general population data. Most of them, however, were not explicitly designed to examine untreated remission but came from projects with other primary aims. This review begins with methodological issues followed by new data on the frequency of natural recovery and factors supporting remission. Finally, suggestions for future research are given.

Methodological Issues

Research over the past years has made new contributions on how sampling methods and definitions of natural recovery alter findings. A comprehensive methodological review on natural recovery research can be found in Sobell, Ellingstad, and Sobell (2000).

Sampling Methods

Most research on causes, conditions, and factors concerning untreated remissions of alcohol and drug use comes from samples recruited via media solicitation. Although a valuable source, such samples may be biased due to special characteristics of remitters responding to such solicitations. The German Transitions in Alcohol Consumption and Smoking (TACOS) study compared media-solicited remitters (n = 176) with those derived from a general population sample (n = 32; Rumpf, Bischof, Hapke, Meyer, & John, 2000). Both groups were fully remitted from alcohol dependence according to DSM-IV criteria for at least 12 months and had received little or no formal help. The samples differed significantly with respect to the amount of drinking and dependence-related variables as well as triggering and maintaining factors for remission. A logistic regression model aiming to explain which variables discriminate best between the samples, and taking interrelationships into account, revealed the following: media-solicited remitters had been more severely dependent, were more often abstinent remitters, were less satisfied with life in several domains, exhibited more health concerns prior to remission, used more coping strategies, and experienced more social pressure. These findings clearly confirm a sample selection bias when recruiting remitters through media solicitation and support the need for general population-based studies.

Definition of the Substance Use Problem

Definitions of a substance use problem in studies of untreated remissions vary widely. Some have used an a priori-defined number of symptoms related to substance use, and others have used the DSM-IV criteria of abuse or dependence. According to a methodological review of the natural recovery research literature, 40% of the studies did not report problem severity (Sobell et al., 2000). Comparability of results requires clear, reproducible, and, when possible, uniform definitions. Alcohol dependence would be considered the most strict definition. Regardless, untreated pathways out of problematic nondependent substance use are worth examining. Although it would be beneficial to have both the dependent and nondependent groups separate, studies often combined the samples. Evidence for this comes from a Canadian study where Cunningham (1999) found a relationship between the severity of drinking problems and the rates of untreated recovery. Using the 1994 Canadian Alcohol and Drug Survey (n = 9,892), he compared groups with one to six lifetime alcohol problems. A total of 885 participants reported at least one problem and had recovered in the past year. Depending on the number of problems, untreated remissions ranged from 87.5% (one problem) to 53.7% (six problems). Thus, findings show that less severe alcohol problems appear to be easier to overcome without treatment. This is an important finding that highlights the need for a clear definition of the problem behavior when studying untreated remissions.

Definition of Treatment

Various definitions of treatment were utilized in previous research on natural recovery, ranging from two self-help group meetings (Sobell, Sobell, Toneatto, & Leo, 1993) to regular self-help group attendance (Humphreys, Moos, & Finney, 1995). In the TACOS study, the impact of different definitions of treatment was analyzed by comparing three groups of media-recruited individuals fully recovered from DSM-IV alcohol dependence: (a) never treated at all (n = 103), (b) minor help (defined as contact with alcohol treatment not exceeding nine self-help group sessions or three counseling sessions with a specialty provider; n = 75), and (c) regular participation in self-help group meetings (n = 50). Findings revealed that remitters from alcohol dependence who received minor help were comparable with remitters who received no help at all, and both groups differed significantly from regular self-help group participants on most triggering and maintenance factors of remission (Bischof, Rumpf, Hapke, Meyer, & John, 2002). These conclusions may have two implications when comparing natural recovery study results. On the one hand, investigations including participants receiving minor help should yield results similar to studies using a more rigorous definition of natural recovery. On the other hand, considering regular self-help group participation as treatment for natural recovery might diminish differences between groups regarding the recovery processes.

Occurrence of Natural Remission in the General Population

Previous studies provide good estimates of the prevalence of remission without formal help (Dawson, 1996; Sobell, Cunningham, & Sobell, 1996). Additional evidence comes from the National Epidemiologic Survey on Alcohol and Related Conditions (NESARC; Dawson et al., 2005). The sample (n = 43,093) is nationally representative of U.S. adults 18 years of age and older. Data were collected through personal interviews conducted in participants' homes. Of the entire sample, 4,422 individuals were classified with DSM-IV alcohol dependence with onset prior to the previous 12 months. From this sample, 25.6% had ever sought help for their alcohol problem. In the last 12 months, only 25% were still dependent, 27.3% were partially remitted (i.e., classified as having alcohol abuse or subthreshold dependence), and 11.8% were at-risk drinkers. Finally, 18.2% were abstinent and 17.7% were low-risk drinkers. Although not explicitly stated, it can be calculated that of those who were fully remitted in the last year (i.e., abstinent or low-risk drinkers), 72.4% did so without formal help (D. A. Dawson, personal communication, November 16, 2006). The percentage of subjects who utilized formal help was distinctly larger in abstinent recoveries (49.3%) compared with nonabstinent recoveries (15.1%). Here, findings confirm a substantial rate of natural recovery that is consistent with previous studies.

Another study examined the rate of untreated remissions among older problem drinkers (Schutte, Moos, & Brennan, 2006). Participants 51 to 65 years old at baseline (n = 1,884) were recruited from a larger community sample. Using data from 4- and 10-year follow-ups, it was found that 73% remitted without any formal help. These findings suggest that rates of untreated remission are similar in older adults as compared with mixed-age samples. However, relative to NESARC data (Dawson et al., 2005), the definition of alcohol problems was more liberal, as evidenced by the use of problem drinking scores. It can be suggested that the rate of untreated remissions would have been lower had DSM-IV alcohol dependence criteria been employed. Evidence for this statement comes from Cunningham's (1999) Canadian report described above. Furthermore, comparisons between remission rates in both studies are complicated by the different time frames used as well as by the use of a retrospective versus a longitudinal design.

In an untreated, mixed sample of 664 individuals who were classified as at-risk drinkers or alcohol dependents or abusers, short-term outcomes after 6, 12, and 18 months were examined (Booth, Fortney, Fortney, Curran, & Kirchner, 2001). Participants were randomly recruited by telephone interviews from the general population in six southern U.S. states. From baseline to the 18-month follow-up, the proportion of alcohol dependent participants decreased from 40.1% to 16.4%, whereas abstinence rose from 0% to 12.9%, and moderate drinking from 19.4% to 31.6%.

As a whole, it can be concluded that the evidence of untreated remission is supported by a substantial body of literature coming from cross-sectional, longitudinal, and short- and long-term databases.

Stability of Untreated Remission

One might argue that remissions without formal help are not stable and, therefore, not worth studying. Thus, data on the stability of untreated remissions are of special interest. In 2006, two studies have been published on this topic. Moos and Moos (2006) recruited problem drinkers who contacted an information and referral center or a detoxification program because of alcohol-related problems and were followed up at 1, 3, 8, and 16 years. Within the first year, 362 participants entered treatment, while 99 did not enter treatment or attend Alcoholics Anonymous (AA). At the 3-year follow-up, 62.4% of the treatment group and 43.4% of the no help group were remitted. At the 16-year follow-up, relapse rates were higher for individuals not utilizing help within the first year (60.5%) compared with those entering treatment or participating in AA (42.9%). The following risk factors for relapse were identified: less education, unemployment, fewer lifetime drinking problems, and more frequent alcohol consumption at the 3-year follow-up. However, group membership was not a significant predictor of relapse. The authors conclude that untreated remissions are frequently followed by relapse. Several limitations of this study are worth mentioning. First, participants initially sought help for their drinking problem (by contacting the treatment facilities) and, therefore, are more likely to differ from those who did not seek treatment. In addition, problems were not restricted to a clearly operationalized alcohol dependence definition. Furthermore, remission was defined as being abstinent or drinking at low risk for a period of 6 months. Finally, the definition of "untreated" was confined to the 1-year period after initial contact, although approximately three-quarters of the participants entered treatment or attended AA by the 8-year follow-up. In sum, the report's definitions of natural recovery and generalizability of data are questionable.

Another study conducted a 2-year follow-up of individuals with fully remitted alcohol dependence according to DSM-IV criteria at baseline (Rumpf, Bischof, Hapke, Meyer, & John, 2006). Participants were recruited by media solicitation ($n = 115$) and additionally from a general population sample ($n = 29$). The latter group fulfilled lifetime alcohol dependence criteria but did not meet the criteria in the past 12 months and had never utilized treatment exceeding two self-help group meetings. Response rate at follow-up was 92.9% and collateral interviews were conducted to corroborate participants' reports. At the 2-year follow-up, 92.3% of participants were in stable remission, 3% were currently alcohol dependent (based on self-report or collateral information; 1.5% each), another 1.5% fulfilled one or two criteria of dependence, and 4.6% had utilized formal help. Although rates of stable remission did not differ significantly between participants recruited through media solicitation compared with those taken from the general population sample, it must be noted that the latter group was rather small. Therefore, further studies are needed to confirm these findings in general population-based samples. In sum, this study suggests that remission from alcohol dependence is not a transient phenomenon. Therefore, findings from cross-sectional studies on natural recovery are not biased by large proportions of remitters who subsequently relapse or seek help.

Both studies cited above differ with respect to their definition of untreated remission. Taken together, evidence suggests that remissions without formal help are very stable when strict definitions of untreated remission are applied. Especially the DSM-IV specifier of full (meeting no dependence criterion) and sustained (at least 1 year) remission should be regarded as crucial for defining stable remission.

Factors Supporting Remission

Studies in the past years can be divided into nonrepresentative (e.g. media-recruited) and representative (general population) samples. Both kinds of designs yield important findings and are reviewed below. Nonrepresentative samples often provide more in-depth analyses whereas representative samples have the advantage of generalizability.

Media-Recruited or Other Nonrepresentative Samples

Moos and Moos (2005) analyzed data from 461 individuals who initially sought help by contacting an information and referral center or a detoxification program because of alcohol-related problems, and were followed-up after 1, 3, 8, and 16 years (as previously described in greater detail). Based on the first-year data, participants were divided into the following three groups: (a) no treatment entry or AA participation ($n = 99$), (b) only AA participation and no treatment entry ($n = 89$), and (c) treatment entry ($n = 273$). For most analyses, the second and third groups were combined. Findings show that all groups improved with respect to a number of variables related to achieving and maintaining remission, such as decline of problem indices and alcohol consumption, increase in self-efficacy to resist alcohol, larger number of friends, more information and problem-solving and coping skills, and decline in avoidance coping and depression. Regarding most factors, the no-help group had somewhat less positive developments than the two helped groups. A stable remission after 8 and 16 years was more frequent among the groups entering treatment or participating in AA by the 1-year follow-up compared with the no help group (42.3% versus 24.2%). In the no-help group, one third entered treatment between the 1- and 8-year follow-up, and 28.3% participated in AA. Interestingly, the groups did not differ significantly from those never seeking formal help in the percentages of stable remission after 8 and 16 years. Data suggest that the group that did not seek help within the first year had a poorer prognosis and subsequent treatment entry within 8 years from baseline did not significantly improve remission rates. One interesting finding comes from a secondary analysis of this same sample using the 3-year follow-up data (Moos & Moos, 2006). Fewer current drinking problems, less negative life events at baseline, and less avoidance coping and drinking to reduce tension were more predictive of remission in the no-help group compared with the help groups. As mentioned earlier, this study has some restrictions with respect to natural recovery research; standards in defining untreated remission have yet to be met and this leads to a reduction in the explanatory power of the report's analyses.

The German TACOS study explored gender differences in a sample of media-recruited, untreated remitters from alcohol dependence (Bischof, Rumpf, Hapke, Meyer, & John, 2000a). Data were assessed in personal interviews using standardized questionnaires. Prior to remission, female remitters ($n = 38$) experienced less social pressure to change their drinking behavior compared with their male counterparts ($n = 106$). In addition, they drove less often while under the influence of alcohol and experienced less satisfaction in different life domains. Female remitters reported a higher impact of health problems on the remission process and, after the resolution, informed fewer individuals about their former drinking problems. More research is needed to determine how men and women differ in their pathways out of alcohol dependence.

Another analysis of the TACOS study focused on maintenance factors of untreated recovery by comparing 92 "natural" remitters with 42 "regular" self-help group participants (Bischof, Rumpf, Hapke, Meyer, & John, 2000b). In sum, more commonalities than differences were found. However, the self-help group attendees informed more individuals about their former alcohol problems (independent of direct self-help group context) and used social support more often as a coping strategy to deal with cravings.

Other differences in coping styles were found in another analysis of the above sample with respect to the role of family and partnership (Rumpf, Bischof, Hapke, Meyer, & John, 2002). Comparing pre- and post-remission periods, remitters with and without self-help group participation showed an increase in support. Those in the helped group experienced more partnership problems prior to their resolution. Greater social support and pressure from family and partners was related to increased cognitive coping efforts in the untreated remitters. An inverse relationship was observed in self-help group participants; higher levels of support and pressure were related to less cognitive coping. Findings suggest that untreated remitters were able to benefit more from social support and pressure, whereas these factors were less effective in self-help group attendees, who might therefore have searched for additional support.

Because social resources have not uniformly been found in the literature as enabling factors for untreated remissions, the existence of subgroups seems plausible. In a cluster-analytical approach using data from the TACOS study, three homogeneous subgroups of natural remitters ($n = 178$) emerged (Bischof, Rumpf, Hapke, Meyer, & John, 2003). Cluster one is characterized by high severity of dependence, low alcohol-related problems, and low social support ("low problems–low support"; $n = 65$), cluster two reveals high severity of dependence, high alcohol-related problems, and medium social support ("high problems–medium support"; $n = 37$), and cluster three includes individuals with high social support, late age of onset, low severity of dependence, and low alcohol-related problems ("low problems–high support"; $n = 76$). Cluster solutions were confirmed using discriminant analyses. The three cluster groups showed considerable differences in sociodemographic variables and subsequent analyses showed considerable differences in triggering and maintaining factors of remission.

A small-size pilot study aimed to prospectively examine the role of motivation and life events in natural recovery (Cunningham, Wild, & Koski-Jännes, 2005). Respondents ($n = 100$) thinking about changing their drinking behavior were recruited through newspaper advertisements. Those who made a serious quit attempt ($n = 53$) were recruited for a 1-year follow-up (58% response rate; $n = 31$). Partial correlations showed relationships between alcohol drinking at follow-up and costs and benefits of reducing drinking, reduction in negative life events, and improvement in positive life events. The study is limited by its small sample size. However, these findings are consistent with previous, retrospective research suggesting that life events and a cognitive appraisal process are important factors of untreated remission.

The only cross-cultural analysis comes from a Canadian and Swiss collaboration (Sobell et al., 2001). It focused on alcohol and drug abusers' perceived reasons for self-change across substances and cultures using computer-assisted content analysis. The Canadian sample consisted of 120 individuals who recovered from alcohol problems as well as 50 participants with former problematic cocaine consumption. The Swiss sample contained naturally recovered alcohol ($n = 30$) and heroin ($n = 30$) respondents. All participants were recruited via media solicitation and data were gathered using narrative interviews. A computer-assisted content analysis program automatically identified words from a content analytical dictionary. With this procedure 11 qualitative word categories were developed. Differences related to substance or country occurred in only 4 of these categories. In the other 7 groupings, words were most frequently related to cognitive evaluations. Therefore, this cognitive appraisal process may be viewed as independent from culture or substance.

Besides the commonality of a cognitive appraisal process, some studies focusing on ethnic subpopulations suggest culture-specific mechanisms of natural recovery (e.g., Cameron, Manik, Bird, & Sinorwalia, 2002; Quintero, 2000).

General Population Samples

Only a few studies on natural recovery have used samples from the general population, but this number is slowly growing. Most of these third generation studies were not specifically designed to examine alcohol and drug remission without formal treatment; therefore, secondary analyses of data gathered for other, more general investigations had to be conducted. One exception comes from the general population arm of the TACOS study. Drawn from a representative sample in northern Germany, 32 untreated recovered alcohol dependent individuals were compared with 25 still-dependent participants (Bischof, Rumpf, Hapke, Meyer, & John, 2001). According to a multivariate analysis, those who achieved remission without formal help showed a higher nonphysiological severity of alcohol dependence, less social pressure to quit drinking, and more incidents of driving while intoxicated. In addition, there was a tendency toward more satisfaction with work and financial situations and living in a stable partnership. These data confirm the concept of social capital (Granfield & Cloud, 1996).

Using the same dataset, the role of psychiatric comorbidity on untreated remissions was examined (Bischof, Rumpf, Meyer, Hapke, & John, 2005). Of the general population sample, 98 participants met criteria for sustained full remission according to the DSM-IV and 36.1% of this group had at least one additional Axis I disorder. The comorbid and non-comorbid groups did not differ significantly in proportions of untreated remission (42.6% versus 36.9%), suggesting that comorbidity has no negative impact on natural recovery.

A more in-depth analysis comes from an untreated, mixed sample of 664 individuals with at-risk drinking or alcohol dependence or abuse (Booth et al., 2001). The following factors were positively associated with a decrease in alcohol-related diagnoses (Booth, Curran, & Han, 2004): female gender, older age, and religiosity. Conversely, negative predictors were recent illegal drug use, negative life events, and social consequences of drinking. Consumption at safe levels at follow-ups was positively correlated with rural residence and religiosity, and negatively related with female gender, negative life events, recent illegal drug use, and social consequences of drinking. Interestingly, comorbidity had only a minimal effect and functioned as a protective factor which is consistent with findings from Bischof et al. (2005). In addition, family history was of no predictive value.

Using a Canadian general population sample, Cunningham (2000) distinguished two large groups who remitted from alcohol dependence or abuse with or without treatment ($n = 589$). One subsample experienced severe alcohol-related problems over a long period in their life and achieved abstinence through utilization of treatment. This is typically the group that can be found in treatment settings. The other group had experienced less drinking-related problems prior to remission, resolved their alcohol problems at a younger age, did not utilize treatment, and currently drank at moderate levels.

Weisner and colleagues compared groups of alcohol dependent individuals from a treatment ($n = 371$) and general population (who had not received formal help within the past year; $n = 111$) sample, both recruited in a California county (Weisner, Matzger, & Kaskutas, 2003). At a 1-year follow-up, the treatment group was 14 times more likely to be abstinent and 7 times more likely to have nonproblematic alcohol use. The only predictors for untreated remission emerging from multivariate analyses were the severity of individuals' drug use and the extent of heavy drinking in their social network; that is, the greater the drug use and heavier the drinking in the social network, the lower the probability of recovery. These findings stress the potential of social network interventions to foster self-change.

With respect to the poorer prognosis of untreated remitters, limitations of this study must be addressed. First, the two groups were recruited in separate samples. It is well established that only a minority of alcohol dependent individuals seek treatment and those in treatment differ from persons in the general population with respect to a multitude of characteristics. Therefore, comparison of the two groups with respect to their remission rates is flawed. In addition, it has to be mentioned that follow-up rates differed, 78% in the treated and 93% in the untreated sample. It is likely that those lost at follow-up elevated the rates of nonremission. Nevertheless, the findings are broadly in concordance with other data revealing that help-seeking plays a significant role in achieving recovery. Dawson, Grant, Stinson, and Chou (2006a) found hazard rate ratios of 1.5 for nonabstinent and 4 for abstinent recovery using retrospective data of the NESARC study. Additional support for the benefits of formal treatment in short-term recovery comes from a Canadian general population survey (Cunningham, 2005).

In the previous literature, the occurrence of life events has been discussed as a trigger for untreated remissions. An analysis of the NESARC data aimed to examine the impact of life events in maturing out of alcohol dependence using data from a large general population sample (Dawson, Grant, Stinson, & Chou, 2006b). In the first step of analysis, this study did not distinguish between respondents with or without a history of treatment. Entry into and exit from a first marriage increased the likelihood of nonabstinent recovery within a period of 3 years after their occurrence. Becoming a parent had only an effect on abstinent recovery. Other life events such as completing school or starting work showed no effect on recovery within 3 years. In the second step, the authors investigated whether treatment had an effect on their results. Such was not the case, suggesting that the life events under study had a similar impact on treated as well as untreated remissions. On the one hand, data confirm the role of life events in overcoming an addiction, yet on the other hand such triggers seem to not be effective for untreated remissions and are important components of remissions following formal treatment. This study clearly has advantages by using a large, representative sample. In addition, it avoids attribution bias by using standardized questionnaires instead of asking participants which events they perceived as influential for their recovery. However, due to its general design and purpose, it does not provide detailed analyses on important factors about the events such as appraisal or coping nor does it address how the event triggered the change processes.

In a study on older adults (51 to 65 years old at baseline), 4- and 10-year follow-ups resulted in the following three groups: (a) 330 untreated remitters, (b) 120 treated remitters, and (c) 130 untreated nonremitters (Schutte et al., 2006). Multivariate logistic regression models revealed that untreated remission was associated with female gender, more schooling, fewer drinking problems, an earlier peak of alcohol consumption, earlier ceasing of new alcohol problems, and less severe depression histories. Furthermore, those remitting without formal help were less often asked to cut down on drinking. The following variables predicted untreated remission compared with untreated nonremission: fewer drinking problems, peak alcohol consumption at an earlier age, and not having received advice as to how to reduce alcohol consumption. Both groups had similar depression histories and experienced comparable health problems, however, untreated remitters were more likely to regard their health problems as a reason for limiting their drinking. These findings replicate earlier data suggesting that remission without formal help is associated with less severe drinking problems and highlights the need to focus on health concerns when fostering self-change in this age group.

Russell and colleagues reinterviewed naturally recovered (n = 83) and hazardous problem drinkers (n = 138) recruited from four population-based samples (Russell et al., 2001). Untreated remitters were more likely to be married, had lower frequencies of intoxication, and had less frequent drug use. Members of their social network drank less and addressed the alcohol problem less often. In addition, natural remission was associated with lower levels of avoidance coping and higher levels of self-esteem. Although derived from community samples, the representativeness of this study is flawed by its low response rates. However, these findings confirm that social resources are influential for untreated remission.

Conclusion and Suggestions for Future Research

In the past several years, research on natural recovery has progressively improved. Using large, general population samples and standardized assessments has improved the generalizability of findings. Unfortunately, most of the representative studies are secondary analyses, and were not specifically designed to examine untreated alcohol and substance use remissions; therefore, more in-depth analyses are sometimes unavailable. As a result, findings from convenience samples are still highly important. Data show that clearly defined criteria for natural recovery are a prerequisite for sound research in this field.

High prevalence rates of untreated recoveries have been confirmed by new studies. In addition, the roles of a cognitive appraisal process, life events, and social capital have found some support; however, some reports show more commonalities than differences between treated and untreated remissions. In addition, findings suggest the existence of subgroups characterized by level of problem severity and social resources. Finally, some evidence exists demonstrating that major mechanisms of untreated remissions are independent of the respective culture.

Looking toward the future, the fourth generation studies should combine both representative samples and detailed datasets. More research is needed with respect to gender differences as well as the interplay of social networks, problem severity, cognition, and motivation. In addition, future research could profit from a broader scientific perspective, which would integrate sociological (e.g., social networks), psychological (e.g., cognition), and biological knowledge (e.g., neurobiological correlates, genetic findings).

References

Bischof, G., Rumpf, H.-J., Hapke, U., Meyer, C., & John, U. (2000a). Gender differences in natural recovery from alcohol dependence. *Journal of Studies on Alcohol, 61*, 783–786.

Bischof, G., Rumpf, H.-J., Hapke, U., Meyer, C., & John, U. (2000b). Maintenance factors of recovery from alcohol dependence in treated and untreated individuals. *Alcoholism: Clinical and Experimental Research, 61*, 783–786.

Bischof, G., Rumpf, H.-J., Hapke, U., Meyer, C., & John, U. (2001). Factors influencing remission without formal help from alcohol dependence in a representative population sample. *Addiction, 96*, 1327–1336.

Bischof, G., Rumpf, H.-J., Hapke, U., Meyer, C., & John, U. (2002). Natural recovery from alcohol dependence: How restrictive should our definition of treatment be? *Journal of Studies on Alcohol, 63*, 229–236.

Bischof, G., Rumpf, H.-J., Hapke, U., Meyer, C., & John, U. (2003). Types of natural recovery from alcohol dependence: A cluster analytic approach. *Addiction, 98*, 1737–1746.

Bischof, G., Rumpf, H.-J., Meyer, C., Hapke, U., & John, U. (2005). Influence of psychiatric comorbidity in alcohol-dependent subjects in a representative population survey on treatment utilization and natural recovery. *Addiction, 100*, 405–413.

Booth, B. M., Curran, G. M., & Han, X. (2004). Predictors of short-term course of drinking in untreated rural and urban at-risk drinkers: Effects of gender, illegal drug use, and psychiatric comorbidity. *Journal of Studies on Alcohol, 65*, 63–73.

Booth, B. M., Fortney, S. M., Fortney, J. C., Curran, G. M., & Kirchner, J. E. (2001). Short-term course of drinking in an untreated sample of at-risk drinkers. *Journal of Studies on Alcohol, 62*, 580–588.

Cameron, D., Manik, G., Bird, R., & Sinorwalia, A. (2002). What may we be learning from so-called spontaneous remission in ethnic minorities? *Addiction Research & Theory, 10*, 175–182.

Cunningham, J. A. (1999). Resolving alcohol-related problems with and without treatment: The effects of different problem criteria. *Journal of Studies on Alcohol, 60*, 463–466.

Cunningham, J. A. (2005). Short-term recovery from alcohol abuse or dependence: Any evidence of a relationship with treatment use in a general population sample? *Alcohol and Alcoholism, 40*, 419–421.

Cunningham, J. A., Lin, E., Ross, H. E., & Walsh, G. W. (2000). Factors associated with untreated remissions from alcohol abuse or dependence. *Addictive Behaviors, 25*, 317–321.

Cunningham, J. A., Wild, T. C., & Koski-Jännes, A. (2005). Motivation and life events: A prospective natural history pilot study of problem drinkers in the community. *Addictive Behaviors, 30*, 1603–1606.

Dawson, D. A. (1996). Correlates of past-year status among treated and untreated persons with former alcohol dependence: United States, 1992. *Alcoholism: Clinical and Experimental Research, 20*, 771–779.

Dawson, D. A., Grant, B. F., Stinson, F. S., & Chou, P. S. (2006a). Estimating the effect of help-seeking on achieving recovery from alcohol dependence. *Addiction, 101*, 824–834.

Dawson, D. A., Grant, B. F., Stinson, F. S., & Chou, P. S. (2006b). Maturing out of alcohol dependence: The impact of transitional life events. *Journal of Studies on Alcohol, 67*, 195–203.

Dawson, D. A., Grant, B. F., Stinson, F. S., Chou, P. S., Huang, B., & Ruan, W. J. (2005). Recovery from DSM-IV alcohol dependence: United States, 2001–2002. *Addiction, 100*, 281–292.

Granfield, R., & Cloud, W. (1996). The elephant that no one sees: Natural recovery among middle-class addicts. *Journal of Drug Issues, 26*, 45–61.

Humphreys, K., Moos, R. H., & Finney, J. W. (1995). Two pathways out of drinking problems without professional treatment. *Addictive Behaviors, 20*, 427–441.

Moos, R. H., & Moos, B. S. (2005). Sixteen-year changes and stable remission among treated and untreated individuals with alcohol use disorders. *Drug and Alcohol Dependence, 80*, 337–347.

Moos, R. H., & Moos, B. S. (2006). Rates and predictors of relapse after natural and treated remission from alcohol use disorders. *Addiction, 101*, 212–222.

Quintero, G. (2000). The lizard in the green bottle: "Aging out" of problem drinking among Navajo men. *Social Science & Medicine, 51*, 1031–1045.

Rumpf, H.-J., Bischof, G., Hapke, U., Meyer, C., & John, U. (2000). Studies on natural recovery from alcohol dependence: Sample selection bias by media solicitation? *Addiction, 95*, 765–775.

Rumpf, H.-J., Bischof, G., Hapke, U., Meyer, C., & John, U. (2002). The role of family and partnership in recovery from alcohol dependence: Comparison of individuals remitting with and without formal help. *European Addiction Research, 8*, 122–127.

Rumpf, H.-J., Bischof, G., Hapke, U., Meyer, C., & John, U. (2006). Stability of remission from alcohol dependence without formal help. *Alcohol and Alcoholism, 41*, 311–314.

Russell, M., Peirce, R. S., Chan, A. W., Wieczorek, W. F., Moscato, B. S., & Nochajski, T. H. (2001). Natural recovery in a community-based sample of alcoholics: Study design and descriptive data. *Substance Use and Misuse, 36*, 1417–1441.

Schutte, K. K., Moos, R. H., & Brennan, P. L. (2006). Predictors of untreated remission from late-life drinking problems. *Journal of Studies on Alcohol, 67*, 354–362.

Sobell, L. C., Cunningham, J. A., & Sobell, M. B. (1996). Recovery from alcohol problems with and without treatment: Prevalence in two population surveys. *American Journal of Public Health, 7*, 966–972.

Sobell, L. C., Ellingstad, T. P., & Sobell, M. B. (2000). Natural recovery from alcohol and drug problems: Methodological review of the research with suggestions for future directions. *Addiction, 95*, 749–764.

Sobell, L. C., Klingemann, H. K., Toneatto, T., Sobell, M. B., Agrawal, S., & Leo, G. I. (2001). Alcohol and drug abusers' perceived reasons for self-change in Canada and Switzerland. *Substance Use and Misuse, 36*, 1467–1500.

Sobell, L. C., Sobell, M. B., Toneatto, T., & Leo, G. I. (1993). What triggers the resolution of alcohol problems without treatment? *Alcoholism: Clinical and Experimental Research, 17*, 217–224.

Weisner, C., Matzger, H., & Kaskutas, L. A. (2003). How important is treatment? One-year outcomes of treated and untreated alcohol-dependent individuals. *Addiction, 98*, 901–911.

5

Natural Recovery from Alcohol and Drug Problems: A Methodological Review of the Literature from 1999 through 2005

José Luis Carballo, José Ramón Fernández-Hermida,
Roberto Secades-Villa, Linda Carter Sobell, Mariam Dum,
and Olaya García-Rodríguez

Introduction

Recognition of the importance of the self-change or natural recovery phenomenon with addictive behaviors has led to a considerable increase in research in recent years. The first major review article on this topic, published in 2000 by Sobell, Ellingstad, and Sobell, reviewed 38 studies of natural recovery that covered almost 40 years of research.

The review by Sobell et al. (2000) discussed a significant number of methodological limitations in addition to future directions for research. The studies, reviewed through 1998, contain the following methodological problems: (a) a lack of demographic data and a family history of substance use, (b) insufficient information about the severity and patterns of addictive behaviors prior to recovery, (c) minimal information on maintenance factors related to the recovery process, (d) limited research on the validity of participants' self-reports, (e) fewer drug (e.g., cocaine, marijuana, polysubstance) than alcohol studies, (f) little information on the stability and patterns of behavioral change associated with natural recovery, and (g) a dearth of cross-cultural studies evaluating cultural determinants of self-change.

Despite the continuing number of published studies documenting the process of self-change with substance abusers (Cohen, Feinn, Arias, & Kranzler, 2007; Dawson et al., 2005; Sobell et al., 2000), there are some who still express doubts about the reliability and stability of recovery for those who report low-risk drinking (Vaillant, 2005).

The intent of this chapter is to review the natural recovery literature from the time of the last major review (Sobell et al., 2000). This chapter reviews studies related to natural recovery of addictive behaviors from 1999 through 2005. As in the previous review, this chapter focuses on the methodology of these articles and the extent to which recent research has addressed the recommendations made by Sobell and her colleagues. Lastly, this chapter will discuss future research directions on natural recovery.

Method

For purposes of maintaining continuity, this chapter reviews studies published from the time of the last review using similar inclusion criteria and variables for analysis. Drawing on the suggestions from the last review (Sobell et al., 2000), new variables were added to the present review.

Studies were identified by (a) searching the Medline and Psychlit databases, (b) reviewing the reference sections of published natural recovery articles, and (c) contacting key researchers in the field. The search and identification criteria included articles published from 1999 through 2005 (the study by Ellingstad, Sobell, Sobell, Eickleberry, & Golden, published in 2006, was included in this review because it was in press in 2005) that contained the term *natural recovery* and other terms reflecting the same phenomenon (e.g., *self-quitters, self-change, natural recovery, natural resolution, spontaneous recovery, spontaneous remission, untreated remission*) for alcohol and other drugs (excluding nicotine).

Once the initial search was completed, all articles had to meet the following inclusion criteria: (a) English-language publications, (b) published or in press in peer-reviewed journals, (c) contained original results (reviews and articles based on case studies or personal stories were excluded), (d) participants must have had a history of alcohol or other drug abuse, and (e) had to include rates of natural recovery.

Twenty-two studies met the criteria for inclusion in the current review. Although primary reference sources provided the majority of the data for the studies, other articles reporting on the same study were consulted when necessary. Primary and secondary references for the studies reviewed are listed in the Appendix.

The following variables were assessed: (a) *participant characteristics*: sociodemographic characteristics during recovery and at the time of the study (e.g., gender, age, education, employment, marital status) and substance use history variables (e.g., years of consumption, diagnosis, problem severity, use of alcohol and other drugs); (b) *study characteristics*: number of participants recovered without formal treatment or help, recruitment and data-collection methods, type of data obtained (i.e., quantitative, qualitative, or mixed), country, reimbursements for interviews, type of study design, recording of interviews, use of control groups, relapse rates, definition of treatment, use of different recovered groups and types of comparison among these groups, and recovery length criterion; (c) *variables related to change*: length of recovery, type of recovery (i.e., abstinence or low-risk use), prior use of treatment or self-help programs, reasons for change, maintenance factors supporting the change, and reasons for not entering treatment; and (d) *study limitations*.

The data were analyzed using SPSS 12.0. Statistical analyses were descriptive and included frequencies and percentages of reported variables in the articles. The results, presented in six tables, compare the present findings with those in the previous review by Sobell et al. (2000).

Results

Table 5.1 shows the percentage of reviewed articles that assessed a variety of study variables. In the current study, the majority (81.8%) of natural recoveries involved alcohol, followed by cannabis (31.8%) and other drugs (e.g., LSD, methamphetamines, sedatives; 27.3%). In the first review, the majority (75%) of natural recoveries also included alcohol.

The mean number (SD) of respondents in the reviewed studies increased from 140.9 (399.2) in the first review to 383.0 (791.3) in the current review. This increase is attributable to several large survey studies. The present review calculated the mean (SD) number of respondents for each substance: (a) alcohol: 215.2 (532.7), (b) heroin: 28.6 (24.0), (c) cocaine: 151.7 (131.6), (d) cannabis: 456.8 (830.8), and (e) polysubstance use: 3 (0.0) respondents.

In the current review, 59% of all studies were conducted in the United States and 23% in Canada, followed by 18% in European countries. The primary recruitment method (45.5%) was surveys, almost a two-fold increase from the past review.

TABLE 5.1. Percentage (*n*) of articles that assessed different study variables.

Variable	Current review (*N* = 22)	Sobell et al. review (*N* = 40)
Substance[a]		
Alcohol	81.8 (18)	75.0 (30)
Heroin	22.7 (5)	22.5 (9)
Cocaine	22.7 (5)	7.5 (3)
Cannabis	31.8 (7)	2.5 (1)
Other drugs	27.3 (6)	12.5 (5)
Mean (SD) number of natural recovery respondents (*n* = 34)	383.0 (791.3)	140.9 (399.2)
Range	12–3177	5–2456
Mean (SD) number of alcohol respondents (*n* = 15)	215.2 (532.7)	
Range	7–2117	
Mean (SD) number of heroin respondents (*n* = 3)	28.6 (24.0)	
Range	4–52	

(*Continued*)

TABLE 5.1. Percentage (*n*) of articles that assessed different study variables.— Cont'd.

Variable	Current review (*N* = 22)	Sobell et al. review (*N* = 40)
Mean (SD) number of cocaine respondents (*n* = 4)	151.7 (131.6)	
Range	26–333	
Mean (SD) number of cannabis respondents (*n* = 6)	456.8 (830.8)	
Range	25–2143	
Mean (SD) number of polydrug respondents (*n* = 1)	3.0 (0.0)	
Range	3	
Mean (SD) number of other illicit drug respondents (*n* = 5)	243.2 (305.6)	
Range	21–766	
Method of recruitment[b]		
Advertisements	40.9 (9)	38.5 (15)
Snowball	9.1 (2)	28.2 (11)
Surveys	45.5 (10)	23.1 (9)
Other	27.3 (6)	17.9 (7)
Incentives/payments	31.8 (7)	20.0 (8)
Method of assessment[c]		
Self-report	100.0 (24)	100.0 (40)
Collaterals	18.2 (4)	30.0 (12)
Type of information		
Quantitative	72.7 (16)	
Mixed (quantitative + qualitative)	27.3 (6)	
Country		
USA	59.1 (13)	59.1 (22)
Canada	22.7 (5)	16.2 (6)
Europe	18.2 (4)	18.9 (7)
Cross-cultural	0.0 (0)	
Definition of treatment	68.2 (15)	82.5 (33)
Study design		
Retrospective	77.3 (17)	
Longitudinal	22.7 (5)	
Interviews recorded	18.2 (4)	32.5 (13)
Control groups included	18.2 (4)	17.5 (7)
Relapse rates assessed	9.1 (2)	5.0 (2)
Use of multiple recovered groups	63.3 (14)	57.5 (23)
Type of recovery comparisons		
Intersubstances	22.7 (5)	
Treated versus untreated	13.6 (3)	
Abstinence versus nonabstinence	4.5 (1)	
Other	22.7 (5)	

[a] Some studies assessed several substances.

[b] Some studies used several methods.

[c] Some studies used several methods.

In addition, advertisements were used for participant recruitment in 40.9% of all studies. The "snowball" technique seems to have lost its popularity since the last review (9.1% in the current study compared to 28.2% in the 2000 review).

There was an increase in the percentage of participants who were paid or given incentives for participating in the studies, rising from 20% in the first review to 31.8% in the present review. In spite of some of the criticisms associated with paying respondents (e.g., validity of the information), this has proven to be an effective recruitment method. Self-report continues to be the main method of data collection for both pre- and post-recovery information. In this regard, several studies have shown that naturally recovered substance abusers provide accurate self-report (Secades-Villa & Fernández-Hermida, 2003; Sobell, Agrawal, & Sobell, 1997; Sobell et al., 2000). The percentage of studies using collaterals' reports to check or verify participants' responses has decreased from 30% to 18%.

In the current review, most researchers reported their results using quantitative data (72.7%). There are slight variations between studies regarding the definition of treatment, but in the present review, treatment generally included the following: Alcoholics Anonymous or other self-help groups; psychological or psychiatric treatment; and advice from medical practitioners, hospitals, or detoxification centers. Attendance of two or three self-help group meetings or one treatment session where the respondents felt that it did not help their recovery were not counted as treatment. Fewer recent studies (68.2%) provided a definition of treatment compared with 82.5% in the first review.

In the previous study, 5% of the reports assessed stability of recovery compared with 9.1% in the current review. The retrospective design continues to be widely used (77.3%) in natural recovery studies. There has also been a slight increase from 57.5% to 63.3% regarding the inclusion of multiple recovery groups. In addition, the most common comparison (23%) has been made between different substances. Comparisons between treated and nontreated respondents were reported in 14% of the studies, while comparative evaluations between abstinence and nonabstinence outcomes accounted for 4% of all studies.

Table 5.2 shows the percentage of articles reporting different sociodemographic characteristics for respondents. Gender (86.4%) and age at the time of the interview (72.7%) continue to be the most widely reported sociodemographic variables. However, in the current review, there has been an increase over the previous study in the reporting of the following variables: (a) occupation (54.5%

TABLE 5.2. Percentage (n) of studies reporting participant sociodemographic characteristics.

Variable	Current review (N = 22)	Sobell et al. review (N = 40)
Age at recovery	27.3 (6)	22.5 (9)
Age at interview	72.7 (16)	62.5 (25)
Education at recovery	13.6 (3)	—
Education at interview	63.6 (14)	45.0 (18)
Gender	86.4 (19)	75.0 (30)
Occupation at recovery	22.7 (5)	10.0 (4)
Occupation at interview	54.5 (12)	47.5 (19)
Marital status at recovery	27.3 (6)	7.5 (3)
Marital status at interview	59.1 (13)	45.0 (18)
Ethnic group	59.1 (13)	37.5 (15)

versus 47.5%), (b) educational level (63.6% versus 45%), (c) marital status (59.1% versus 45%), and (d) reference to ethnic origin (59.1% versus 37.5%). The percentage of studies reporting sociodemographic variables for respondents when interviewed versus at the time of recovery continues to be much higher in both reviews.

The profile of respondents in the recent natural recovery studies is quite similar to that of the previous review: (a) mean (SD) age of respondents when interviewed was 41.4 (7.5) years versus 40.5 (9.1) in the past review and (b) males comprised the majority in both studies.

Table 5.3 shows the percentages of studies that report data for substance use history and recovery variables. In the current review, almost 78% of the studies reported problem severity and more than 85% reported a history of use compared with 60% and 47.5%, respectively, in the first review. Reporting the length of respondents' substance use history prior to recovery increased from 45% to 68.2%. Multiple drug use, including nicotine, was reported in 72.7% of all studies. In the majority of these reports, the second drug was nicotine. In both reviews, abstinence recoveries were provided in all studies. The reporting of low-risk drinking increased from 78.6% to 86.6% for all studies.

Table 5.4 presents descriptive statistics for problem recovery length and substance use characteristics for the studies in the two reviews. The data in Table 5.4 are similar for both reviews. For example, the mean (SD) number of years respondents had a problem prior to their recovery was 12.8 (4.9) years in the current study and 10.9 (4.0) years in the first review. The mean minimum required recovery length for studies in both reviews was similar, averaging 1.2 years in the present review and 1.4 in the previous review. The mean (SD) length of recovery among respondents was 8.0 (2.7) years in the current review and 6.3 (2.3) years in the first review. Both reviews suggest that respondents' recoveries are very stable and enduring. The percentages of studies reporting abstinent and low-risk recoveries in both reviews were very similar.

Table 5.5 shows the percentage of studies reporting reasons for change, maintenance factors, and barriers to treatment for the two reviews. Reasons for recovery

TABLE 5.3. Percentage (*n*) of studies reporting substance use history and recovery variables.

Variable	Current review (*N*=22)	Sobell et al. review (*N*=40)
Problem length prior to recovery	68.2 (15)	45.0 (18)
Problem severity or consequences	77.3 (17)	60.0 (24)
Prerecovery substance use	86.4 (19)	47.5 (19)
Minimum recovery length required	77.3 (17)	80.0 (32)
Recovery length	36.4 (8)	60 (24)
Type of alcohol recovery[a]		
Abstinence	100.0 (18)	100.0 (28)
Low-risk drinking	86.6 (13)	78.6 (22)
Prior treatment or self-help attendance	100.0 (22)	90.0 (36)
Use of multiple drugs	72.7 (16)	—

[a] Alcohol studies only; current review, *n* = 15; Sobell et al. review, *n* = 28.

TABLE 5.4. Problem recovery length and substance use characteristics for studies in the two reviews.

Variable	Current review	Sobell et al. 2000 review
Mean (SD) problem length prior to recovery (years)	12.8 (4.9)	10.9 (4.0)
Range	6.0–19.7	5.0–17.0
Mean (SD) minimum recovery length required (years)	1.2 (0.7)	1.4 (0.8)
Range	0.2–3.0	0.5–3.3
Mean (SD) recovery length (years)	8.0 (2.7)	6.3 (2.3)
Range	3.0–11.5	0.4–11.7
Type of alcohol recovery[a]		
Abstinence (range)	56.6% (29.9%–100%)	59.7% (3.0%–100.0%)
Low risk drinking (range)	43.4% (0.0%–70.1%)	40.3% (0.0%–97.0%)

[a] Alcohol studies only; current review, $n = 15$; Sobell et al. review, $n = 28$.

were reported for close to two thirds of all respondents in both reviews (current review, 63.6%; past review, 62.5%). Overall, while similar reasons for change were reported in both reviews, the percentage of studies reporting these reasons were different. In the review by Sobell et al. (2000), health was the most frequently reported reason for change (42.5%), while in the present review the most frequently reported reason was family-related (54.5%), followed closely by health (50%) and financial matters (50%).

In the current review, maintenance factors were reported by close to two-thirds (59.1%) of all studies, whereas in the first review, they were reported in only 45% of the studies. In the current study, the two most widely mentioned factors contributing to maintenance continue to be social support and family support, with 54.5% and 45.5%, respectively. These two factors were also the highest in the first review. The current studies also found avoidance of substance-use situations reported by over one third of all respondents (36.4%), followed closely by self-control (31.8%) and religion (34.6%) as important factors influencing maintenance.

Finally, in terms of barriers to treatment, a low percentage of studies reported similar difficulties in both reviews (current, 13.6%; past, 22.5%). The barrier most frequently reported in the current review was the belief that treatment was unnecessary or that the substance use problem was not very serious (13.6%), followed by 9.1% for all other barriers.

In the first review, although Sobell et al. (2000) discussed several study limitations, they did not assess whether studies actually reported any limitations. The current review examined articles for limitations reported by authors (see Table 5.6). A large number (95.5%) of the studies reported at least one limitation. The two most common limitations (54.5%) concerned retrospective designs (e.g., reliability of information, difficulties in distinguishing cause and effect) and the generalization of results to addictive behaviors and extrapolation of results to substance abuse treatment. Close to one quarter (27.3%) of the studies reported concerns about bias when recruiting respondents through advertisements.

TABLE 5.5. Percentage (*n*) of studies reporting reasons for change, maintenance factors, and barriers to treatment.

Variable	Current review (*N*=22)	Sobell et al. review (*N*=40)
Reasons for recovery	63.6 (14)	62.5 (25)
Family-related	54.5 (12)	22.5 (9)
Health-related	50.0 (11)	42.5 (17)
Finance-related	50.0 (11)	30.0 (12)
Negative personal effects	45.5 (10)	30.0 (12)
Related to significant other	45.5 (10)	25.0 (10)
Social-related	45.5 (10)	20.0 (8)
Legal issues	40.9 (9)	20.0 (8)
Religious reasons	40.9 (9)	17.5 (7)
Viewed substance use differently	36.4 (8)	27.5 (11)
Work-related	31.8 (7)	15.0 (6)
Fear of consequences	22.7 (5)	12.5 (5)
Lifestyle changes	18.2 (4)	15.0 (6)
Change in living arrangements	13.6 (3)	15.0 (6)
Seeing negative effects of use on others	13.6 (3)	10.0 (4)
Maintenance factors	59.1 (13)	45.0 (18)
Social support/change in social group	54.5 (12)	32.5 (13)
Significant other/family	45.5 (10)	27.5 (11)
Avoidance of substance use situations	36.4 (8)	17.5 (7)
Religion	36.4 (8)	15.0 (6)
Self-control or will power	31.8 (7)	15.0 (6)
Positive personal attributes	31.8 (7)	12.5 (5)
Development of non substance- related interests	27.3 (6)	20.0 (8)
Work-related	27.3 (6)	17.5 (7)
Health	22.7 (5)	12.5 (5)
Lifestyle change	22.7 (5)	17.5 (7)
Finances	22.7 (5)	12.5 (5)
Change in living arrangements	13.6 (3)	15.0 (6)
Barriers to treatment	13.6 (3)	22.5 (9)
Belief that treatment is not necessary or problem not severe enough	13.6 (3)	12.5 (6)
Stigma-labeling associated with treatment	9.1 (2)	20.5 (8)
Negative beliefs or experiences in relation to treatment	9.1 (2)	15.0 (6)
Privacy, not wanting to share problems	9.1 (2)	10.0 (4)
Financial costs	9.1 (2)	5.0 (2)
Inconvenience	9.1 (2)	5.0 (2)

TABLE 5.6. Percentage (*n*) of the 22 studies in the current review that reported limitations.

Variable	
Reported at least one limitation	95.5 (21)
Limitations of retrospective reports	54.5 (12)
Generalization and extrapolation of the findings	54.5 (12)
Recruitment bias	27.3 (6)
Superficiality of analyses	18.2 (4)
Scarcity of information on drug use history and problem severity	18.2 (4)
Sample size	9.1 (2)

In this regard, one study (Rumpf, Bischof, Hapke, Meyer, & John, 2000) found differences in dependence and recovery length between respondents recruited through advertisements and those recruited in general population surveys.

Discussion and Conclusions

Since the last major review, there has been a substantial increase in the number of published studies of naturally recovered substance abusers. Over 7 years (1999–2005), 22 studies met the same criteria used in the first review (Sobell et al., 2000), where 38 articles were published during 38 years (1960–1997). Changes from the 2000 review to the current are not very significant, except for the substantial increase in the number of studies on natural recovery, as well as the increase in number of studies examining drugs other than alcohol.

One of the central aspects of research in the natural recovery field is the analysis of the reasons for change and factors influencing maintenance of change. Notable among the reasons for change is a concept referred to as a "cognitive appraisal" of the "pros and cons" of continuing to use versus stopping or changing one's use (Klingemann et al., 2001; Sobell et al., 2001). Recovery is thought to occur when people who have engaged in a cognitive evaluation of their substance use see the "cons" outweighing the "pros." Unfortunately, at this time, it is unclear why this occurs at a particular moment in a person's life.

In the present review, family-related reasons were the most frequently reported reasons for changing compared with health in the first review. The decrease in the number of studies providing health-related reasons for change from the first to the current review may relate to the increase in the number of drug studies.

One of the objectives of this review was to evaluate the extent to which the changes proposed by Sobell et al. (2000) for natural recovery studies have been implemented. With respect to sociodemographic characteristics at the time of recovery, there has been a slight increase in the percentage of studies reporting such variables, but this is still very small compared with the percentage reporting these variables at the time of the interview. This needs to change as variables such as age, occupation, and educational level may be crucial to the initiation of the self-change process. In past studies, now classic in the substance abuse field (Cahalan, 1970), age has played an important role in natural recoveries. Specifically, age and age-related responsibilities (e.g., starting a job, having children) have provided explanations for self-change (i.e., maturation of the individual; Drew, 1968; Winick, 1962). With respect to gender, natural recoveries are still higher among males, which is not surprising given the higher percentage of males with substance abuse problems. In a recent natural recovery study (Bischof, Rumpf, Hapke, Meyer, & John, 2000), it was reported that while no significant differences were found, women tended to report keeping their alcohol problem hidden more as compared with men. The women also perceived less pressure and social support for stopping drinking. For these reasons, gender cannot be overlooked as an important variable in the recovery process (Bischof et al., 2000).

There has also been an increase in the reporting of past substance use, in addition to studies evaluating natural recovery from drugs other than alcohol. The exploration of recovery from multiple substances, including nicotine, may serve to improve knowledge of this phenomenon (Sobell, Sobell, & Agrawal, 2002). While several studies have examined the prevalence of natural recovery from illicit drugs (Cunningham, 1999; Price, Risk, & Spitznagel, 2001), they have not examined patterns of multiple drug use and recovery. Information about whether recovery from multiple substances occurs at the same time, or whether recovery from one substance predicts cessation or continued use of other substances is currently lacking. Studies in this area are sorely needed.

This review demonstrates, as have almost all natural recovery studies of alcohol and drug abusers, that people who recover naturally have less serious substance abuse histories compared with those who seek treatment (Bischof, Rumpf, Hapke, Meyer, & John, 2002; Carballo et al., under review; Chitwood & Morningstar, 1985; Cunningham, Lin, Ross, & Walsh, 2000; Sobell, Cunningham, & Sobell, 1996; Sobell et al., 2000, 2001; Weisner, Matzger, & Kaskutas, 2003). In addition, the consequences of substance abuse and the deterioration produced by alcohol and drug use appear to occur less in naturally recovered individuals than in those participating in treatment studies. This, however, does not imply that the severity profiles for those who change on their own are the same. For example, in a recent study severity of addiction has been used as one of the variables for establishing types of natural recovery from alcohol abuse (Bischof, Rumpf, Hapke, Meyer, & John, 2003). In this study, types of natural recovery were established on the basis of a cluster analysis. The first type corresponded to cases of low dependence, few alcohol-related problems, and little social support. The second was characterized by high dependence, many alcohol-related problems, and moderate social support. The third was defined by high social support, low dependence, and few alcohol-related problems. This group was also characterized by late alcohol problem onset (Bischof et al., 2003).

With regard to the development of more detailed analyses of the processes and determinants of self-change (Sobell et al., 2000), some researchers have recently begun to use novel qualitative types of data analysis. While the majority of studies continue to use quantitative information, more researchers are using computer programs to evaluate qualitative data from taped interviews. Using qualitative data, researchers can assess aspects of natural recovery (e.g., reasons for change, maintenance factors) more thoroughly. However, qualitative analyses are often thought of as complementary to quantitative data analyses (Ellingstad et al., 2006; Hanninen & Koski-Jännes, 1999; Koski-Jännes, 2002; Sobell et al., 2001).

Sobell et al. (2000) also recommended that studies use additional data sources (e.g., official reports or interviews with collaterals) to corroborate respondents' self-reports. The current review found that the percentage of studies presenting such data is still small (less than one third of all studies). The previous review also discussed the importance of asking respondents about maintenance factors related to recovery. The present review reported an increase in the percentage of studies reporting such factors. Especially important among the maintenance factors found in the current review were those relating to social and family support received by the respondents. In both reviews, this factor was reported most commonly by respondents as helping them maintain their change. In this regard, the increase of social capital and the improvement of social functioning may play important roles in the success of the recovery process (Granfield & Cloud, 2001).

Natural recovery studies with cocaine, cannabis, and polysubstance abusers were identified in the Sobell et al. (2000) review as another area needing to be addressed. While there has been a slight increase in the number of studies focusing on substances other than alcohol, the vast majority still involve alcohol abusers. Additional natural recovery studies are needed to learn about the process of self-change with other drugs and whether the processes and determinants of natural recovery with alcohol abusers are similar for other drugs. As discussed in other chapters of this book, natural recoveries occur in addictive behaviors unrelated to substance use (e.g., pathological gambling, eating disorders). Future research needs to examine rates of these behaviors and what drives this change process (Carballo-Crespo, Secades-Villa, Fernández-Hermida, García-Rodríguez, & Sobell, 2004; Hodgins & el-Guebaly, 2000).

The 2000 review recommended setting a minimum recovery criterion of 5 years because this interval reflects stable recoveries. While the majority of studies in the current review used at least a 1-year recovery criterion, the mean number of years of recovery for respondents was about 7 years. Thus, although the stricter criterion of 5 years was not used, a majority of the respondents would be considered stably recovered. Because the stability of the recovery process has only been assessed in a few studies (Rumpf, Bischof, Hapke, Meyer, & John, 2006; Sobell, Sobell, & Kozlowski, 1995), more longitudinal research is needed. Finally, given the limitations referred to in the studies themselves, future research should: (a) use longitudinal designs to minimize difficulties with retrospective approaches when possible, (b) carry out more in-depth analyses of the interview data using, for example, qualitative data analysis methods, (c) use large sample sizes, (d) minimize recruitment biases through the use of multiple recruitment methods, (e) compare different types of recoveries (e.g., treated versus nontreated) and different substances (e.g., cocaine versus cannabis), and (f) evaluate variables that are thought to be associated with the process of self-change (e.g., age, gender, problem severity). Last, future research needs to include cross-cultural designs that contribute to an understanding of the differences and similarities between natural recoveries in different cultures and countries. Based on this suggestion in the first review, two studies of natural recovery with Spanish-speaking respondents are being conducted in Spain and the United States. These studies are evaluating the processes and determinants that affect self-change, and comparing the findings with those obtained from Anglo-Saxon respondents. As in previous studies, Spanish self-changers have a less severe addiction history than substance abusers who recover through treatment (Carballo et al., under review).

In summary, having analyzed natural recovery studies with alcohol and drug abusers published from 1999 through 2005, and having compared these results with those of Sobell et al. (2000), it is clear that recent natural recovery studies have not addressed most of the issues raised in the first review and have failed to implement the proposed design changes, with the exception of a few studies. Therefore, it is strongly urged that researchers conducting studies in this area incorporate the proposed recommendations from the current review as well as those discussed in the first review.

Acknowledgment. This work was supported by grant MCYT-03-BSO-00732 (Ministerio de Cienciay Tecnología – Ministry of Science and Technology, Spain).

References

Bischof, G., Rumpf, H.-J., Hapke, U., Meyer, C., & John, U. (2000). Gender differences in natural recovery from alcohol dependence. *Journal of Studies on Alcohol, 61,* 783–786.

Bischof, G., Rumpf, H.-J., Hapke, U., Meyer, C., & John, U. (2002). Remission from alcohol dependence without help: How restrictive should our definition of treatment be? *Journal of Studies on Alcohol, 63,* 229–236.

Bischof, G., Rumpf, H.-J., Hapke, U., Meyer, C., & John, U. (2003). Types of natural recovery from alcohol dependence: A cluster analytic approach. *Addiction, 98,* 1737–1746.

Cahalan, D. (1970). *Problem drinkers: A national survey.* San Francisco: Jossey-Bass.

Carballo, J. L., Fernández-Hermida, J. R., Sobell, L. C., Dum, M., Secades-Villa, R., García-Rodríguez, O., et al. (under review). Process of change among Spanish alcohol and drug abusers who recovered on their own and through treatment.

Carballo-Crespo, J. L., Secades-Villa, R., Fernández-Hermida, J. R., García-Rodríguez, O., & Sobell, L. (2004). Recuperación de los problemas de juego patológico con y sin tratamiento. *Salud y Drogas, 4*(61–78).

Chitwood, D. D., & Morningstar, P. C. (1985). Factors which differentiate cocaine users in treatment from nontreatment users. *International Journal of Addiction, 20,* 449–459.

Cohen, E., Feinn, R., Arias, A., & Kranzler, H. R. (2007). Alcohol treatment utilization: Findings from the National Epidemiologic Survey on Alcohol and Related Conditions. *Drug and Alcohol Dependence 86(2-3):* 214–221.

Cunningham, J. A. (1999). Untreated remissions from drug use: The predominant pathway. *Addictive Behaviors, 24,* 267–270.

Cunningham, J. A., Lin, E., Ross, H. E., & Walsh, W. E. (2000). Factors associated with untreated remissions from alcohol abuse or dependence. *Addictive Behaviors, 25,* 317–321.

Dawson, D. A., Grant, B. F., Stinson, F. S., Chou, P. S., Huang, B., & Ruan, W. J. (2005). Recovery from DSM-IV alcohol dependence: United States, 2001–2002. *Addiction, 100,* 281–292.

Drew, L. R. H. (1968). Alcoholism as a self-limiting disease. *Quarterly Journal of Studies on Alcohol, 29,* 956–967.

Ellingstad, T. P., Sobell, L. C., Sobell, M. B., Eickleberry, L., & Golden, C. J. (2006). Self-change: A pathway to cannabis abuse resolution. *Addictive Behaviors, 31,* 519–530.

Granfield, R., & Cloud, W. (2001). Social context and "natural recovery": The role of social capital in the resolution of drug-associated problems. *Substance Use & Misuse, 36*, 1543–1570.

Hanninen, V., & Koski-Jännes, A. (1999). Narratives of recovery from addictive behaviours. *Addiction, 94*, 1837–1848.

Hodgins, D. C., & el-Guebaly, N. (2000). Natural and treatment-assisted recovery from gambling problems: A comparison of resolved and active gamblers. *Addiction, 95*, 777–789.

Klingemann, H., Sobell, L. C., Barker, J., Blomqvist, J., Cloud, W., Ellingstad, T. P., et al. (2001). *Promoting self-change from problem substance use: Practical implications for policy, prevention and treatment*. Boston: Kluwer Academic Publishers.

Koski-Jännes, A. (2002). Social and personal identity projects in the recovery from addictive behaviours. *Addiction Research & Theory, 10*, 183–202.

Price, R. K., Risk, N. K., & Spitznagel, E. L. (2001). Remission from drug abuse over a 25-year period: Patterns of remission and treatment use. *American Journal of Public Health, 91*, 1107–1113.

Rumpf, H. J., Bischof, G., Hapke, U., Meyer, C., & John, U. (2000). Studies on natural recovery from alcohol dependence: Sample selection bias by media solicitation? *Addiction, 95*, 765–775.

Rumpf, H. J., Bischof, G., Hapke, U., Meyer, C., & John, U. (2006). Stability of remission from alcohol dependence without formal help. *Alcohol and Alcoholism, 41*, 311–314.

Secades-Villa, R., & Fernández Hermida, J. R. (2003). The validity of self-reports in a follow-up study. *Addictive Behaviors, 28*, 1175–1182.

Sobell, L. C., Agrawal, S., & Sobell, M. B. (1997). Factors affecting agreement between alcohol abusers' and their collaterals' reports. *Journal of Studies on Alcohol, 58*, 405–413.

Sobell, L. C., Cunningham, J. A., & Sobell, M. B. (1996). Recovery from alcohol problems with and without treatment: Prevalence in two population surveys. *American Journal of Public Health, 86*, 966–972.

Sobell, L. C., Ellingstad, T. P., & Sobell, M. B. (2000). Natural recovery from alcohol and drug problems: Methodological review of the research with suggestions for future directions. *Addiction, 95*, 749–764.

Sobell, L. C., Klingemann, H. K., Toneatto, T., Sobell, M. B., Agrawal, S., & Leo, G. I. (2001). Alcohol and drug abusers' perceived reasons for self-change in Canada and Switzerland: Computer-assisted content analysis. *Substance Use & Misuse, 36*, 1467–1500.

Sobell, L. C., Sobell, M. B., & Agrawal, S. (2002). Self-change and dual recoveries among individuals with alcohol and tobacco problems: Current knowledge and future directions. *Alcoholism: Clinical Experimental Research, 26*, 1936–1938.

Sobell, M. B., Sobell, L. C., & Kozlowski, L. T. (1995). Dual recoveries from alcohol and smoking problems. In J. B. Fertig & J. A. Allen (Eds.), *Alcohol and tobacco: From basic science to clinical practice* (pp. 207–224). Rockville, MD: National Institute on Alcohol Abuse and Alcoholism.

Vaillant, G. (2005). Secrets and lies: Comments on Dawson et al. (2005). *Addiction, 100*, 294.

Weisner, C., Matzger, H., & Kaskutas, L. A. (2003). How important is treatment? One-year outcomes of treated and untreated alcohol-dependent individuals. *Addiction, 98*, 901–911.

Winick, C. (1962). Maturing out of narcotic addiction. *Bulletin on Narcotics, 14*, 1–10.

Appendix

Primary References

Bezdek, M., Croy, C., & Spicer, P. (2004). Documenting natural recovery in American-Indian drinking behavior: A coding scheme. *Journal of Studies on Alcohol, 65,* 428–433.

Blomqvist, J. (2002). Recovery with and without treatment: A comparison of resolutions of alcohol and drug problems. *Addiction Research & Theory, 10,* 119–158.

Boyd, S. J., Tashkin, D. P., Huestis, M. A., Heishman, S. J., Dermand, J. C., Simmons, M. S., et al. (2005). Strategies for quitting among non-treatment-seeking marijuana smokers. *American Journal of Addiction, 14,* 35–42.

Cameron, D., Manik, G., Bird, R., & Sinorwalia, A. (2002). What may we be learning from so-called spontaneous remission in ethnic minorities? *Addiction Research & Theory, 10,* 175–182.

Cunningham, J. A. (1999). Untreated remissions from drug use: The predominant pathway. *Addictive Behaviors, 24,* 267–270.

Cunningham, J. A. (2000). Remissions from drug dependence: Is treatment a prerequisite? *Drug and Alcohol Dependence, 59,* 211–213.

Cunningham, J. A., Blomqvist, J., Koski-Jannes, A., Cordingley, J., & Callaghan, R. (2004). Characteristics of former heavy drinkers: Results from a natural history of drinking general population survey. *Contemporary Drug Problems, 31,* 357–369.

Cunningham, J. A., Cameron, T., Koski-Jännes, A., Cordingley, J., & Toneatto, T. (2002). A prospective study of quit attempts from alcohol problems in a community sample: Modeling the processes of change. *Addiction Research & Theory, 10,* 159–173.

Cunningham, J. A., Koski-Jännes, A., & Toneatto, T. (1999). Why do people stop their drug use? Results from a general population sample. *Contemporary Drug Problems, 26,* 695–710.

Cunningham, J. A., Lin, E., Ross, H. E., & Walsh, W. E. (2000). Factors associated with untreated remissions from alcohol abuse or dependence. *Addictive Behaviors, 25,* 317–321.

Dawson, D. A., Grant, B. F., Stinson, F. S., Chou, P. S., Huang, B., & Ruan, W. J. (2005). Recovery from DSM-IV alcohol dependence: United States, 2001–2002. *Addiction, 100,* 281–292.

Ellingstad, T. P., Sobell, L. C., Sobell, M. B., Eickleberry, L., & Golden, C. J. (2006). Self-change: A pathway to cannabis abuse resolution. *Addictive Behaviors, 31,* 519–530.

Finfgeld, D. L., & Lewis, L. M. (2002). Self-resolution of alcohol problems in young adulthood: A process of securing solid ground. *Qualitative Health Research, 12,* 581–592.

Granfield, R., & Cloud, W. (2001). Social context and "natural recovery": The role of social capital in the resolution of drug-associated problems. *Substance Use & Misuse, 36,* 1543–1570.

Koski-Jännes, A., & Turner, N. (1999). Factors influencing recovery from different addictions. *Addiction Research, 6,* 469–492.

Price, R. K., Risk, N. K., & Spitznagel, E. L. (2001). Remission from drug abuse over a 25-year period: Patterns of remission and treatment use. *American Journal of Public Health, 91,* 1107–1113.

Rumpf, H. J., Bischof, G., Hapke, U., Meyer, C., & John, U. (2000). Studies on natural recovery from alcohol dependence: Sample selection bias by media solicitation? *Addiction, 95*, 765–775.

Russell, M., Peirce, R. S., Chan, A. W., Wieczorek, W. F., Moscato, B. S., & Nochajski, T. H. (2001). Natural recovery in a community-based sample of alcoholics: Study design and descriptive data. *Substance Use & Misuse, 36*, 1417–1441.

Tucker, J. A., Vuchinich, R. E., & Rippens, P. D. (2002). Environmental contexts surrounding resolution of drinking problems among problem drinkers with different help-seeking experiences. *Journal of Studies on Alcohol, 63*, 334–341.

Vik, P. W., Cellucci, T., & Ivers, H. (2003). Natural reduction of binge drinking among college students. *Addictive Behaviors, 28*, 643–655.

Weisner, C., Matzger, H., & Kaskutas, L. A. (2003). How important is treatment? One-year outcomes of treated and untreated alcohol-dependent individuals. *Addiction, 98*, 901–911.

Secondary References

Bischof, G., Rumpf, H. J., Hapke, U., Meyer, C., & John, U. (2000). Maintenance factors of recovery from alcohol dependence in treated and untreated individuals. *Alcoholism: Clinical and Experimental Research, 24*, 1773–1777.

Bischof, G., Rumpf, H.-J., Hapke, U., Meyer, C., & John, U. (2000). Gender differences in natural recovery from alcohol dependence. *Journal of Studies on Alcohol, 61*, 783–786.

Bischof, G., Rumpf, H.-J., Hapke, U., Meyer, C., & John, U. (2001). Factors influencing remission from alcohol dependence without formal help in a representative population sample. *Addiction, 96*, 1327–1336.

Bischof, G., Rumpf, H.-J., Hapke, U., Meyer, C., & John, U. (2002). Remission from alcohol dependence without help: How restrictive should our definition of treatment be? *Journal of Studies on Alcohol, 63*, 229–236.

Bischof, G., Rumpf, H.-J., Hapke, U., Meyer, C., & John, U. (2003). Types of natural recovery from alcohol dependence: A cluster analytic approach. *Addiction, 98*, 1737–1746.

Bischof, G., Rumpf, H.-J., Meyer, C., Hapke, U., & John, U. (2005). Influence of psychiatric comorbidity in alcohol-dependent subjects in a representative population survey on treatment utilization and natural recovery. *Addiction, 100*, 405–413.

Cunningham, J. A., Blomqvist, J., Koski-Jännes, A., & Cordingley, J. (2005). Maturing out of drinking problems: Perceptions of natural history as a function of severity. *Addiction Research & Theory, 13*, 79–84.

Cunningham, J. A., Wild, T. C., & Koski-Jännes, A. (2005). Motivation and life events: A prospective natural history pilot study of problem drinkers in the community. *Addictive Behaviors, 30*, 1603–1606.

Hanninen, V., & Koski-Jännes, A. (1999). Narratives of recovery from addictive behaviours. *Addiction, 94*, 1837–1848.

Koski-Jännes, A. (2002). Social and personal identity projects in the recovery from addictive behaviours. *Addiction Research & Theory, 10*, 183–202.

Rumpf, H.-J., Bischof, G., Hapke, U., Meyer, C., & John, U. (2002). The role of family and partnership in recovery from alcohol dependence: Comparison of individuals remitting with and without formal help. *European Addiction Research, 8*, 122–127.

Tucker, J. A., Vuchinich, R. E., & Rippens, P. D. (2002). Predicting natural resolution of alcohol-related problems: A prospective behavioral economic analysis. *Experimental & Clinical Psychopharmacology, 10*, 248–257.

6
Self-Change in a Broader Context: Beyond Alcohol and Drugs

6.1
Self-Change: The Rule among Smokers

Stephanie Flöter and Christoph Kröger

Epidemiology of Smoking and Quitting

In 2000, 23.3% of adults in the United States were current smokers and approximately 70% of them reported the desire to quit smoking completely. Among the estimated 42.4% ever-smokers, 50.6% were former smokers (Centers for Disease Control and Prevention [CDC], 2002). In other words, about one-half of U.S. ever-smokers become nonsmokers during their lives (Hughes, Keely, & Naud, 2004).

In Germany, the proportion of ex-smokers in the adult population is 24.2% (Augustin, Metz, Heppekausen, & Kraus, 2005). Whereas the highest prevalence of smoking and the lowest number of ex-smokers can be found in the young adult cohort (41.3% current smokers, 6.7% ex-smokers), the number of smokers is decreasing with increases in age, first slowly, then progressively more rapidly. At the same time, the proportion of ex-smokers is continuously increasing (Augustin et al., 2005; Lampert & Burger, 2004). The declining prevalence of smoking is the result both of the elevated mortality rate among smokers (see Doll, Peto, Boreham, & Sutherland, 2004) and of the increase in smokers becoming nonsmokers. The quit rate, defined as the ratio of ex-smokers to the sum of all individuals who have ever smoked, is increasing with age. In the cohort of persons aged over 65 years, the rate is 73.8% for women and 77% for men (Lampert & Burger, 2004); this means that in Germany three-quarters of the ever-smokers have quit smoking at some point.

Several quit attempts are typically necessary before lifelong success (Hughes et al., 2004). In the course of 1 year, approximately one third of smokers in Germany and the United Kingdom (Junge & Nagel, 1999; West, McEwen, Bolling, & Owen, 2001), and about 40% of smokers in the United States and Australia (CDC, 2002; Trotter & Letcher, 2000) report having tried to quit smoking for at least 1 day. However, only a small proportion is able to maintain abstinence for a sustained period; the medium-term success rate for a given attempt is about 3–5% (CDC, 2002; Meyer, Rumpf, Schumann, Hapke, & John, 2003; West et al., 2001). From their review of studies on unaided quitting, Hughes et al. (2004) conclude that for a typical U.S. smoker it may take 10–14 attempts before a smoker stops. However, this interpretation assumes that the success rate does not vary across attempts and that most successful smokers never access treatment.

Self-Quitting

As the existing evidence suggests, most quitters do not utilize any aids for smoking cessation. The first systematic analysis of the use of assistance for smoking cessation in the general population was published by Fiore et al. (1990). They found that, in the 10 years preceding the survey, about 15% of respondents used assistance in at least one of their quit attempts and that only 7.9% reported using any aid in their most recent attempt. That means that over 90% of smokers who quit at that time did so on their own. Since this seminal paper, much has occurred in the field of tobacco control and new aids for smoking cessation have been developed. A number of studies since then have investigated what methods are used by smokers in quit attempts. They differ in many methodological aspects. Some ask open-ended questions about methods used for quitting while other studies have participants choose from a list of possible aids. No consensus exists regarding what is actually considered an "aid" (e.g., in one study "support from family or friends" was included in the list of aids for quitting; Buck & Morgan, 2001). Therefore, the resulting proportions of individuals who tried to quit smoking in the course of 1 year and used at least one form of assistance vary to some extent and range between approximately 15% and 30% (Buck & Morgan, 2001; Cokkinides, Ward, Jemal, & Thun, 2005; Hammond, McDonald, Fong, & Borland, 2004; Meyer, Rumpf, Hapke, & John, 2000; Westmaas & Langsam, 2005; Zhu, Melcer, Sun, Rosbrook, & Pierce, 2000). While it can be concluded that the use of assistance has somewhat increased in the last decade, the overall result remains that most smokers quit on their own.

Interestingly, most studies consistently found that aids are more often used in unsuccessful than in successful quit attempts (Doran, Valenti, Robinson, Britt, & Mattick, 2006; Fiore et al., 1990; Kraus & Augustin, 2001; Meyer et al., 2000). There has been much discussion about the meaning of this finding. One could conclude that quitting without external help is the best strategy to become a nonsmoker. Yet, this would contrast sharply with the findings from effectiveness studies indicating that smokers who engage in strategies such as counseling, nicotine replacement therapies, or other pharmacological aids show much higher success rates than control groups (Lancaster, Stead, Silagy, & Sowden, 2000). Therefore, authors are forced to come up with different explanations for the lower utilization rate among former smokers. In one study, the episode of active smoking dated back much further for ex-smokers not having used any help (Meyer et al., 2000). Regarding the increase in available aids in the last decade, there could have been an overall lower utilization rate among smokers at the time these individuals made their quit attempt.

There is also the possibility of a growing recall bias, with more time having passed since quitting. Another explanation could lie in the special characteristics of help-seeking smokers. Some studies found that those seeking assistance were heavier smokers (Fiore et al., 1990; Meyer et al., 2000) with a longer duration of smoking and higher nicotine dependence (Meyer et al., 2000) and had made more cessation attempts than those who quit unaided (Fiore et al., 1990). Therefore, as Zhu et al. (2000) state, perhaps "the potential advantages of assistance did not overcome the initial disadvantages of those who sought help" (p. 305). In their study, the individuals who used assistance had more than double the long-term cessation rate of those who quit without assistance (15.2% versus 7.0%). This effect may at least in part be due to different characteristics of the study sample; those who sought help in the Zhu et al. study smoked much less than, for example, those in the Fiore et al. study.

Success in a Given Self-Quit Attempt

There are two major reviews concerning the success of a given quit attempt in self-quitters (Cohen et al., 1989; Hughes et al., 2004). Both come to the conclusion that success rates for self-quitting are very low. Cohen et al. (1989), in their summary of 10 prospective studies, found a median long-term prolonged abstinence (LTPA) rate of 5% for 6-month and 4% for 12-month follow-ups. The studies published since then and reviewed in the paper by Hughes et al. (2004) replicate these results and conclude "that the 6-month LTPA rate for a given quit attempt among untreated smokers appears to be between 3 and 5%" (p. 35). In addition, Hughes et al. (2004) looked at the shape of the relapse curve and found that the majority of initial quitters relapsed within the first 8 days following their quit date. Thus, it appears that the main problem in stopping smoking by oneself is initiating a period of abstinence rather than late relapse. Even if the observed outcomes of self-quit attempts do not appear very promising, one must bear in mind that the evaluation of a single quit attempt may not necessarily be a good predictor of the probability of quitting over a lifetime (Schachter, 1982). Additionally, despite the relatively low abstinence rates in quit attempts, the overall volume of self-quitting is enormous and, thus, unaided quitting has the greatest impact on smoking prevalence in the population (Shiffman, Mason, & Henningfield, 1998).

Reduction as Outcome

If one looks at "self-change" rather than "self-healing," one also must consider reduction of tobacco consumption as an outcome. Attempts to reduce the amount of cigarettes smoked are at least as common as quit attempts.

In a British study with a representative sample of the adult population, 51% of smokers said they had attempted to cut down in a 1-year period (West et al., 2001). In a German sample, 39.4% reported a serious reduction attempt during a period of 30 months (Meyer et al., 2003), and data from the Community Intervention Trial for smoking cessation in the United States suggest that 40% of smokers had reduced their smoking by at least 5% during a 2-year period (Hughes, Cummings, & Hyland, 1999). Quit and reduction attempts overlap to a great extent; for example, Meyer et al. (2003) found that among participants who tried to reduce, 56.5% reported a quit attempt as well. The likelihood of maintaining reduction is at least equal to the likelihood of maintaining abstinence. In the study by Hughes et al. (1999), 21% of assessed smokers succeeded in reducing their cigarette consumption and maintained this reduction for at least 2 years. In the German study, 15% of all still-smoking participants managed to maintain their achieved reduction (Meyer et al., 2003). Concerns that reduction undermines the probability of later quit attempts are not supported by current studies, but neither is the fact that reduction attempts enhance the probability of quitting (Hughes et al., 1999; Meyer et al., 2003).

Reasons for Quitting

Existing studies often fail to probe influences that trigger the self-change process. Nevertheless, some data are available on reasons for quitting and quit attempts cited by current and former smokers. The social environment seems to have a strong impact on the smoker. A German study suggests that during the past 12 months smokers were most frequently urged to quit smoking by family or friends, mainly by their spouse or partner (34%; Kraus & Augustin, 2001). In addition, 20% of men and about 15% of women were advised by their physician to quit smoking. Hyland et al. (2004) reported that, compared with an earlier study (Hymowitz et al., 1997), the percentage of participants reporting pressure to quit from family, friends, and doctors has increased with time. The most common reason given for quitting smoking is concern for one's own health (Grotvedt & Stavem, 2005; Hyland et al., 2004; Hymowitz et al., 1997; Larabie, 2005; West et al., 2001), followed by reasons such as wanting to improve physical fitness, disliking addiction, expense, and concern for the effect on others (Grotvedt & Stavem, 2005; Hyland et al., 2004; Hymowitz et al., 1997). The priorities tend to change somewhat with age and gender. While the wish to improve physical fitness is particularly important among young men, women tend to quit more often out of consideration for their children or for aesthetic reasons. In addition, quitting because of an existing illness or as the result of advice from a physician increases with age (Grotvedt & Stavem, 2005). (See L. Sobell's chapter on conceptual issues in self-change in this book for a discussion of whether brief physician advice constitutes treatment rather than a mere trigger for self-change.)

Predictors of Successful Self-Quitting

Determining what factors predict successful smoking cessation, specifically in self-quitters, is a complex task limited by the difficulties of comparing studies (e.g., predictor variables assessed differ across studies, definitions and time frames for short- and long-term maintenance are not standardized, and few studies compare factors related to short- and long-term outcomes within the same study; Ockene et al., 2000). One finding across studies is that variables that predict short-term success do not seem to be the same as those related to long-term maintained abstinence (Garvey, Bliss, Hitchcock, Heinold, & Rosner, 1992; Gulliver, Hughes, Solomon, & Dey, 1995; Marlatt, Curry, & Gordon, 1988; Westmaas & Langsam, 2005).

In their review of 11 prospective studies of self-quitters, Ockene et al. (2000) found the following variables to be consistently predictive of maintained abstinence for at least 6 months: higher education, greater confidence in ability to stay quit (i.e., self-efficacy), lighter smoking, less alcohol consumption, fewer cigarettes smoked per day, and fewer slips in current quit attempt. In conclusion, more studies are needed to overcome the methodological obstacles prevalent in the existing research in order to determine what factors are important in successfully quitting smoking by oneself.

References

Augustin, R., Metz, K., Heppekausen, K., & Kraus, L. (2005). Tabakkonsum, Abhängigkeit und Änderungsbereitschaft. Ergebnisse des Epidemiologischen Suchtsurvey 2003 [Tobacco use, dependency and readiness to change. Results of the 2003 Epidemiological Survey of Substance Abuse]. *Sucht, 51*, 40–48.

Buck, D., & Morgan, A. (2001). Smoking and quitting with the aid of Nicotine Replacement Therapies in the English adult population. *European Journal of Public Health, 11*, 211–217.

Centers for Disease Control and Prevention. (2002). Cigarette smoking among adults: United States, 2000. *MMWR, 51*, 642–645.

Cohen, S., Lichtenstein, E., Prochaska, J. O., Rossi, J. S., Gritz, E. R., Carr, C. R., et al. (1989). Debunking myths about self-quitting. Evidence from 10 prospective studies of persons who attempt to quit smoking by themselves. *American Psychologist, 44*, 1355–1365.

Cokkinides, V. E., Ward, E., Jemal, A., & Thun, M. J. (2005). Under-use of smoking-cessation treatments: Results from the National Health Interview Survey, 2000. *American Journal of Preventive Medicine, 28*, 119–122.

Doll, R., Peto, R., Boreham, J., & Sutherland, I. (2004). Mortality in relation to smoking: 50 years observations on male British doctors. *British Medical Journal, 328*, 1519.

Doran, C. M., Valenti, L., Robinson, M., Britt, H., & Mattick, R. P. (2006). Smoking status of Australian general practice patients and their attempts to quit. *Addictive Behaviors, 31*, 758–766.

Fiore, M. C., Novotny, T. E., Pierce, J. P., Giovino, G. A., Hatziandreu, E. J., Newcomb, P. A., et al. (1990). Methods used to quit smoking in the United States: Do cessation programs help? *Journal of the American Medical Association, 263*, 2760–2765.

Garvey, A. J., Bliss, R. E., Hitchcock, J. L., Heinold, J. W., & Rosner, B. (1992). Predictors of smoking relapse among self-quitters: A report from the Normative Aging Study. *Addictive Behaviors, 17*, 367–377.

Grotvedt, L., & Stavem, K. (2005). Association between age, gender, and reasons for smoking cessation. *Scandinavian Journal of Public Health, 33*, 72–76.

Gulliver, S. B., Hughes, J. R., Solomon, L. J., & Dey, A. N. (1995). An investigation of self-efficacy, partner support, and daily stresses as predictors of relapse to smoking in self-quitters. *Addiction, 90*, 767–772.

Hammond, D., McDonald, P. W., Fong, G. T., & Borland, R. (2004). Do smokers know how to quit? Knowledge and perceived effectiveness of cessation assistance as predictors of cessation behaviour. *Addiction, 99*, 1042–1048.

Hughes, J. R., Cummings, K. M., & Hyland, A. (1999). Ability of smokers to reduce their smoking and its association with future smoking cessation. *Addiction, 94*, 109–114.

Hughes, J. R., Keely, J., & Naud, S. (2004). Shape of the relapse curve and long-term abstinence among untreated smokers. *Addiction, 99*, 29–38.

Hyland, A., Li, Q., Bauer, J. E., Giovino, G. A., Steger, C., & Cummings, K. M. (2004). Predictors of cessation in a cohort of current and former smokers followed over 13 years. *Tobacco Control, 6*, 363–369.

Hymowitz, N., Cummings, K. M., Hyland, A., Lynn, W. R., Pechacek, T. F., & Hartwell, T. D. (1997). Predictors of smoking cessation in a cohort of adult smokers followed for five years. *Tobacco Control, 6*, 57–62.

Junge, B., & Nagel, M. (1999). Das Rauchverhalten in Deutschland [Smoking behavior in Germany]. *Gesundheitswesen, 61*, 121–125.

Kraus, L., & Augustin, R. (2001). Repräsentativerhebung zum Gebrauch psychoaktiver Substanzen bei Erwachsenen in Deutschland 2000 [Population survey on the consumption of psychoactive substances in the German adult population 2000]. *Sucht, 47*, 5–87.

Larabie, L. C. (2005). To what extent do smokers plan quit attempts? *Tobacco Control, 14*, 425–428.

Lampert, T., & Burger, M. (2004). Rauchgewohnheiten in Deutschland - Ergebnisse des telefonischen Bundes-Gesundheitssurveys 2003 [Smoking habits in Germany—Results of the German National Telephone Health Survey 2003]. *Gesundheitswesen, 66*, 511–517.

Lancaster, T., Stead, L. F., Silagy, C., & Sowden, A. (2000). Effectiveness of interventions to help people stop smoking: Findings from the Cochrane Library. *British Medical Journal, 321*, 355–358.

Marlatt, G. A., Curry, S., & Gordon, J. R. (1988). A longitudinal analysis of unaided smoking cessation. *Journal of Consulting and Clinical Psychology, 56*, 715–720.

Meyer, C., Rumpf, H.-J., Hapke, U., & John, U. (2000). Inanspruchnahme von Hilfen zur Erlangung der Nikotin-Abstinenz [Utilization of aids for smoking cessation]. *Sucht, 46*, 398–407.

Meyer, C., Rumpf, H.-J., Schumann, A., Hapke, U., & John, U. (2003). Intentionally reduced smoking among untreated general population smokers: Prevalence, stability, prediction of smoking behavior change and differences between subjects choosing either reduction or abstinence. *Addiction, 98*, 1101–1110.

Ockene, J. K., Emmons, K. M., Mermelstein, R. J., Perkins, K. A., Bonollo, D. S., Voorhees, C. C., et al. (2000). Relapse and maintenance issues for smoking cessation. *Health Psychology, 19*, 17–31.

Schachter, S. (1982). Recidivism and self-cure of smoking and obesity. *American Psychologist, 37*, 436–444.

Shiffman, S., Mason, K. M., & Henningfield, J. E. (1998). Tobacco dependence treatments: Review and prospectus. *Annual Review of Public Health, 19*, 335–358.

Trotter, L., & Letcher, T. (2000). *Quit evaluation studies No. 10*. Melbourne, Australia: Victorian Smoking and Health Program.

West, R., McEwen, A., Bolling, K., & Owen, L. (2001). Smoking cessation and smoking patterns in the general population: A 1-year follow-up. *Addiction, 96*, 891–902.

Westmaas, J. L., & Langsam, K. (2005). Unaided smoking cessation and predictors of failure to quit in a community sample: Effects of gender. *Addictive Behaviors, 30*, 1405–1424.

Zhu, S. H., Melcer, T., Sun, J., Rosbrook, B., & Pierce, J. P. (2000). Smoking cessation with and without assistance: A population-based analysis. *American Journal of Preventive Medicine, 18*, 305–311.

6.2
Natural Recovery from Problem Gambling

Tony Toneatto and Jachen C. Nett

With the growing accessibility to and availability of a wide range of gaming activities throughout North America, there is growing concern over the increasing number of individuals who are seeking treatment for problem gambling. This issue has received the greatest systematic attention in North America (Arseneault, Ladouceur, & Vitaro, 2001; Kallick, Suits, Dielman, & Hybels, 1979; Ladouceur, Jacques, Ferland, & Giroux, 1999; Moore, 2001; Volberg & Steadman, 1989; Welte, Barnes, Wieczorek, Tidwell, & Parker, 2001). Prevalence rates ranging from 1% to 2% throughout most North American jurisdictions have been widely reported, with rates several times greater when subclinical gamblers are included (Rush & Moxam, 2001; Shaffer, Hall, & Vander Bilt, 1999).

In recent years, the global impact of gambling problems has become evident. Studies in Australia (Dickerson & Hinchy, 1988; Productivity Commission, 1999), New Zealand (Abbott & Volberg, 2000; Problem Gambling Foundation of New Zealand, 2003), South Africa (Collins & Barr, 2003), and throughout Europe—in particular, Great Britain (Fisher, 1999; Orford, Sproston, Erens, White, & Mitchell, 2003), Norway (Götestam & Johansson, 2003), Sweden (Rönnberg, 2001; Volberg, Abbott, Rönnberg, & Munck, 2001), Switzerland (Bondolfi, Osiek, & Ferrero, 2000; Molo Bettelini, Alippi, & Wernli, 2000), and Spain (Baacke, 1997; Becoña, 1996; Legarda, Babio, & Abreu, 1992)—have shown similar rates of gambling problems.

Several sources of evidence suggest that recovery from a gambling problem may not always be mediated through contact with the formal treatment system, but may reflect natural recovery processes paralleling the results found with untreated recovery from substance dependencies (e.g., Blomqvist, 2002; Klingemann, 1992; Sobell et al., 2001; Stewart, 1999; Toneatto, Sobell, Sobell, & Rubel, 1999). Epidemiological studies of gambling prevalence frequently identify significant numbers of "former gamblers." For example, Hodgins, Wynne, and Makarchuk (1999) found that over one-third of life-time gamblers surveyed reported no problems in the previous year. Similarly, Bland, Newman, Orn, and Stebelsky (1993) found that only about 50% of those with lifetime pathological gambling problems continued to have such problems in the 6 months prior to the interview in a population survey of psychiatric patients. In a study of two large representative national surveys in the United States, Slutske (2006) found that only 36–39% of individuals who had reported a lifetime history of DSM-IV pathological gambling reported any gambling symptoms in the previous year. Since only 7–12% had sought formal treatment or had attended Gamblers Anonymous, the study's findings suggest that about one-third of problem gamblers may have naturally recovered.

In addition, the number of treatment-seeking gamblers is often considerably below what would be expected based on the point prevalence data. The National Gambling Impact Study Commission (1999) estimated that less than 3% of pathological gamblers have sought formal treatment. In Ontario, Canada, for example, the number of individuals seeking treatment (a few thousand per year) is well below what the prevalence data would indicate (i.e., approximately 340,000 Ontarians with at-risk or problem gambling; Rush & Moxam, 2001). A Swiss study (Künzi, Fritschi, & Egger, 2004) found approximately 1,000 to 1,500 (or between 2.8 and 3.1%) of the estimated 35,000 to 48,000 problem gamblers (based on a prevalence rate ranging between 0.62 and 0.84%; Bondolfi, Osiek, & Ferrero, 2000) sought treatment in Switzerland in 2003.

These findings suggest that alternative recovery pathways may be more common than believed. The natural recovery from gambling as an alternative pathway has been studied in a small number of studies. In one study, Hodgins and el-Guebaly (2000) found gambling severity to predict treatment entry, with less severe problem gamblers being more likely to prefer natural recovery. These results were largely replicated by Toneatto et al. (in press) and Nett, Schatzmann, Klingemann, and Gerber (2003) who showed that treated gamblers had a longer problem gambling duration, greater gambling severity, more gambling symptoms (e.g., feelings of despair, panic, suicide), and more gambling-related negative consequences (e.g., higher financial losses, more severe family and health problems) compared with the naturally recovered gamblers. There is also some evidence that comorbidity with problematic substance use is relatively more pronounced among treated gamblers (Nett et al., 2003). Finally, according to Turner (2000) there is a correlation between self-recovery from gambling and a deeper understanding of the nature of randomness and the principles of probability. He suggests that teaching people about randomness may be an important part of both treatment and prevention of problem gambling.

Similar to untreated recovery from addictions, natural recovery from problem gambling appears to involve a cognitive evaluation process focused on the detrimental impact of gambling on individuals' core values, as well as an accumulation of gambling-related negative consequences (Hodgins, 2001; Hodgins, Makarchuk, el-Guebaly, & Peden, 2002; Toneatto et al., in press). Hodgins et al. (2002), for example, identified negative emotional states, financial crisis, interpersonal distress, and conflict as frequently mentioned reasons for resolving a gambling problem. Additionally, Nett et al. (2003) noted that before a change in gambling behavior, there is usually a "spontaneous" decision to do so. Such change was rarely preceded by a gradual decision-making process.

Hodgins (2001) and Hodgins and el-Guebaly (2000) found that the change strategies that naturally recovering gamblers reported were generally practical and action-oriented. Such strategies included stimulus control, avoidance, instituting desirable lifestyle changes, and maintaining an acute ongoing awareness of gambling-related negative consequences (see also Nett et al., 2003). Toneatto et al. (in press) found that the most common change strategies during the year postresolution included stimulus control, adoption of a gambling-incompatible lifestyle, limited access to money, self-disclosure to others of the commitment to stop gambling, and an acute awareness of gambling-related negative consequences. As suggested by Nett et al. (2003), a well-planned modification of social and leisure activities is an important element to be considered when an attempt to quit gambling is undertaken.

Toneatto et al. (in press) also asked recovered gamblers to suggest effective ways other gamblers might succeed if they chose untreated recovery. About half of the sample said that there was "nothing" that could be done to trigger the recovery process; however, those who made suggestions pointed to the importance of raising awareness of the negative consequences of problem gambling and arousing cognitive dissonance between the individual's values and the consequences of continued gambling. A controlled gambling goal was generally advised against by about half of the sample, 80% of whom had chosen abstinence from gambling. For those who might choose nonabstinence, limiting time and amount spent gambling and adopting gambling-incompatible lifestyles were advocated by the recovered gamblers.

In summary, Hodgins and el-Guebaly (2000) and Toneatto et al. (in press) suggest that severity of problem gambling may be the primary variable distinguishing those who choose to recover from gambling without treatment from those who seek treatment. Most studies of natural recovery from gambling (e.g., Hodgins et al., 2002), like those of substance dependence, identify a crisis in self-image or values, accompanied by multiple gambling-related negative consequences; these consequences thus precipitate a reevaluation process of the role of gambling in their lives. Hodgins (2001), Hodgins and el-Guebaly (2000), Toneatto et al. (in press), and Nett et al. (2003) reported similar change strategies by their recovered gamblers consisting primarily of limit-setting, stimulus control, and the adoption of a gambling-incompatible lifestyle.

Additional research is needed to better understand the methods that initiate and maintain natural recovery as an important and alternative pathway to recovery from gambling. Such knowledge may influence educational and prevention strategies as well as inform treatment for problem gamblers.

References

Abbott, M. W., & Volberg, R. A. (2000). *Taking the pulse on gambling and problem gambling in New Zealand: A report on the phase one of the 1999 National Prevalence Survey.* Wellington: The Department of Internal Affairs, New Zealand.

Arseneault, L., Ladouceur, R., & Vitaro, F. (2001). Gambling and psychotropic substance consumption: Prevalence, coexistence and consequences. *Canadian Psychology-Psychologie Canadienne, 42,* 173–184.

Baacke, D. (1997). *Medienkompetenz.* Tübingen: Niemeyer.

Becoña, E. (1996). Prevalence surveys of problem and pathological gambling in Europe: The cases of Germany, Holland and Spain. *Journal of Gambling Studies, 12,* 179–192.

Bland, R. C., Newman, S. C., Orn, H., & Stebelsky, G. (1993). Epidemiology of pathological gambling in Edmonton. *Canadian Journal of Psychiatry, 38,* 108–112.

Blomqvist, J. (2002). Recovery with and without treatment: A comparison of resolutions of alcohol and drug problems. *Addiction Research & Theory, 10,* 119–158.

Bondolfi, G., Osiek, C., & Ferrero, F. (2000). Prevalence estimates of pathological gambling in Switzerland. *Acta Psychiatrica Scandinavica, 101,* 473–475.

Collins, P., & Barr, G. (2003). *Gambling and problem gambling in South Africa: A national study.* Cape Town: National Centre for the Study of Gambling at the University of Cape Town.

Dickerson, M., & Hinchy, J. (1988). The prevalence of excessive and pathological gambling in Australia. *Journal of Gambling Behavior, 4,* 135–151.

Fisher, S. (1999). A prevalence study of gambling and problem gambling in British adolescents. *Addiction Research, 7,* 509–538.

Götestam, K. G., & Johansson, A. (2003). Characteristics of gambling in the Norwegian context: A DSM-IV based telephone interview. *Addictive Behaviors, 28,* 189–197.

Hodgins, D. C. (2001). Processes of changing gambling behavior. *Addictive Behaviors, 26,* 121–128.

Hodgins, D. C., & el-Guebaly, N. (2000). Natural and treatment-assisted recovery from gambling problems: A comparison of resolved and active gamblers. *Addiction, 95,* 777–789.

Hodgins, D., Makarchuk, K., el-Guebaly, N., & Peden, N. (2002). Why problem gamblers quit gambling: A comparison of methods and samples. *Addiction Research Theory, 10,* 203–218.

Hodgins, D., Wynne, H., & Makarchuk, K. (1999). Pathways to recovery from gambling problems: Follow-up from a general population survey. *Journal of Gambling Studies, 15,* 93–104.

Kallick, M., Suits, D., Dielman, T., & Hybels, J. A. (1979). *A survey of American gambling attitudes and behavior.* Ann Arbor: Institute for Social Research, University of Michigan.

Klingemann, H. (1992). Coping and maintenance strategies of spontaneous remitters from problem use of alcohol and heroin in Switzerland. *The International Journal of the Addictions, 27,* 1359–1388.

Künzi, K., Fritschi, T., & Egger, T. (2004). *Glücksspiel und Spielsucht in der Schweiz.* Bern: Büro für Arbeits- und sozialpolitische Studien.

Ladouceur, R., Jacques, C., Ferland, F., & Giroux, I. (1999). Prevalence of problem gambling: A replication study 7 years later. *Canadian Journal of Psychiatry-Revue Canadienne De Psychiatrie, 44,* 802–804.

Legarda, J. J., Babio, R., & Abreu, J. M. (1992). Prevalence estimates of pathological gambling in Seville (Spain). *British Journal of Addiction, 87*, 767–770.

Molo Bettelini, C., Alippi, M., & Wernli, B. (2000). *An investigation into pathological gambling.* Mendrisio: Centre for Documentation and Research, OSC, Accento.

Moore, T. L. (2001). *The prevalence of disordered gambling among adults in Oregon: A secondary analysis of data.* Wilsonville: Oregon Gambling Addiction Treatment Foundation.

National Gambling Impact Study Commission. (1999). *Final report.* Washington, DC: U.S. Government Printing Office.

Nett, J. C., Schatzmann, S., Klingemann, H., & Gerber, M. (2003). *Forschungsbericht - Spielbankengesetzgebung und 'Selbstheilung' von der Spielsucht.* Bern: Institut für Sozialplanung und Sozialmanagement ISS, Hochschule für Sozialarbeit HSA Bern.

Orford, J., Sproston, K., Erens, B., White, C., & Mitchell, L. (2003). *Gambling and problem gambling in Britain.* New York: Brunner-Routledge.

Problem Gambling Foundation of New Zealand. (2003). *Supporting the well-being of young people in relation to gambling in New Zealand. Final report and recommendations.* Epsom: Author.

Productivity Commission. (1999). *Australia's gambling industries. Report No. 10. Chapter 6 What is problem gambling & Appendix F, National Gambling Survey* (No. 10). Canberra: AusInfo.

Rönnberg, S. (2001). Die schwedische Prävalenzstudie zum pathologischen Glücksspielen (J. Petry, Trans.). In I. Füchtenschnieder & K. Hurrelmann (Eds.), *Glücksspiel in Europa- Vom Nutzen und Schaden des Glücksspiels im europäischen Vergleich* (pp. 1–144). Geesthacht: Neuland.

Rush, B., & Moxam, R. S. (2001). *Treatment of problem gambling in Ontario: Service utilization and client characteristics.* Ontario: Center for Addiction and Mental Health.

Shaffer, H. J., Hall, M. N., & Vander Bilt, J. (1999). Estimating the prevalence of disordered gambling behavior in the United States and Canada: A research synthesis. *American Journal of Public Health, 89*, 1369–1376.

Slutske, W. S. (2006). Natural recovery and treatment-seeking in pathological gambling: Results of two U.S. national surveys. *American Journal of Psychiatry, 163*, 297–302.

Sobell, L. C., Klingemann, H. K. H., Toneatto, T., Sobell, M. B., Agrawal, S., & Leo, G. I. (2001). Alcohol and drug abusers' perceived reasons for self-change in Canada and Switzerland: Computer-assisted content analysis. *Substance Use & Misuse, 36*, 1467–1500.

Stewart, C. (1999). Investigation of cigarette smokers who quit without treatment. *Journal of Drug Issues, 29*, 167–186.

Toneatto, T., Cunningham, J., Hodgins, D., Adams, M., Turner, N., & Koski-Jännes, A. (in press). Recovery from problem gambling without formal treatment. *Addiction Research and Theory.*

Toneatto, T., Sobell, L. C., Sobell, M. B., & Rubel, E. (1999). Natural recovery from cocaine dependence. *Psychology of Addictive Behaviors, 13*, 259–268.

Turner, N. E. (2000). Randomness, does it matter? *Journal of Gambling Issues*(2). Retrieved from: http://www.camh.net

Volberg, R. A., Abbott, M., Rönnberg, S., & Munck, I. (2001). Prevalence and risks of pathological gambling in Sweden. *Acta Psychiatrica Scandinavica, 104*, 250–256.

Volberg, R. A., & Steadman, H. J. (1989). Prevalence estimates of pathological gambling in New Jersey and Maryland. *American Journal of Psychiatry, 146,* 1618–1619.

Welte, J., Barnes, G., Wieczorek, W., Tidwell, M. C., & Parker, J. (2001). Alcohol and gambling pathology among US adults: Prevalence, demographic patterns and comorbidity. *Journal of Studies on Alcohol, 62,* 706–712.

6.3
The Natural Course and Outcome of Eating Disorders and Obesity

Janet Polivy

The natural course of recovery from eating disorders and obesity has not received much attention; in part because once a diagnosable disorder is identified the individual is generally put into some form of treatment. Thus, most examinations of the course and outcome of these disorders rely on studies of patients who are receiving or have received treatment for the problem rather than a "natural (untreated) course." This makes it difficult to determine whether therapy is actually helpful in alleviating eating disorders or obesity. Is symptomatic improvement in some individuals a result of treatment or part of the natural course of the disorders? Are those who receive treatment representative of patients with the disorders, or do they represent a biased sample? Does therapy increase the number of people who improve or does treatment have either no effect or a negative effect on ultimate outcomes? These questions need to be addressed with respect to eating disorders. What has been addressed, in part, is the extent to which individuals recover from the disorder (with or without treatment), and, to a lesser degree, the general progression of the disorder (at least with respect to eating disorders, though not obesity).

In reviewing the literature on outcomes in eating disorders, Pike (1998) noted that "there is no predictable or normative long-term course associated with anorexia nervosa. Some individuals achieve complete recovery, others are ravaged by a chronic disorder, and some die from it" (p. 447). Thus, she suggested that researchers integrate findings from both treatment outcome and naturalistic follow-up studies. A more recent review (Steinhausen, 2002) concluded that for anorexia nervosa, there is a high rate of mortality, and less than one-half of those who survive recover fully from the disorder.

From the current literature it seems there may be a natural progression among the eating disorders from anorexia nervosa (AN) to bulimia nervosa (BN) or eating disorder not otherwise specified (EDNOS), although this does not imply that all eating disorder patients ever had AN or more than one disorder. For example, 51 teenaged patients diagnosed with AN in a community screening were compared with 51 controls, and reexamined 6 years later (Råstam, Gillberg, & Gillberg, 1995). Although most of the anorexic cases no longer fulfilled the criteria for the diagnosis of AN, many currently met the diagnostic criteria for BN or EDNOS, and so were not free of eating disorder symptoms. Another study found that 2 years after inpatient treatment, 22% of AN patients had developed BN (Fichter & Quadflieg, 1996). After 6 years, there were still 27% with AN, 10% had developed BN, and 2% had EDNOS (Fichter & Quadflieg, 1999). Similarly, approximately 6 years after diagnosis and treatment, 8 of 43 AN patients who were reexamined had developed EDNOS, 5 had BN, 3 had both AN and BN, while only 4 still suffered from AN (Schulze et al., 1997). By 5 years after treatment for AN, 30% of the patients had developed BN (Strober, Freeman, & Morrell, 1997), although by 7 years three quarters of patients were deemed fully recovered from their AN. Another 7-year follow-up of AN patients indicated that of 34 patients, 7 still had AN, 4 had developed BN, and 10 were diagnosed with EDNOS. By 10 years after initial treatment, 1 of 39 AN patients still exhibited AN, and 2 had BN (Herpertz-Dahlmann et al., 2001). Thus, it seems that although one-half to three quarters of AN patients recover from the disorder over several years, a large number progress to develop another eating disorder or remain anorectic.

Looking more broadly at eating disorder patients following treatment, studies find that the majority no longer meet diagnostic criteria for an eating disorder, but many continue to have serious problems. For example, a prospective, naturalistic study following 225 women with AN, BN, and mixed AN and BN found that although nearly one-half of the initially anorexic and mixed diagnosis individuals no longer met full eating disorder diagnostic criteria during the first-year posttreatment follow-up, the recovery rate of bulimics was significantly better than that of anorexic or mixed diagnosis cases (Herzog et al., 1993). Herzog (1993) interviewed 33 women with sub-diagnostic AN and/or BN who were seeking treatment for eating disorder, and reexamined them 24 and 52 months afterwards. During the initial follow-up period, 15 of the 33 developed a fully diagnosable eating disorder. At the final assessment, 4 continued to have a diagnosable disorder, 22 were subdiagnostic, and 6 had recovered. In a different group of participants, 2 years after treatment, 50% of BN patients continued to have the full BN syndrome, 3.1% fulfilled criteria for AN, and 46.9% were below threshold for a diagnosis of AN or BN (Fichter & Quadflieg, 1996). In this same study, 30% of AN patients continued to have AN and 22% had developed BN, while the remaining 48% no longer had an eating disorder. After 6 years, of the original BN patients, 22% were still bulimic, 3.7% had AN, 2% had EDNOS, and two died. Most of these individuals (72%), though, had no diagnosable eating disorder (Fichter & Quadflieg, 1997). As mentioned earlier, the AN patients studied by this team did not improve as much over 6 years, with 39% still having an eating disorder, and six patients (6%) had died; however, the majority (55%) no longer had an eating disorder (Fichter & Quadflieg, 1999). Patients who presented with binge eating disorder (BED) tended to do well 3 to 6 years after treatment, with only 1 death out of 68 patients, 4 maintaining their BED, 5 moving to BN, and 5 developing EDNOS; this left 77% with no remaining disorder (Fichter, Quadflieg, & Gnutzmann, 1998). After 12 years, almost 8% of the patients had died and 39% had a negative outcome. While 56% were no longer diagnosed with an eating disorder, about one-half remained somewhat symptomatic (Fichter, Quadflieg, & Hedlund, 2006). Negative predictors of outcome included sexual problems, impulsivity, longer duration of inpatient treatment, and long duration of an eating disorder. During a 7-year follow-up at another center, 15 of 34 patients still fulfilled criteria for an eating disorder diagnosis, and 21 qualified for some other psychiatric diagnosis (Herpertz-Dahlmann, Wewetzer, Hennighausen, & Remschmidt, 1996). A more recent follow-up of a large number (246) of AN and BN patients found that the full recovery rate after 7 years was significantly higher for BN (74%) than for AN (33%; Herzog et al., 1999).

The order in which symptoms remit over time was examined in treated patients with AN and BN (Clausen, 2004). Similar patterns emerged for recovery from the two disorders; physical symptoms remitted before psychological symptoms of both AN and BN, while psychological symptoms such as obsession with weight and shape were the last to remit.

The progression of eating disorder symptomatology in treated individuals is instructive, but does not necessarily indicate the true course of the disorder. In order to determine whether eating disorders spontaneously remit, or are resolved only after treatment, the progression of symptoms in untreated individuals who either have the disorders or seem to be developing them needs to be examined. To this end, several studies have screened community samples of women (and occasionally men) and followed them over time. Joiner, Heatherton, and Keel (1997) screened over 400 female students from Harvard University while they attended college and again 10 years later, and found that bulimic symptoms were remarkably stable over the interval, and that initial scores on symptom indices predicted later pathology. Over a 6-month period, a group of women whose self-reports indicated that they suffered from BED reported decreased symptomatology to the extent that 10 of 21 were in at least partial remission (Cachelin et al., 1999). Adult women self-reported their eating attitudes and pathological eating behaviors twice, and reported fewer symptomatic behaviors 6 years later, but increased disturbances of eating-related attitudes (Rizvi, Stice, & Agras, 1999). Two community-based groups of women with BN or BED were assessed every 15 months for 5 years (Fairburn, Cooper, Doll, Norman, & O'Connor, 2000). In both samples, participants reported improvements in symptoms over time, particularly those with a diagnosis of BED; only 18% continued to have any form of an eating disorder after 5 years (although 39% became obese). Comparatively, one-half to two thirds of the BN patients continued to have a diagnosable disorder. A later report on the BN sample indicated that 44% could be considered as remitted over the course of 5 years, 51% persisted in their binge eating, 56% continued in compensatory behaviors, and the remaining women fell between cured and persisting in pathology (Fairburn et al., 2003). Finally, the natural course of BN and EDNOS was assessed over a 2-year period, and, as in previous studies, it was found that the probability of remission was higher for EDNOS (59%) than for BN (40%), and that those with BN took longer for their symptoms to remit (Grilo et al., 2003).

Because disordered eating often emerges during the first year of university (e.g., Striegel-Moore, Silberstein, Frensch, & Rodin, 1989), college students have been studied over time to determine whether those who begin with evidence of eating pathology improve over time or go on to develop a clinical disorder. A number of female and male undergraduate students at Harvard University were assessed as students and again 10 years later (Heatherton, Nichols, Mahamedi, & Keel, 1995). Almost all measures indicated improvements in disordered eating attitudes and behaviors over the course of 10 years, with 33% of those who initially appeared to have BN scoring as nondisordered at follow-up. Binge eating and related pathological behaviors declined, dieting became less frequent, and body image improved. More recently, students entering university were given self-report questionnaires, and subgroups that scored especially high or low in terms of eating pathology were interviewed every 6 months for 2 years (Mills & Polivy, 2005). Self-reported eating pathology decreased over the 2 years, although dietary restraint and body dissatisfaction did not change. Participants who had been identified as potentially eating-disordered at the beginning of the study generally showed evidence of improvement in eating pathology, including being less upset by out-of-control and overeating episodes by the last assessment. Those who scored highest on pathology at the start of the study, however, were least likely to improve over time, and weight and shape continued to play a major role in self-evaluation and interfered with their ability to feel good about themselves.

Finally, patients newly admitted for treatment for AN were asked what variables they thought were most conducive to recovery (Tozzi, Sullivan, Fear, McKenzie, & Bulik, 2003). The three most commonly mentioned factors were supportive relationships outside the family, therapy, and maturation.

The research thus suggests that different eating disorders have different courses, with AN being the most recalcitrant and having the highest mortality, BN being somewhat less refractory than AN, but more so than EDNOS or BED. Moreover, the latter two disorders appear most likely to remit over time. Subclinical pathological eating attitudes and behaviors such as those seen in many university students appear to improve naturally over time, but in more severe instances they seem likely to progress to full-blown pathology.

Comparing treated and nontreated individuals who recover from eating disorders, it appears that treated patients are more likely to recover fully from the disorder. Studies generally find that a majority of treated patients recover over the long term, but somewhat less than half of untreated patients seem to recover on later assessment. Before concluding that treatment is more effective than self-change, however, more research is needed to determine whether self-selection factors such as becoming motivated to seek treatment (and presumably giving up one's eating disorder symptoms) account for the observed differences in recovery among those with eating disorders. The natural course of obesity is difficult to study because the emphasis on slimness in current Western society mandates that anyone who is not fashionably svelte should at least attempt to lose weight (i.e., treat the condition of obesity; e.g., Polivy & Herman, 1987). *Consumer Reports* asked their readership to describe their experiences with weight loss, and found that of over 32,000 readers who replied to the survey, nearly 25% lost 10% of their initial weight and maintained the loss for at least 1 year (Anonymous, 2002). Half of these people actually maintained a mean loss of 37 pounds (more than 10% of their weight) for 5 years or more. More than 80% of the individuals who reported losing weight claimed to have done so on their own, without treatment.

Tinker and Tucker (1997 a,b) interviewed and assessed 21 adults who had lost significant amounts of weight without treatment, and maintained the loss over a period of 4.5 years. These individuals viewed weight loss treatments in a negative manner, and utilized procedures such as making healthier food choices and increasing exercise in order to decrease their weight. Similarly, the individuals who comprise the National Weight Control Registry[1] (e.g., Klem, Wing, McGuire, Seagle, & Hill, 1997, 1998; Phelan, Hill, Lang, Dibello, & Wing, 2003; Wing & Hill, 2001), just over one-half of whom indicated that they had lost the weight without formal treatment (Klem et al., 1997), report having used similar techniques to meet the minimum standards required for entry into the Registry. Moreover, the converse behaviors of decreasing one's level of exercise and increasing the level of fat that one consumes were associated with weight regain during the year after entering the Registry in the 35% who regained weight (McGuire, Wing, Klem, Lang, & Hill, 1999).

This raises the question of whether instituting one's own regimen of changed eating habits and exercising in order to lose weight constitutes treatment (even if it is self-cure) as opposed to the natural course of the condition, in the way that eating disorders may remit "naturally" without treatment. There may be a difference between the "natural course" of a disorder (which can include a degree of spontaneous remission), and what is being called "natural recovery" from conditions such as obesity (e.g., Tinker & Tucker, 1997 a, b) or alcohol (e.g., Sobell et al., 2001) wherein the individual undergoes "self-change." The latter involves a decision to change followed by a self-initiated effort to alter the maladaptive behaviors that sustain the unwanted condition. Presumably, those focused on promoting self-change are interested in natural recovery rather than spontaneous remission that occurs without motivation or intentional behavior change on the part of the individual.

---

[1] The National Weight Control Registry was begun in the United States a decade ago in order to study people who have managed to lose weight successfully and maintain the loss for at least a year. More than 4,000 participants were enrolled in the registry as of 2003 (Phelan et al., 2003).

References

Anonymous. (2002, June). The truth about dieting: You can win for losing. *Consumer Reports*, pp. 26–31.

Cachelin, F. M., Striegel-Moore, R. H., Elder, K. A., Pike, K. M., Wilfley, D. E., & Fairburn, C. G. (1999). Natural course of a community sample of women with binge eating disorder. *International Journal of Eating Disorders, 25*, 45–54.

Clausen, L. (2004). Time course of symptom remission in eating disorders. *International Journal of Eating Disorders, 36*, 296–306.

Fairburn, C. G., Cooper, Z., Doll, H. A., Norman, P. A., & O'Connor, M. E. (2000). The natural course of bulimia nervosa and binge eating disorder in young women. *Archives of General Psychiatry, 57*, 659–665.

Fairburn, C. G., Stice, E., Cooper, Z., Doll, H. A., Norman, P. A., & O'Connor, M. E. (2003). Understanding persistence in bulimia nervosa: A 5-year naturalistic study. *Journal of Consulting and Clinical Psychology, 71*, 103–109.

Fichter, M. M., & Quadflieg, N. (1996). Course and two-year outcome in anorexic and bulimic adolescents. *Journal of Youth and Adolescence, 25*, 545–562.

Fichter, M. M., & Quadflieg, N. (1997). Six-year course of bulimia nervosa. *International Journal of Eating Disorders, 22*, 361–384.

Fichter, M. M., & Quadflieg, N. (1999). Six-year course and outcome of anorexia nervosa. *International Journal of Eating Disorders, 26*, 359–385.

Fichter, M. M., Quadflieg, N., & Gnutzmann, A. (1998). Binge eating disorder: Treatment outcome over a 6-year course. *Journal of Psychosomatic Research, 44*, 385–405.

Fichter, M. M., Quadflieg, N., & Hedlund, S. (2006). Twelve-year course and outcome predictors of anorexia nervosa. *International Journal of Eating Disorders, 39*, 87–100.

Grilo, C. M., Sanislow, C. A., Shea, M. T., Skodol, A. E., Stout, R. L., Pagano, M. E., et al. (2003). The natural course of bulimia nervosa and eating disorder, not otherwise specified is not influenced by personality disorders. *International Journal of Eating Disorders, 34*, 319–330.

Heatherton, T. F., Nichols, P., Mahamedi, F., & Keel, P. (1995). Body weight, dieting, and eating disorder symptoms among college students, 1982 to 1992. *American Journal of Psychiatry, 152*, 1623–1629.

Herpertz-Dahlmann, B. B., Hebebrand, J., Muller, B., Herpertz, S., Heussen, N., & Remschmidt, H. (2001). Prospective 10-year follow-up in adolescent anorexia nervosa: Course, outcome, psychiatric comorbidity, and psychosocial adaptation. *Journal of Child Psychology and Psychiatry and Allied Disciplines, 42*, 603–612.

Herpertz-Dahlmann, B. B., Wewetzer, C., Hennighausen, K., & Remschmidt, H. (1996). Outcome, psychosocial functioning, and prognostic factors in adolescent anorexia nervosa as determined by prospective follow-up assessment. *Journal of Youth and Adolescence, 25*, 455–471.

Herzog, D. B. (1993). A follow-up study of 33 subdiagnostic eating disordered women. *International Journal of Eating Disorders, 14*, 261–267.

Herzog, D. B., Dorer, D. J., Keel, P. K., Selwyn, S. E., Ekeblad, E. R., Flores, A. T., et al. (1999). Recovery and relapse in anorexia and bulimia nervosa: A 7.5-year follow-up study. *Journal of the American Academy of Child and Adolescent Psychiatry, 38*, 829–837.

Herzog, D. B., Sacks, N. R., Keller, M. B., Lavori, P. W., von Ranson, K. B., & Gray, H. M. (1993). Patterns and predictors of recovery in anorexia nervosa and bulimia nervosa. *Journal of the American Academy of Child and Adolescent Psychiatry, 32*, 835–842.

Joiner, T. E., Heatherton, T. F., & Keel, P. K. (1997). Ten-year stability and predictive validity of five bulimia-related indicators. *American Journal of Psychiatry, 154*, 1133–1138.

Klem, M. L., Wing, R. R., McGuire, M. T., Seagle, H. M., & Hill, J. O. (1997). A descriptive study of individuals successful at long-term maintenance of substantial weight loss. *American Journal of Clinical Nutrition, 66*, 239–246.

Klem, M. L., Wing, R. R., McGuire, M. T., Seagle, H. M., & Hill, J. O. (1998). Psychological symptoms in individuals successful at long-term maintenance of weight loss. *Health Psychology, 17*, 336–345.

McGuire, M. T., Wing, R. R., Klem, M. L., Lang, W., & Hill, J. O. (1999). What predicts weight regain in a group of successful weight losers? *Journal of Consulting and Clinical Psychology, 67*, 177–185.

Mills, J. S., & Polivy, J. (2005, October). *The natural course of eating pathology in female college students*. Poster session presented at the annual convention of the Eating Disorders Research Society, Toronto.

Phelan, S., Hill, J. O., Lang, W., Dibello, J. R., & Wing, R. R. (2003). Recovery from relapse among successful weight maintainers. *American Journal of Clinical Nutrition, 78*, 1079–1084.

Pike, K. M. (1998). Long-term course of anorexia nervosa: Response, relapse, remission, and recovery. *Clinical Psychology Review, 18*, 447–475.

Polivy, J., & Herman, C. P. (1987). The diagnosis and treatment of normal eating. *Journal of Consulting and Clinical Psychology, 55*, 635–644.

Råstam, M., Gillberg, I. C., & Gillberg, C. (1995). Anorexia nervosa 6 years after onset: Part II. Comorbid psychiatric problems. *Comprehensive Psychiatry, 36*, 70–76.

Rizvi, S. L., Stice, E., & Agras, W. S. (1999). Natural history of disordered eating attitudes and behaviors over a 6-year period. *International Journal of Eating Disorders, 26*, 406–413.

Schulze, U., Neudorfl, A., Krill, A., Warnke, A., Remschmidt, H., & Herpertz-Dahlmann, B. (1997). Early-onset anorexia nervosa: Course and outcome. *Zeitschrift Fur Kinder - und Jugendpsychiatrie und Psychotherapie, 25*, 5–16.

Sobell, L. C., Klingemann, H., Toneatto, T., Sobell, M. B., Agrawal, S., & Leo, G. (2001). Alcohol and drug abusers' perceived reasons for self-change in Canada and Switzerland: Computer-assisted content analysis. *Substance Use and Misuse, 36*, 1467–1500.

Steinhausen, H. C. (2002). The outcome of anorexia nervosa in the 20th century. *American Journal of Psychiatry, 159*, 1284–1293.

Striegel-Moore, R., Silberstein, L., Frensch, P., & Rodin, J. (1989). A prospective study of disordered eating among college students. *International Journal of Eating Disorders, 8*, 499–509.

Strober, M., Freeman, R., & Morrell, W. (1997). The long-term course of severe anorexia nervosa in adolescents: Survival analysis of recovery, relapse, and outcome predictors over 10–15 years in a prospective study. *International Journal of Eating Disorders, 22*, 339–360.

Tinker, J. E., & Tucker, J. A. (1997a). Environmental events surrounding natural recovery from obesity. *Addictive Behaviors*, *22*, 571–575.

Tinker, J. E., & Tucker, J. A. (1997b). Motivations for weight loss and behavior change strategies associated with natural recovery from obesity. *Psychology of Addictive Behaviors*, *11*, 98–106.

Tozzi, F., Sullivan, P. F., Fear, J. L., McKenzie, J., & Bulik, C. M. (2003). Causes and recovery in anorexia nervosa: The patient's perspective. *International Journal of Eating Disorders, 33*, 143–154.

Wing, R. R., & Hill, J. O. (2001). Successful weight loss maintenance. *Annual Review of Nutrition, 21*, 323–341.

6.4
Spontaneous Desistance from Crime

Jukka-Pekka Takala

> The plot of a recent motion picture is based on a comparison of
> two boys engaged in theft. When discovered, one ran more rapidly,
> escaped, and became a priest; the other ran less rapidly, was caught
> and committed to a reformatory, and became a gangster. In other
> circumstances, the one who ran more rapidly might have become
> the gangster and the one who ran less rapidly the priest.
>
> Sutherland, 1939, p. 4

Sutherland does not give the name of the movie, but it is more than likely
"Angels with Dirty Faces" (1938) directed by Michael Curtiz and starring
James Gagney as the gangster and Pat O'Brien as his law-abiding brother.
Edwin Sutherland's brief mention of the developmental plot of the film, in
the third edition of his classic textbook *Criminology*, captured in a nutshell
some of the problems of criminal careers and desistance from crime.

The plot actually used in the film illustrates insights and suggestions from
the criminological labeling theory, which came of age in the 1950s and 1960s.
The one caught became a serious criminal, presumably (partly or mainly)
because he was labeled as a criminal and because other careers closed for him
(or at least became more difficult). The one who got away desisted from crime
because other career possibilities remained open for him. Labeling theory
emphasizes these kinds of pathways. Thus, from this point of view, the best
intervention in crime may be no intervention at all, and spontaneous desistance from crime seems the most reliable and successful road to a noncriminal
way of life.

However, as Sutherland (1939) suggested in the quotation above, an oppo-
site turn of the plot would have been just as plausible. The futures of the
brothers could have been reversed. This idea gets support from some modern studies. In a follow-up study of a youth cohort in Edinburgh, young
people who were caught by the police were more likely to persist in their
offending than those who offended at a similar level (as measured by self-
report) but who were not caught (Smith, 2006). However, getting caught is
unlikely to be random. Thus, the study design leaves room for doubts about
conclusions on causality. In some cases, an early warning or punishment
seems to help the offender mend his ways. Furthermore, several former criminals have regretted that no one confronted them early and firmly enough

to guide them away from crime before they developed a serious career in crime. In an English study interviewing probationers and probation officers on the issues of criminal career and desistance, Sue Rex (1999) gained the impression that the offenders were willing to take more direction than the probation officers gave.

What Is to Stop Crime Spontaneously?

In "Angels with Dirty Faces," the O'Brien character abstained from crime without having been caught or punished. Was he a spontaneous desister? The criminal justice system is built on the assumption that people choose their actions freely, at least to some extent, and therefore either the threat of punishment or the imposing of punishment is expected to set them straight. In principle, there is no requirement or expectation that the offender should receive some therapy or treatment to make him or her stop offending. Of course, there are shades to this picture. Many jurisdictions try to combine punishment with behavior-altering therapies. This is as it should be, but these therapies are usually something added on, or something extra. The principle is that people should learn from the blame and threat of punishment, or, at the very least, from the punishment imposed on them. Of course, this process does not always work as intended, but several natural experiments in which the police, or the criminal justice system more generally, have stopped functioning for a while (because of a police strike, for instance) have convinced most observers that the system works at least to some extent. Of course, some people dispute the need or even minor efficacy of any kind of punishment, but they are a definite minority.

Researchers have used somewhat varying definitions of desistance from crime depending on how exactly they have tackled questions such as the following:

• What counts as crime?
• Is offending measured by official records, self-reported crime, or some other method? How long must one be free of crime to be a desister?
• Is decrease in frequency or seriousness of offenses taken into account?

Using the term *spontaneous* desistance adds further definitional issues. Is it required that the person has received no specific behavior-altering therapy to qualify as *spontaneous* stopping of crime? Under this definition, probably most recorded offenders have later spontaneously desisted, since such treatment is relatively rare. Or is a stricter definition used, so that it is also required that they have never been caught or punished for their offenses? If so, do we count only measures by the police and other criminal justice system agencies or do we include actions by other authorities, or even informal sanctions? A very strict definition might also require that the offender has not even met with any *informal* sanctions or penalties for the offenses.

There are interesting phenomena under all definitions. Some kinds of crime are wide ly considered to be hard to drop without therapy or treatment, such as persistent sexual offending. Recently, claims have also been made that domestic violence is impossible to stop without professional intervention, usually meaning some kind of therapy or violence-stopping program for the male perpetrator.

Most phenomena under the other definition (i.e., stopping offending without official punishment) may seem trivial. Based on surveys of self-reported crime, we know that most young people commit offenses and that almost all of them stop doing so (in any serious frequency) irrespective of whether they are caught or punished (e.g., Mulvey et al., 2004). Males commit more crimes than females, and the criminal activities of both groups seem to peak at around 16–17 years of age; thereafter, the majority engages in crime less frequently as they age. Population surveys seem to show that the number of people who report having committed crimes at some point in the past but not for a considerable period of time before the survey is much larger than the number of people who have been caught by the police (e.g., Budd, Sharp, & Mayhew, 2005).

Thus, one can state that most people who commit crime stop without any intervention by the criminal justice system or behavior-altering treatment. However, this may not be very interesting since it concerns fairly minor crimes (e.g., shoplifting, petty theft, minor criminal damage, minor assaults, occasional use of forbidden substances). It is true that such processes involve a very large number of people, and one could think that a greater understanding of the process of desistance might bring tangible benefits. Nevertheless, understanding desistance from more serious crime seems more important. During their criminally active stage, the most active offenders are responsible for a great proportion of the most serious crime that takes place in society.

Even young males who engage in serious types of crimes, such as burglary or assault, do so infrequently and do not persist at it for a long period of time. By their mid-20s, many prolific young offenders no longer accumulate serious criminal charges (Shover, 1996). Even in these cases, stopping crime is usually no dramatic or memorable event, and no reasons or causes are investigated.

Unfortunately, knowledge of spontaneous desistance from serious, persistent crime is not very well-developed. There are, to begin with, no reliable estimates on how many persistent serious offenders are never caught and yet, at some point, discontinue offending. Strictly speaking, only they would be considered spontaneous desisters from serious crime. More is known about some of those persistent offenders who have been caught and punished and then at some later point stop. One could use the results from those studies and make reasonable estimates as to what extent the results would apply to spontaneous desisters under the strict definition. A supplementary approach would be to do the same type of exploratory research on spontaneous remission from different addictions (e.g., alcoholism, drug dependence), as studies suggest that there are many commonalities in desistance from addictions and desistance from crime. Laub and Sampson (2001) mention such common elements as "the decision or motivation to change, cognitive restructuring, coping skills, continued monitoring, social support, and general lifestyle change, especially new social networks" (p. 38).

Correlates of Desistance and the Desistance Process

From the literature on desistance from crime, a number of factors emerge as clear correlates of desistance: a good marriage and family, change from association with deviant people to associating with law-abiding persons, cutting down on alcohol or drug use, stable employment, and change or maturation of identity. Their causal role in bringing an end to criminal activities is more open to question, because most studies are unable to distinguish other causal pathways, such as the selection effect, from the effect of factors leading to desistance (e.g., those who desist are more likely to be able to start a good marriage). However, some studies (Laub & Sampson, 2001) support the idea that, to some extent, there is a true causality between these factors and desistance.

The Edinburgh study (Smith, 2006) lends support to the idea that social structure and social context are more important for growing out of delinquency than the circumstances of the individual family. Bonds with family and school are important, but it is likely that the neighborhood context has an influence on the formation of these bonds. In-depth studies of criminal careers and desistance tend to find that desistance is a process that can occur in multiple stages. Various authors denote and name them somewhat differently, but all schemes seem to include similar sets of core elements. First, there is a stage of growing awareness of the problems caused by offending, or a growing motivation to find another way of life. Second, there is some conscious decision to stop; the decision or intention can become more "fixed" by publicly announcing it to one's friends or in front of a larger audience, which can also involve a change of personal identity in some dramatic way (e.g., religious conversion). Third, there is maintenance of the nonoffending behavior. This may involve a variety of conscious or unconscious actions that lead to dropping old relations and building new ones, and forming new daily routines that provide less tempting opportunities for crime. Fourth, there may or may not be lapses and relapses to criminal behavior, but, in a successful process, they will be limited in time and severity.

In terms of gender differences, females commit far less serious offenses than males and it is not surprising that research on their desistance from crime has been more limited than research on male desistance. Studies using quantitative data (Uggen & Kruttschnitt, 1998) have found that the correlates for desistance for females are similar to those for males. Age, marriage and family, and stable employment are positively correlated with desistance.

In qualitative studies, differences between male and female desistance have been found. For instance, becoming a mother seems to be more reliably linked with desistance from crime than becoming a father.

In Stephen Farrall's study of English probationers (2003), desistance was linked to the number of problems that probation officers saw in their probationers. Specifically, as the number of an individual offender's problems (e.g., family, finances, substance use) increased, the likelihood that he or she was able to desist decreased. Among those who had problems, desistance was linked to probation officers' estimates as to how well their probationers would be able to cope with those problems.

Maturation and Morality

As mentioned above, the peak of criminal activity for most people is in adolescence. Some years into adulthood a clear majority has stopped committing crimes. Hence, growing older is closely linked to desisting. The mechanisms that transmit this change, however, are open to debate. One possibility is that developmental change in late adolescence and early adulthood facilitates the acquisition or refinement of competencies and values that make criminal behavior less attractive or less acceptable to one's self. Most people mature with age and, as they do so, they gain greater control over their impulses and begin to value achievements that criminal activity would jeopardize. In other words, their values or goals change so that crime becomes less acceptable for them. Emotional, intellectual, and moral development is linked to this. As people age, they tend to turn toward more socially desirable, long-term goals. They may also gain competencies that make conventional alternatives to crime more attractive; for example, they pay more in terms of money, satisfaction, or acceptance by valued others.

In the British offending survey (Budd et al., 2005), the two most commonly cited reasons for stopping crime were that "I knew it was wrong" and "I grew up and/or settled down" (p. 50). These reasons were more often given by those who had been engaged in "traditional" crimes such as theft and damage to property, and somewhat less so by drug dealers.

Only a quarter of former drug sellers said they gave up dealing because 'I knew it was wrong', while for other offences between 42 per cent and 59 per cent said this. Conversely, while a third of drug sellers said stopping using drugs was a reason why they gave up selling, this was mentioned by a very small proportion for property and violent offences. (Budd et al., 2005, p. 51)

If most people mature to be more law-abiding after adolescence, then it also means that their same-age peers are less delinquent than they used to be. Hence, if everybody becomes law-abiding, it is difficult to distinguish peer influence from the aggregate effects of all individuals growing older. However, research does suggest that peers have independent influence.

First, not everybody drops crime; some maintain a criminally active way of life. Second, qualitative studies suggest that losing delinquent friends and gaining conventional ones is often important for desistance and may require work and effort.

Growing Aversion for Risk

For most people, appetite for risk diminishes with age after adolescence. This tends to diminish their taste for crime as well, as most serious crime carries a heightened risk of negative consequences. Physical prowess also starts to decline after young adulthood, and one is less able to endure physical exertion or to function on very little sleep. These kinds of reasons come up in interviews with older long-career offenders. They get tired of the physical and psychological demands of crime.

Some adopt a new approach to the possibility of getting caught: that is, they do not want to be exposed to the risk of getting caught (Shover, 1996). They also adjust their mode of operation toward less risky directions. Maximum risks are present when society's condemnations are at their most severe and the chances of getting caught are the highest. Background operations are often safer than being a front-line actor. Hence, some offenders first start avoiding the highest risks and might, in the process, gain positions and qualifications that make it easier to phase out crime altogether, even if the latter transition may not seem to be a dramatic one. Some may also gain business partners in crime and, with some of them, it is possible to develop a wholly legitimate gainful cooperation, although little is known on this subject.

Changes in Adult Life

Some may "drift" back into normalcy without any serious decision to do so when their circumstances, their acquaintances, or the persons they socialize with change, or when new possibilities appear. A pattern of daily activities may develop that leaves little time for crime. The context of their lives may change so that noncriminal ways of achieving their goals are easier to follow. This occurs through the acquisition of adult roles that are often associated with familial and occupational responsibilities. Such roles make it less possible and less useful to engage in criminal activities. Of course, they are far from failsafe methods. Much depends on the quality and details of these matters. While getting married or falling in love will generally stop or reduce offending, it does not do so in every case. The spouses or lovers can be partners in crime and when the spouse encourages or condones offending behavior, it may be difficult for the other to abstain from crime. Findings from studies conducted in the United States suggest that while marriage correlates with reduction of or desistance from crime, cohabitation does not. It would be interesting to know whether this holds true for those European countries where cohabitation is more common than in the United States. In terms of occupational responsibilities, having a daily schedule can be an influential factor. Working in a place that is supervised or controlled during the day, and spending evenings and weekends with a spouse and children leaves little time to commit crime. This also changes the type of people one has a chance to meet and leads to less contact with active criminals.

Childhood antisocial behavior predicts adolescent offenses, which in turn predicts adult offending, but not very strongly. Depending on the study and the definition used for crime and desistance, the figures for those that continue engaging in serious offenses range from very few to a large majority. Also, a great proportion of adult offenders, sometimes over one-half, have not been recorded for committing crimes before adulthood. Laub and Sampson's (2001) research suggests that changes in one's adult life are important for changes in a criminal career, irrespective of childhood and adolescent factors and the general effects of growing older. For instance, a good marriage and stable employment enhance the probability of desistance.

Turning Points: Inside and Outside Views

Many reformed offenders cite a memorable event in their lives as a turning point. It can be a dramatic change in one's interpersonal circles such as a birth in the family, death of a friend, divorce, falling in love, or a religious experience (Gadd & Farrall, 2004; Mulvey et al., 2004). The accounts by former offenders tend to emphasize their own conscious decisions, while accounts by social workers and probation officers often put more emphasis on changes in external circumstances or the possibility for offenders to use their personal talents and strong suits. It is uncertain, however, to what extent these are somewhat arbitrary reconstructions of the past, or to what extent true causes pushed the development in the law-abiding direction.

One possibility of stopping crime is to turn a deviant career into an asset where it can be used as a partial fulfillment of the qualifications of some jobs (Klingemann, 1999). These positions typically have to do with reintegration of criminals into society or as an information source for methods geared toward harm reduction. In most, if not all, countries, there are a number of prominent ex-criminals who have started a successful career in philanthropic work, rehabilitation, or running halfway houses for people struggling with alcohol or other drug problems. It also appears that almost all of these individuals have adopted a strong religious identity.

While it is certainly true that any former offender can, in principle, help society by altruistic acts, it is also probable that there are only a limited number of niches in which this can be turned into a positive, full-time career. Klingemann (1999) also points out that some can continue parallel careers in both a deviant and non-deviant world.

Against All Odds

A Swedish team (Haggård, Gumbert, & Grann, 2001) studied four former serious violent offenders who had been at a serious risk of reoffending, but "against all odds" had not done so. The offenders had been sentenced to prison several times for violent and other offenses, and they had received very high scores on tests that predict violence (Psychopathy Checklist Revised PCL-R, and the historical subset H.10 of the Historical-Clinical-Risk Management Model-20). However, they had not been reconvicted for any crimes for 10 years, even if they had spent at least the last 5 years outside of prisons and forensic hospitals. In their accounts of their desistance from crime, all four emphasized one specific event or factor that they saw as a turning point that had taken them from their criminal career to a law-abiding way of life. For three of them, it was linked to a conscious decision. For one of the three, it was the negative experience of the forensic psychiatric hospital where he was committed. Another spoke about his being arrested and how he had had time to think about his behavior. The third attributed his desistance from crime to the relationship with the woman he lived with (a contextual, social support factor) as well as his unpleasant experience at the forensic hospital. The fourth, a former sex-offender, attributed his desistance to an understanding psychiatrist who prescribed him anti-androgen medication. The fact that two of the men were physically disabled may have also contributed to their desistance.

All four offenders reported that they had stopped or decreased their use of narcotics and alcohol. However, two of them still occasionally used drugs but, on these occasions, they isolated themselves so as not to get into trouble. This links to a more general finding: contrary to standard accounts of desistance, these men did not reestablish links with conventional society (except for families for some of them). "The violent and highly antisocial men interviewed in this study had to isolate themselves in their efforts to live as noncriminals. The reason was that they did not feel comfortable or safe with others; they were unsure of their own reactions to different situations and others' responses to them" (Haggård et al., 2001, p. 1061).

Family Violence and Question of Change without Treatment

There is a popular view that domestic violence cannot be stopped unless the perpetrator undergoes treatment or a violence-stopping program. Challenging men and their alleged ideologies of male domination has been proffered as the most (and only) promising form of intervention that could stop their violence. Without this, the cycle of violence would keep repeating.

It is true that domestic violence is *often* repeated and prolonged. Many cases, generally, do conform to the famous Duluth Wheel of Abuse, with cyclically alternating periods of violence and tranquility (Pence & Paymar, 1993). However, these conclusions are drawn primarily from clinical samples of women in shelters, who have experienced severe and prolonged forms of violence. The picture changes when samples more representative of the victims of all levels of violence are investigated (Johnson, 1995).

The major aspects of domestic violence that are reported in general population surveys on violence against women *do not* conform to the Duluth Wheel. For instance, Feld and Straus (1990) compared the 1985 U.S. National Family Violence Survey and the 1986 reinterviews of married respondents and found that a large proportion of abusers had discontinued their violence. One third of those who had committed three or more acts of severe violence in the first year committed no violence in the second year, 10% used minor violence, and 57% continued using severe violence. The majority (58%) of those who committed one or two severe acts in Year 1, used no violence in Year 2.

Other surveys have had similar findings. In the Finnish National Survey on Violence Against Women, among those women in a long-term relationship whose first violent victimization by their partner had occurred more than 10 years earlier, only 26% reported a violent episode from the most recent year (Heiskanen & Piispa, 1998). Taking into account the sizable missing data, this means that violence discontinued in 40 to 74% of these relationships. Presumably, very few of the men who had stopped using violence had attended any treatment for their violence. Similarly, using data from the U.S. National Youth Survey, Wofford, Elliott, and Menard found that almost one-half (48%) of offenders suspended violence in their marital relationships 3 years later (as cited in Laub & Sampson, 2001, p. 31). Using data from a community-based sample, Quigley and Leonard (as cited in Laub & Sampson, 2001, p. 31) found that about one-quarter (24%) of those men who had been aggressive during the first year of marriage had not been violent during the following 2 years. However, those engaged in serious violence were less likely to stop, as only 14% of them desisted at Year 2 and 3.

Recent research from industrialized countries demonstrates that the forms of partner violence are not uniform. There is the classic, severe, and escalating form of violence characterized by multiple physical and psychological forms of abuse and threats combined with increasingly possessive and controlling behavior on the part of the abuser. However, there is also a more moderate form of relationship violence, where continuing frustration and anger occasionally erupt into physical aggression (Johnson, 1995; Krug et al., 2002).

Thus, it is clear that some portion of domestic violence against women stops without any therapy or antiviolence educational programs for the perpetrator, and some of it also ends without any criminal justice intervention. On the other hand, surprisingly little is reliably known on the effectiveness of different treatments and reeducation programs for domestic violence reoffenders. There are only a couple of randomized controlled experiments, which show no differences, but their weight as general evidence *against* treatment programs is compromised by other problems (see Wathen & MacMillan, 2003). In quasi-controlled experiments, such programs tend to fare better (Babcock, Green, & Robie, 2004), but they, of course, leave more room for possible selection biases (e.g., those who are more likely to desist because of some yet unknown background reason are more likely to enter and stay in an antiviolence program). The most consistent predictor of continued violence is severity at the time of prediction. Other predictors often found are psychological abuse, attempts at isolation of the partner, and the youth of the perpetrator (Johnson, 2003).

Conclusion

In short, a simplistic lesson from the movie "Angels with Dirty Faces" might be that no intervention is the best intervention in crime *overall*. However, this would be going too far and would also ignore the possibilities of general prevention and vicarious deterrence. That is, it is not quite true that the eventual law-abiding brother in the movie had no experience with the criminal justice system. He was *almost* caught, and he experienced his brother being caught. It may be that in some cases, near-misses and experiences that happen to individuals' loved ones are effective turning points in the development from criminal to noncriminal behavior.

In the British offending survey, it was found that being caught by the police, or fear that this could happen and the likely sentence that would result, was given as one reason for stopping crime by a substantial number of those who had not offended for the past year. The proportion varied from 5% to 33% by crime type and was largest among those who had admitted burglary, vehicle-related thefts, shoplifting, and drug selling (Budd et al., 2005). The authors note that the impact of an official sanction in deterring offenders appears to be "relatively strong, but certainly not the main factor" (pp. 50–51).

Punishment and its threat, then, seem to have an effect on desistance from crime. However, they should be used wisely and moderately. They should express blame but not make it more difficult for the offender to go back to a noncriminal way of life. Furthermore, they should not prevent the operation of the processes of spontaneous desistance.

References

Babcock, J. C., Green, C. E., & Robie, C. (2004). Does batterers' treatment work? A meta-analytic review of domestic violence treatment. *Clinical Psychology Review* 23(8), 1023–1053.

Budd, T., Sharp, C., & Mayhew, P. (2005). *Offending in England and Wales: First results from the 2003 Crime and Justice Survey.* London: Home Office.

Feld, S. L., & Straus, M. A. (1989). Escalation and desistance of wife assault in marriage. *Criminology, 27*(1), 141–161.

Gadd, D., & Farrall, S. (2004). Criminal careers, desistance and subjectivity. *Theoretical Criminology, 8*(2), 123–156.

Haggård, U., Gumpert, C. H., & Grann, M. (2001). Against all odds: A qualitative follow-up study of high-risk violent offenders who were not reconvicted. *Journal of Interpersonal Violence, 16*(10), 1048–1065.

Heiskanen, M., & Piispa, M. (1998). *Faith, hope, battering.* Helsinki: Statistics Finland.

Johnson, H. (2003). The cessation of assaults on wives. *Journal of Comparative Family Studies, 34*(1), 75–91.

Johnson, M. P. (1995). Patriarchal terrorism and common couple violence: Two forms of violence against women. *Journal of Marriage & the Family, 57*(2), 283–295.

Klingemann, H. (1999). Addiction careers and careers in addiction. *Substance Use & Misuse, 34*(11), 1505–1526.

Krug, E. G., Dahlberg, L. L., Mercy, J. A., Zwi, A. B., & Lozano, R. (Eds.). (2002). *World report on violence and health.* Geneva: World Health Organization.

Laub, J. H., & Sampson., R. J. (2001). Understanding desistance from crime. In M. Tonry (Ed.), *Crime and justice: A review of research* (Vol. 28, pp. 1–69). Chicago: University of Chicago Press.

Mulvey, E. P., Steinberg, L., Fagan, J., Cauffman, E., Piquero, A. R., Chassin, L., et al. (2004). Theory and research on desistance from antisocial activity among serious adolescent offenders. *Youth Violence and Juvenile Justice, 2*, 213–236.

Pence, E., & Paymar, M. (1993). *Education groups for men who batter: The Duluth model.* New York: Springer.

Rex, S. (1999). Desistance from offending: Experiences of probation. *The Howard Journal of Criminal Justice, 38*(4), 366–383.

Shover, N. (1996). *Great pretenders: Pursuits and careers of persistent thieves.* Boulder, CO: Westview Press.

Smith, D. (2006). *Social inclusion and early desistance from crime* (The Edinburgh Study of Youth Transitions and Crime, No. 12). Edinburgh: Centre for Law and Society, The University of Edinburgh.

Sutherland, E. H. (1939). *Criminology* (3rd ed.). Philadelphia: Lippincott.

Uggen, C., & Kruttschnitt, C. (1998). Crime in the breaking: Gender differences in desistance. *Law and Society Review, 32*, 339–366.

Wathen, C. N., & MacMillan, H. L. (2003). Interventions for violence against women: Scientific review. *Journal of the American Medical Association, 289*(5), 589–600.

6.5
Self-Change from Stuttering: An Overview

Patrick Finn

What Is Stuttering?

Stuttering is a highly variable disorder characterized by involuntary disruptions in speech fluency that usually consist of sound or word repetitions, sound prolongations, and momentary blocks during which no or very little sound is emitted. These disruptions are often marked by noticeable struggle, effort, and muscle tension. Debilitating feelings about communication and oneself as a speaker often develop, as well as avoidance behaviors related to speaking, especially in certain situations such as talking on the telephone or speaking to strangers. Onset of stuttering is usually between the ages of 2 and 5 years, with more males than females presenting with long-term symptoms. Prevalence, or the number of cases at a given time, is 5% and incidence, or average life frequency, is 1% (Bloodstein, 1995). Current theories and research suggest that stuttering is a genetically predisposed, neurophysiological speech disorder (Brown, Ingham, Ingham, Laird, & Fox, 2005; Felsenfeld et al., 2000).

Natural Recovery during Early Childhood Stuttering

Most preschool and early school age children who stutter recover without treatment usually within the first few years of onset, with reported rates ranging from 50% to 74% (Brosch, Haege, Kalehne, & Johannsen, 1999; Mansson, 2000; Yairi & Ambrose, 1999). This recovery is often sufficiently complete that the children's recovered speech is perceptually indistinguishable from that of normally fluent children (Finn, Ingham, Ambrose, & Yairi, 1997). The mechanisms underlying early childhood recovery are still unclear. However, there is evidence to suggest that genetic factors may play a role because many children who recover without treatment are more likely to report a family history of recovery than children who continue to stutter (Ambrose, Cox, & Yairi, 1997). There are indications that environmental factors may also be important in promoting natural recovery. Parents whose children recovered without treatment often reported that they encouraged their child to "slow down" or "stop and say it over" whenever stuttered speech occurred (Lankford & Cooper, 1974; Wingate, 1976).

Treatment studies suggest that, in fact, these parental admonishments may have had an ameliorative effect. Pointing to the natural recovery research as the basis for their treatment approach, Reed and Godden (1977), using an ABA study design, demonstrated that when two preschool children who stuttered were simply instructed by the clinician to "slow down" contingent on a moment of stuttering, their stuttering frequency was essentially reduced to zero and maintained for up to 8 months after treatment was terminated. Similarly, the Lidcombe program, which was also influenced by the natural recovery literature (Onslow, Costa, & Rue, 1990), developed a parent-administered, operant treatment for preschool children who stutter. Parents were trained to provide correction to their child contingent on a moment of stuttering (e.g., "Whoops, that was a bumpy word, can you say it nice and smooth?") and reinforce stutter-free speech (e.g., "Good talking, no bumpy words!"). Over 10 years of clinical research trials have provided compelling evidence for the efficacy of this approach, demonstrating long-term treatment gains with speech behavior that is stutter-free and comparable to normal peers (Onslow, Packman, & Harrison, 2003).

Treatment Approaches for Managing Stuttering After Childhood

For children who continue to stutter into their elementary school years and beyond, it is widely believed that the longer they live with the disorder, the more persistent and chronic it will become (Guitar, 1998). As a result, approaches to managing persistent forms of stuttering are usually more complex and place a greater emphasis on self-control or self-regulation. The two best-known approaches for addressing persistent stuttering are generally referred to as stutter modification, or attitude therapy, and speech modification, or behavior modification therapy.

The stutter modification approach is based on the premise that clients must learn to accept their stuttering and self-regulate their reactions to stuttering, such as minimizing or eliminating their avoidance and struggle behaviors (Manning, 2001). Thus, treatment goals focus on self-acceptance of one's stuttering and reducing negative attitudes toward oneself as a communicator. The speech modification approach is based on the view that replacement of stuttered with stutter-free speech depends on how well the clients can learn to self-manage and self-evaluate their speech behavior (Ingham, 1999). As a result, treatment goals are directed toward natural-sounding, stutter-free speech behavior and the development of self-measurement skills for evaluating that speech.

The evidence base to support these two approaches differs markedly. Although the stutter modification approach has existed for over 60 years and has been widely advocated (Cordes, 1998), there have been few scientifically rigorous studies to evaluate its efficacy, and the few that have been conducted provided negative support (Blomgren, Roy, Callister, & Merrill, 2005). In contrast, the speech modification approach has considerable supportive evidence as demonstrated in both systematic reviews (Bothe, Davidow, Bramlett, & Ingham, 2006) and meta-analysis studies (Andrews, Guitar, & Howie, 1980). Regardless, there continues to be much dissatisfaction among clinicians concerning both approaches for managing stuttering, as expressed by their lack of confidence in their ability to implement the therapies and their doubts about their clinical effectiveness (Blaker, Harbaugh, & Finn, 1996–1997).

The Phenomenon of Untreated Recovery after Childhood

The conventional wisdom is that untreated recovery becomes increasingly less likely after childhood and the need for treatment becomes increasingly more likely (e.g., Guitar, 1998). Nonetheless, there is research suggesting that persistent stuttering is not always as intractable as widely believed. Review of the past research literature on untreated recovery shows that on average, 70.7% (range = 56.9–90%) of subjects estimated that their age of recovery was during adolescence or adulthood and that much of this improvement occurred without the benefit of professional help (Finn, 2004). More recent findings based on a sample of 103 adult participants, the largest sample of persons who recovered from stuttering without treatment, found that 57% reported that they had recovered at or after the age of 12 years, with an average age of recovery being 17.7 years of age (range = 12–35 years of age; Finn & Felsenfeld, 2006). It should be cautioned, however, that these studies perhaps underestimated the rate of early recovery because many adults who recovered during their preschool years are unlikely to recall that they ever stuttered.

Although untreated late recovery appears to be a well-documented phenomenon, the most widely used textbooks on stuttering (Ratner, 2001), while citing rates of early childhood recovery, rarely mention late recovery. It is unclear why this phenomenon has been essentially overlooked, but some authorities have argued that because these findings have often challenged long-held, widely favored views about persistent stuttering as an intractable disorder, they have basically been ignored or suppressed (Ingham, 1983; Wingate, 1976). The potential problem with ignoring the evidence that recovery occurs after childhood is that an incomplete, one-sided view of persistent stuttering is likely to prevail and have negative implications for theoretical and clinical perspectives of the disorder. For example, it is argued that adults who have recovered from stuttering without treatment might serve as a behavioral, cognitive, and neurophysiological benchmark for evaluating treatments for adolescents and adults who continue to stutter, while helping to identify the limits of recovery from a persistent disorder (Ingham, Finn, & Bothe, 2005).

Findings from Late Recovery Research

Methodological Challenges

The importance of investigating late recovery without treatment is sometimes overshadowed by troublesome methodological challenges. Retrospective designs have been the main approach for investigating late recovery. Because research subjects are being investigated when they are no longer presenting with stuttered speech behaviors, there have been questions concerning the validity of participants' claims that they did, in fact, once have a clinically valid stuttering problem (Ingham, 1983). Furthermore, it is important to establish that their recovery was reasonably independent of any formal treatment that might have been received for their stuttering. Obviously, if recovery was clearly linked to formal treatment, then it is no longer a valid sample of untreated recovery.

These two concerns have been recently addressed in the literature. First, since past speech behavior such as stuttering cannot be verified directly, the most practical approach for cross-checking participants' claims that they used to stutter is to obtain the judgments of persons who knew the participant in the past when they did exhibit a stuttering problem, such as a parent, sibling, or friend. At the same time, it is unclear if such nonprofessionals are capable of making correct judgments whether a person had a clinically valid stuttering problem. Finn (1996), however, demonstrated that nonprofessionals were able to reliably identify speech-related behaviors in participants' past speech that were consistent with behaviors reported in the extant stuttered speech of persons verified as individuals with persistent stuttering. In contrast, these behaviors were never reported in the speech of persons verified as normally fluent speakers. Thus, obtaining collateral reports is a viable method for independently verifying untreated recovered stutterers' claims that they used to stutter. In addition, because the speaker-based experiences of stuttering are sufficiently unique in terms of struggled speech and avoidance behavior, the recovered stutterers' self-reports of their past stuttering can provide further supportive evidence that their claims of past stuttering are valid.

Second, many late recovered stutterers report that they did receive some treatment for their stuttering when they were children, usually when they were in elementary or middle school. Almost always, they have reported that this treatment was ineffectual or, if it did have any benefit, it was short-lived and their recovery did not occur until several years later when they were adolescents or older. This alone, in most cases, is supportive evidence that their recovery occurred independent of treatment because there is no reason to believe that unsuccessful treatment would somehow result in benefits several years later. In addition, treatment outcome studies have shown that most relapses from treatment gains usually take place within 6 months following the termination of treatment (Finn, 1998). Thus, even when exposed to formal treatment, recovery that occurs several years later is most likely independent of that treatment. More importantly, when such untreated recovery does occur, the recovered speakers often attribute improvement to their own efforts or self-change.

Mechanisms of Self-change

Self-change as a possible mechanism for late untreated recovery from stuttering has been recognized for centuries. Bormann (1969), for example, described an account of the seventeenth century Colonial American clergyman and author, Cotton Mather, who self-managed his stuttering when he was 18 years old by practicing speaking slowly and deliberately. An early report by Heltman (1941) presented an account of a male who, during his high school and college years, overcame his severe stuttering by developing public speaking skills and actively competing in speaking contests and debates. Freund (1970) described a self-improvement program that he began when he was 35 years old that included practicing speaking in a smooth, melodic manner in various situations that led to reductions in his avoidance behavior. More recently, Anderson and Felsenfeld (2003) detailed three individuals who recovered after childhood without the benefit of treatment and categorized their reasons for recovery as a conscious decision to change, an increase in self-confidence, and active changes in speech behavior.

The most convincing accounts, however, have emerged from several surveys of recovered speakers. Finn (2004) examined these findings by focusing on the subjects' explanations as to why their late recovery from stuttering occurred without treatment. The results of this review revealed that self-change was the most frequently reported reason for recovery. Table 6.5.1 lists these reports along with the percentage of subjects who reported self-change. Self-change was defined in this review as recovered stutterers who managed or modified their own behavior, thoughts, or feelings in order to control or eliminate their stuttering without the benefit of professional help. Some examples of subjects' statements regarding the reasons for their untreated recovery are provided in Table 6.5.2. As these brief statements suggest, late recovered subjects describe a clear motivation to change, a shift toward a more positive attitude concerning their speaking abilities or themselves, and a conscious or willful change in their manner of speaking.

TABLE 6.5.1. Percent of subjects reporting self-change as a basis for late recovery.

Author(s)	Total N	Self-change
Johnson (1950)	$N = 23$	60.8%
Shearer & Williams (1965)	$N = 58$	69.0%
Wingate (1964)	$N = 50$	66.0%
Martyn & Sheehan (1968)	$N = 48$	62.5%
Quarrington (1977)	$N = 27$	74.0%
Finn (1996)	$N = 15$	78.6%

TABLE 6.5.2. Examples of respondents' statements when asked for reasons for untreated late recovery.

Respondent 1:

"I finally just told myself 'Enough of that' and sat back down and never looked up the rest of the period. And went home after school. And I can't tell you how long I sat in front of that mirror but it was a long time. And there at the end I made a decision that instead of hiding behind this problem I was gonna fight it. I was gonna be the first one to raise my hand and just work my way through it."

Respondent 2:

"I don't know, but I think I can guess a little bit. I think it's as I became more mature, and as I became more in control of my emotions, I think that contributed to it. And I think as I got older and I became more self-confident, I think that contributed to it. I also employed sometimes a little technique, and I have done this in later years, more recent years, and that is to increase the volume of my speech. And whether that creates a bit more airflow or more deliberacy or whatever, it seems to help. Not that I need that much help these days at all. But that could help."

Respondent 3:

"So to overcome it I decided that I would teach myself, prove to myself that I could pronounce every sound in the English language. So I wrote a vast chart of sounds, like B-A-T would be bate, bat, bought, bot. And I practiced saying them until I could say the Bs."

Are These Accounts of Self-Change Credible?

The fact that subjects may attribute their recovery to self-management of their own speech behavior or thoughts and feelings related to speaking does not necessarily mean that this is the actual reason for their improvement. However, these descriptions of recovery by self-directed means are often remarkably similar to the clinical routines clients are instructed to follow in many well-known treatment programs (Finn, 2004; Ingham et al., 2005). In fact, systematic changes in speech behavior such as slowing down are well-established as effective treatment agents for long-term clinical reductions in stuttering (Bothe et al., 2006; Cordes, 1998) and there are compelling theoretical reasons (Perkins, 1989), as well as empirical evidence from treatment outcome research (Craig, 1998), to suggest that changes in attitude, especially increased self-confidence, are critical to long-term maintenance of treatment gains. Perhaps, most important of all, self-management and self-evaluation have been key features of several successful treatment outcome studies (Bothe et al., 2006; Craig, 1998; Finn, 2007). Thus, while it may be difficult to establish a direct link between reports of self-management and improvements in stuttering without treatment, it appears likely that these are credible accounts for late recovery until research suggests otherwise.

Outcomes of Self-Managed Late Recovery

How long do the gains from late recovery without treatment endure? The answer to this question is limited to only two studies; however, the findings from these reports indicate that recovery associated with self-change is remarkably long. Finn and Felsenfeld (2006) reported that the average duration of late recovery for subjects ($n = 103$) who had recovered during adolescence (i.e., recovered at or after age 12 years) was 20.9 years with a range of 1 to 65 years. Finn, Howard, and Kubala (2005) also found a long duration of recovery of 31.4 years with a range of 13 to 68 years (this finding is based on 14 of the 15 subjects in this report as the one remitted subject recovered during early childhood). Moreover, this investigation also included speech behavior measures and self-report outcomes for untreated recovery, which will be described below.

Based on investigator judgment or subject self-report, outcomes of late recovery without treatment have suggested that the subjects' speech behavior is normally fluent in most cases, but there still may be an occasional tendency to stutter (see for review, Finn, 2004). The percentage of subjects reporting a tendency to still stutter ranged across early studies from 9% (Johnson, 1950) to 64% (Shearer & Williams, 1965). Findings from more recent studies, however, have been more consistent with a range of 60% (Finn, 1997) to 72.8%, with the latter based on a sample size of 103 subjects (Finn & Felsenfeld, 2006).

Listener judgments of the speech behavior of late recovered speakers, based on videotaped speech samples, have revealed that their speech is perceptually distinguishable from normal controls (Finn, 1997; Finn et al., 2005). Not surprisingly, it is the speakers who still report an occasional tendency to stutter that contributes to this perceptual difference. In contrast, those speakers who no longer reported a tendency to stutter were indistinguishable from the normally fluent speakers. Nonetheless, the speech quality of all the recovered speakers was rated by listeners as more natural sounding than the speech of clients who had been successfully treated for their stuttering (Finn, 1997).

Based on self-report data, Finn et al. (2005) have also found that self-managed late recovered stutterers no longer experienced the pervasive negative attitudes commonly reported by persistent stutterers or any overwhelming barriers to communication. Perhaps most importantly, they appeared to be confident that whenever stuttering did occur they would be able to regain their fluent speech. They also seemed especially sensitive to mental states or feelings that might prompt stuttering. Yet, when they found themselves in these circumstances, they thought of implementing strategies for dealing with or repairing any possible stuttering. This finding replicated the results reported by Anderson and Felsenfeld (2003), that recovered stutterers indicate that some ongoing level of vigilance is required for maintaining fluency despite the fact that they had been recovered for many years. It is also consistent with reports in the behavior modification literature suggesting that client vigilance and implementation of proactive strategies are important for managing lapses in order to ensure long-term maintenance of treatment gains for chronic problems (Kirschenbaum & Tomarken, 1982).

Recent Findings and Future Directions

As this overview has suggested, self-managed late recovery from persistent forms of stuttering is possible and this recovery is often enduring. It is also clear, however, that improvement is not always complete. Some late recovered speakers continue to have residual stuttering, and although it is infrequent and readily controllable, they also report that they do not experience any sense of handicap and are essentially completely functional as everyday communicators (Finn et al., 2005). Future research will need to examine why some individuals are able to self-manage a complete recovery and others are not. Two hypotheses appear to be plausible. The first is that residual stuttering may represent the limits of any recovery, treated or untreated, because the diminished capacity for neural plasticity in adulthood may place constraints on expectations for producing a completely normally fluent speaker (Ingham et al., 2005). Related to this are recent findings that there may be a significant genetic factor that governs recovery from stuttering without treatment (Felsenfeld & Finn, 2003); thus, there may be some genetic component that places limits on recovery. The second hypothesis is that self-managed recovery may be imperfect, at least for some individuals, because they are nonprofessionals and further improvement could be possible with formal treatment (Finn, 2004).

Recently published findings related to the neurophysiological aspects of recovery, based for the most part on speakers who had recovered without treatment after childhood, have all suggested that these speakers' neurological systems have not completely normalized (Forster & Webster, 2001; Ingham, Ingham, Finn, & Fox, 2003; Mouradian, Paslawski, & Shuaib, 2000). Interestingly, some of these speakers (see Ingham et al., 2003) were also self-managed late recovered speakers who no longer reported a tendency to stutter, had been judged by listeners to be indistinguishable from normally fluent controls, and from an experiential perspective, also reported complete recovery from stuttering (see Finn et al., 2005). Yet, the neurophysiological evidence based on brain imaging findings suggested that although their neural systems no longer resembled those of adults who still stutter, they also did not function in the same manner as normal controls (Ingham et al., 2003). Clearly, further research is necessary to determine the impact of neurological normalcy and the relationship between normalcy and behavior. Self-managed late recovered speakers may provide one avenue for looking at these relationships.

Finally, it is clear that self-managed late recovered speakers are achieving long-term improvements in their stuttering that even clinicians would envy. Thus, it would seem logical that future research needs to further investigate what this population can tell us about procedures that can be incorporated into interventions for helping those who continue to stutter.

References

Ambrose, N. G., Cox, N. J., & Yairi, E. (1997). The genetic basis of persistence and recovery in stuttering. *Journal of Speech, Language, and Hearing Research, 40*, 567–580.

Anderson, T. K., & Felsenfeld, S. (2003). A thematic analysis of late recovery from stuttering. *American Journal of Speech-Language Pathology, 12*, 243–253.

Andrews, G., Guitar, B., & Howie, P. (1980). Meta-analysis of the effects of stuttering treatment. *Journal of Speech and Hearing Disorders, 45*, 287–307.

Blaker, K., Harbaugh, D., & Finn, P. (1996–1997). Clinician attitudes toward stuttering: A survey of New Mexico. *Texas Journal of Audiology and Speech-Language Pathology, 22*, 109–114.

Blomgren, M., Roy, N., Callister, T., & Merrill, R. M. (2005). Intensive stuttering modification therapy: A multidimensional assessment of treatment outcomes. *Journal of Speech, Language, and Hearing Sciences, 48*, 509–523.

Bloodstein, O. (1995). *The handbook of stuttering* (5th ed.). San Diego: Singular.

Bormann, E. G. (1969). Ephphatha, or, some advice to stammerers. *Journal of Speech and Hearing Research, 12*, 453–461.

Bothe, A. K., Davidow, J. H., Bramlett, R. E., & Ingham, R. J. (2006). Stuttering treatment research 1970–2005: I. Systematic review incorporating trial quality assessment of behavioral, cognitive, and related approaches. *American Journal of Speech-Language Pathology, 15*, 321–341.

Brosch, S., Haege, A., Kalehne, P., & Johannsen, H. S. (1999). Stuttering children and the probability of remission—The role of cerebral dominance and speech production. *International Journal of Pediatric Otorhinolaryngology, 47*, 71–76.

Brown, S., Ingham, R. J., Ingham, J. C., Laird, A. R., & Fox, P. T. (2005). Stuttered and fluent speech production: An ALE meta-analysis of functional neuroimaging studies. *Human Brain Mapping, 25*, 105–117.

Cordes, A. K. (1998). Current status of the stuttering treatment literature. In A. K. Cordes & R. J. Ingham (Eds.), *Treatment efficacy for stuttering: A search for empirical bases* (pp. 117–144). San Diego: Singular.

Craig, A. R. (1998). Relapse following treatment for stuttering: A critical review and correlative data. *Journal of Fluency Disorders, 23*, 1–30.

Felsenfeld, S., & Finn, P. (2003, August). *Examining recovery from stuttering using a population-based twin sample*. Paper presented at the 4th World Congress International Fluency Association, Montreal, Canada.

Felsenfeld, S., Kirk, K. M., Zhu, G., Statham, D. J., Neale, M. C., & Martin, N. G. (2000). A study of the genetic and environmental etiology of stuttering in a selected twin sample. *Behavior Genetics, 30*, 359–366.

Finn, P. (1996). Establishing the validity of recovery from stuttering without treatment. *Journal of Speech and Hearing Research, 39*, 1171–1181.

Finn, P. (1997). Adults recovered from stuttering without formal treatment: Perceptual assessment of speech normalcy. *Journal of Speech, Language, and Hearing Research, 40*, 821–831.

Finn, P. (1998). Recovery without treatment: A review of conceptual and methodological considerations across disciplines. In A. K. Cordes & R. J. Ingham (Eds.), *Treatment efficacy for stuttering: A search for empirical bases* (pp. 3–28). San Diego: Singular.

Finn, P. (2004). Self-change from stuttering during adolescence and adulthood. In A. K. Bothe (Ed.), *Evidence-based treatment of stuttering: Empirical bases and applications* (pp. 117–136). Mahwah, NJ: Lawrence Erlbaum Associates.

Finn, P. (2007). Self-regulation and the management of stuttering. In E. G. Conture & R. F. Curlee (Eds.), *Stuttering and related disorders of fluency* (3rd ed., pp. 342–359). New York: Thieme

Finn, P., & Felsenfeld, S. (2006, November). *A life-span perspective of stuttering and recovery*. Paper presented at the Annual Convention of the American Speech-Language-Hearing Association, Miami, FL.

Finn, P., Howard, R., & Kubala, R. (2005). Unassisted recovery from stuttering: Self-perceptions of current speech behavior, attitudes, and feelings. *Journal of Fluency Disorders, 30*, 281–305.

Finn, P., Ingham, R. J., Ambrose, N., & Yairi, E. (1997). Children recovered from stuttering without formal treatment: Perceptual assessment of speech normalcy. *Journal of Speech, Language, and Hearing Research, 40*, 867–876.

Forster, D. C., & Webster, W. G. (2001). Speech-motor control and interhemispheric relations in recovered and persistent stuttering. *Developmental Psychology, 19*, 125–145.

Freund, H. (1970). Self-improvement after unsuccessful treatments. In M. Fraser (Ed.), *To the stutterer* (pp. 49–53). Memphis, TN: Speech Foundation of America No. 9.

Guitar, B. (1998). *Stuttering: An integrated approach to its nature and treatment.* (2nd ed.). Baltimore: Williams & Wilkins.

Heltman, H. J. (1941). History of recurrent stuttering and recovery in twenty-five year old post graduate college student. *Journal of Speech Disorders, 6*, 49–50.

Ingham, R. J. (1983). Spontaneous remission of stuttering: When will the emperor realize he has no clothes on? In D. Prins & R. J. Ingham (Eds.), *Treatment of stuttering in early childhood* (pp. 113–140). San Diego: College-Hill Press.

Ingham, R. J. (1999). Performance-contingent management of stuttering. In R. F. Curlee (Ed.), *Stuttering and related disorders of fluency* (2nd ed., pp. 139–159). New York: Thieme.

Ingham, R. J., Finn, P., & Bothe, A. (2005). Roadblocks revisited: Neural change, stuttering, and recovery from stuttering. *Journal of Fluency Disorders, 30*, 91–107.

Ingham, R. J., Ingham, J. C., Finn, P., & Fox, P. (2003). Towards a functional neural systems model of developmental stuttering. *Journal of Fluency Disorders, 28*, 297–318.

Johnson, P. A. (1950). *An exploratory study of certain aspects of the speech histories of twenty-three former stutterers.* Unpublished master's thesis, University of Pittsburgh.

Kirschenbaum, D. S., & Tomarken, A. J. (1982). On facing the generalization problem: The study of self-regulatory failure. In P. C. Kendall (Ed.), *Advances in cognitive-behavioral research and therapy* (Vol. 1, pp. 119–200). New York: Academic Press.

Lankford, S. D., & Cooper, E. B. (1974). Recovery from stuttering as viewed by parents of self-diagnosed recovered stutterers. *Journal of Communication Disorders, 7*, 171–180.

Manning, W. H. (2001). *Clinical decision making in fluency disorders* (2nd ed.). San Diego: Singular/Thomson Learning.

Mansson, H. (2000). Childhood stuttering: Incidence and development. *Journal of Fluency Disorders, 25*, 47–57.

Martyn, M. M., & Sheehan, J. G. (1968). Onset of stuttering and recovery. *Behaviour Research and Therapy, 6*, 295–307.

Mouradian, M. S., Paslawski, T., & Shuaib, A. (2000). Return of stuttering after stroke. *Brain and Language, 73*, 120–123.

Onslow, M., Costa, L., & Rue, S. (1990). Direct early intervention with stuttering: Some preliminary data. *Journal of Speech and Hearing Disorders, 55*, 405–416.

Onslow, M., Packman, A., & Harrison, E. (2003). *The Lidcombe program of early stuttering intervention: A clinician's guide.* Austin, TX: Pro-Ed.

Perkins, W. H. (1989). Why do stutterers stop stuttering: What experts will think in 2010. *Seminars in Speech and Language, 10*, 122–127.

Quarrington, B. (1977). How do the various theories of stuttering facilitate our therapeutic approach? *Journal of Communication Disorders, 10*, 77–83.

Ratner, N. B. (2001). The syllabus project. *Special Interest Division 4: Fluency and Fluency Disorders, 11*(4), 16–18.

Reed, C. G., & Godden, A. L. (1977). An experimental treatment using verbal punishment with two preschool stutterers. *Journal of Fluency Disorders, 2*, 225–233.

Shearer, W. M., & Williams, J. D. (1965). Self-recovery from stuttering. *Journal of Speech and Hearing Disorders, 30*, 288–290.

Wingate, M. E. (1964). Recovery from stuttering. *Journal of Speech and Hearing Disorders, 29*, 312–321.

Wingate, M. E. (1976). *Stuttering: Theory and treatment*. New York: Irvington.

Yairi, E., & Ambrose, N. G. (1999). Early childhood stuttering I: Persistency and recovery rates. *Journal of Speech, Language, and Hearing Research, 42*, 1097–1112.

7
One Way to Leave Your Lover: The Role of Treatment in Changing Addictive Behaviors

Mark B. Sobell

> The problem is all inside your head she said to me.
> The answer is easy if you take it logically...
> There must be fifty ways to leave your lover.
>
> Paul Simon, "50 Ways to Leave Your Lover," 1975

Whether the topic is addictive behaviors, infections, or fractures, the traditional view of treatment in a medical model is that it addresses the cause of the disorder and either returns the person to normal functioning or helps the individual achieve a reasonable accommodation to a disability. For treatment of withdrawal symptoms, the medical model is defensible—the disorder has a known physiological basis, the treatment derives from that knowledge, and the treatment is reliably effective. For other aspects of addictive behavior, especially compulsive use, the model's fit is highly questionable. The basis for the behavior is neither understood nor necessarily physiological (although drug effects have a physiological basis, that does not mean that the "cause" of their use is physiological).

Meaningful Explanations of Change in Addictive Behavior

Tucker and King (1999) have noted that the effects of treatments and other interventions for addictive behaviors typically are associated with short-term benefits but are plagued by problem recurrence. This occurs despite the being based on highly divergent assumptions (e.g., learned behavior, disease) and having different characteristics (e.g., lengths). Moreover, outcomes are positively associated with an individual's resources and with environmental variables following treatment. When these facts are collectively taken into account, along with evidence that many people recover from substance abuse problems without intervention (Sobell, Ellingstad, & Sobell, 2000), the utility of the traditional perspective becomes very doubtful. Natural recoveries often are not reactions to specific precipitating events but rather follow cognitive reappraisals (i.e., the individual weighs the pros and cons and makes a decision to change; Sobell, Sobell, Toneatto, & Leo, 1993; also reviewed in Sobell & Sobell, 2000). In turn, this suggests that the critical ingredient for precipitating change is one's commitment (i.e., motivation) to change. This is not to deny that psychoactive substances affect the individual's physiology. However, that is a separate issue from explaining what drives continued use despite the likelihood of negative consequences, the essence of addictive behavior. The viewpoint adopted in this chapter is that any meaningful explanation of change in addictive behavior (i.e., recovery) must be able to explain all varieties of change, including those stimulated by environmental events, those that have been described as the result of a "maturing out" process, and other natural recoveries.

Fifty Ways to Leave Your Lover

> **Recovered Alcohol Abuser**
> "I wasn't a human being as I intended to be. I had reached a point where I felt trapped by alcohol. It was my mistress…"

An individual's attraction to their drug of choice can be understood as a love relationship (Saunders & Allsop, 1985; Stewart, 1987). Taking this analogy one step further, there are many ways that the dissolution of a relationship can be achieved—many ways to leave one's lover. That there are multiple routes to recovery from substance abuse problems becomes easier to understand when the full range of problems is considered rather than an isolated focus on severe cases (Institute of Medicine, 1990). This issue has been best addressed for alcohol problems, where epidemiological findings have indicated that the population of individuals with severe problems far outnumbers those with less severe problems. The Institute of Medicine, in its 1990 report to the National Institute on Alcohol Abuse and Alcoholism, estimated the ratio to be four not severely dependent alcohol abusers for every severely dependent case (Institute of Medicine, 1990). Most people do not find it surprising that individuals with minor alcohol problems often overcome their problems without the assistance of others. Likewise, it is common knowledge that most people who stop smoking do so on their own (Fiore et al., 1990; Orleans et al., 1991). Also, like treated alcohol abusers, ex-smokers in treatment are more dependent than the average smoker, and before stopping smoking ex-smokers were less dependent on nicotine than are current smokers (Fagerström et al., 1996). Time and again, the most intuitive conclusion is that change can be achieved through many routes and that the most important precipitant of change is the decision to change. In short, if individuals are strongly motivated to change, they will find a way to do so.

Tucker (1999) has compellingly argued for viewing recovery within an individual's total life context as it evolves over time. From this perspective,

---

Recovered Alcohol Abusers

Example 1:
"Well, basically you have to want to stop. You have to recognize that you have a problem then you have to really want to stop. I guess there's a thing I refer to as self-esteem and if you don't have that then I think you're lost. It's going to be a barrier so you must feel that you're a good person and you can do it."

Example 2:
"Well, I think I had the feeling that if I'm gonna beat this thing, it's up to me, and nobody else is going to make me stop drinking. It's my problem and I have to resolve it myself. Why should I go to, and ask somebody else and put my problems on their shoulders, when it's one of my own."

Example 3:
"I was supposed to take her to a Sunday School picnic in the afternoon, on that Saturday afternoon, and on that Saturday morning I got juiced up and I was unable to take her. So the next day I had a terrible feeling of guilt and remorse and I guess maybe I had one or two beers left, I gulped that, and I said this is it. That's the end of that nonsense and I've never had a drink since. Well, it just happened that this was the last straw I guess. I made up my mind that I'm going to beat this thing and this is the end of it. Good-bye! I was going to beat it. I felt so badly about it."

---

behavior change is not necessarily seen as an isolated event; it can also be the endpoint of a process that takes place over time. The onset and offset of substance abuse problems can be viewed as phases in one's career. The remainder of this chapter will consider why some individuals utilize treatment services as part of their attempts to change, while others do not.

Figure 7.1 presents a hypothetical overview of the behavior change process. Although it will be discussed with regard to addictive behaviors, the same model could be used to describe different types of behavior change. The early part of the change process (i.e., becoming committed to change) has recently become a topic of considerable research in the addiction field. Research on motivation was fueled by Prochaska and DiClemente's (DiClemente, Prochaska, & Gibertini, 1985; Prochaska & DiClemente, 1986) extension of Prochaska's transtheoretical model of change in psychotherapy to the addiction field. The model breaks down the change process into a set of hypothetical stages. While the model has been the subject of considerable criticism and controversy recently (Bandura, 1997; Carey, Purnine, Maisto, & Carey, 1999; Davidson, 1998; Sutton, 2001; West, 2005), a review of these issues is beyond the scope of this chapter. The important features of this model for the present consideration are: (a) that it postulates that motivation is a state variable (i.e., changeable) and as such should be addressed in treatment, and (b) that it is nonsensical to conduct therapy intended to help an individual change if the person is not committed to changing.

Whereas the stages of change (transtheoretical) model evoked a plethora of research and comment, including the advent of motivational interviewing as an alternative approach to dealing with individuals in substance abuse treatment (Miller & Rollnick, 1991; Substance Abuse and Mental Health Administration, 1999), research on how change occurs, the help-seeking process, and the role

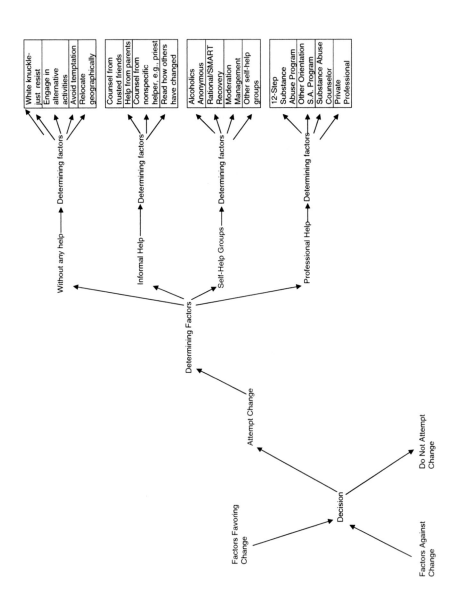

FIGURE 7.1. Overview of the behavior change process.

of treatment in change has been neither plentiful nor well organized. This hypothetical process, as presented in Figure 7.1, can be viewed as involving the following two phases: (a) deciding on the general route of change to be followed and (b) deciding on the specific route of change. Although research and common sense make clear that alternative routes to recovery exist and are used, studies are seriously deficient concerning the sets of variables labeled as "Determining Factors" in Figure 7.1. This diagram considers the change process from the standpoint of the individual, not from the perspective of the treatment professional. Thus, the necessary research does not consist of matching studies aimed at identifying what types of individuals will do best in what types of treatment (e.g., Project MATCH Research Group, 1997), but rather on how people decide how they will attempt to change, whether they will seek help, what type of help they will seek, and why.

Because the focus of this chapter is on the role of treatment in change, the existing literature on factors affecting help seeking will not be reviewed here. Moreover, reviews of that literature are already available (Aday & Andersen, 1974; Becker & Maiman, 1975; Hasin & Grant, 1995; Simpson & Tucker, 2002; Thom, 1986; Thom, Brown, Drummond, Edwards, & Mullan, 1992). Instead, the current discussion will be largely conceptual, with an emphasis on identifying areas of research likely to illuminate influences on change decisions.

Factors Influencing Route of Change

Although there has been a dearth of research on how people choose their route of attempted recovery, this does not mean that the boxes labeled "Determining factors" in Figure 7.1 are black boxes. As some relevant research has reported there are several factors that logically belong within the boxes' content. Table 7.1 presents a conceptual listing of factors likely to influence an individual's decision about what recovery route to pursue. These factors, which operate in selecting the general route of change and the specific method within that route, range from personal beliefs and experiences, to practical issues, to community structure and attitudes.

Having made a decision to attempt to change, the ways in which an individual can approach this objective must start from one's knowledge about how to change and what assistance might be available. It should be noted that this knowledge derives not only from general information and help that is available but also from vicariously knowing about the experiences of others. In terms of community health service planning, it is obvious that using services efficiently will begin with the population being aware of cost-effective services and, importantly, being aware that many individuals are able to recover without the help of formal services. Because traditional substance abuse programs tend to be intensive and costly (Institute of Medicine, 1990; Klingemann & Hunt, 1998), at least in the United States, it would be highly advisable to embark on a campaign to make the general population aware of multiple routes to recovery.

TABLE 7.1. Factors likely to influence decisions about what route of change to pursue.

Information/knowledge
  Treatment programs
  How others have changed
  Self-help group existence and local availability
  Trusted others available to provide informal counsel
  Professional services available
  How people recover from substance abuse
Environmental factors
  Availability of self-help groups, treatment programs, professionals
  Access to services (e.g., waiting lists, transportation)
  Community attitudes toward problems, recovery, etc.
Personal situation/pragmatic factors
  Cost of treatment programs, professional services
  Interference with other responsibilities (e.g., work, child care)
Psychological factors
  Attitude toward independence
  Trust of others to give aid
  Beliefs about how one should recover
  Past experiences

Finally, there are two ways by which information plays a role in determining the route of recovery. First, it serves to constrain alternatives. People cannot be expected to adopt alternatives that they do not know exist. Besides knowing that options are available, a second and even more important issue is that individuals should also have accurate information in order to make decisions among those alternatives. For example, in North America it is commonly believed that Alcoholics Anonymous and 12–Step programs have been demonstrated to be the most effective approaches to recovery, although this is at odds with the empirical literature (Miller et al., 1995). Thus, an additional prerequisite for achieving efficient use of community services is the dissemination of accurate information about all available routes of recovery.

Environmental factors also influence decisions about which recovery routes to select. Starting with differences such as urban and rural environments, the setting will place real limits on the substance abuser's options (Marlatt, 1999; Tucker, Vuchinich, & Rippens, 2002). Environmental considerations can be greatly affected by the availability of treatment programs as well as helping professionals, since even small communities tend to have self-help groups available. However, in very small communities if privacy is important, then this may serve as a barrier to using self-help groups.

> **Recovered Alcohol Abuser**
>
> "He said, 'You're known as a town drunk.' Now there were other things that had happened as well....But that was the cruncher. I was really blew my lid when he said that. When he said that I was known as a town drunk, no son of mine or family has to put up with that from me."

Another important aspect of the environment that impacts choosing a route of change relates to access to services (Kavanagh, Sitharthan, Spilsbury, & Vignaedra, 1999; Tucker & Davison, 2000). Factors such as convenience or difficulty accessing services or length of time until services are available (e.g., waiting lists) may not be tolerable and may ultimately affect a person's decision to change. Also, the environment acts as a source of collective social influence (Pescosolido, 1991; Tucker & Davison, 2000). The individual's social network not only provides support and advice but also a context of beliefs, attitudes, and hearsay about methods of change. To the extent that social approval is important to the individual, social context is bound to influence decisions about change routes.

Recovered Alcohol Abuser

"You know, one of the greatest things that happened was that [name deleted] never drank very much, but she quit and supported me.... So she decided then that 'hey, you know, I am not going to drink either.' And from that moment neither of us drank anything. Yes, cause it's a social thing."

Individualized factors will also impact choice of alternatives. Many of the change routes extract personal costs that the individual may or may not find worthwhile. These range from the monetary cost of treatment programs or professional services, to the investment of time (e.g., inpatient treatment to attending weekly self-help group meetings), to competing with responsibilities (e.g., at home or work) and activities (e.g., hobbies, gardening).

Lastly, central to choosing change routes will be psychological factors. The other elements discussed so far serve to make the individual aware of a menu of choices and a set of costs and benefits related to each choice. However, the resultant choice is made against the backdrop of psychological factors. Individual differences in traits, attitudes, backgrounds, preferences, values, and the other factors that combine to yield idiosyncratic identities will ultimately serve as the filtering mechanism through which choice emerges. Some of these factors may include the stigma that often surrounds issues of substance abuse as well as a general fear of or unwillingness to engage in treatment. The latter issue also affects help seeking for many health problems that are not stigmatizing, such as heart disease (Tucker & Davison, 2000). Such factors have long been ignored despite their obvious importance to understanding how people decide what methods to use in attempting to change. Understanding how people choose what route to try to change is extremely important for health care planning. It is clear that if all individuals with substance abuse problems were to seek to use treatment services, the amount of resources available would be woefully inadequate. Thus, while this area of research begins with observational and descriptive studies, ultimately the goals would be to: (a) encourage those individuals who can achieve self-change or recovery through self-help programs to do so and (b) promote a set of empirically based interventions by which substance abusers could identify the services likely to be necessary to resolve their problem.

The Role of Treatment in Changing Addictive Behavior

This section focuses on the role of treatment in changing addictive behavior and assumes that other community level interventions are necessary to achieve the dual goals of (a) increasing the use of treatment where necessary and (b) decreasing unnecessary use of treatment. Given the above context for help seeking, what should be the role of treatment in changing addictive behavior? One aspect of the role is to just "be there." For treatment to be a route to change, opportunities for treatment must exist. In an ideal world, it would be sufficient to make a variety of services available which could be utilized according to need. However, need for assistance in changing may be only one reason why people utilize clinical services. For example, F. C. Breslin (personal communication, November 1999) found that several participants who had successful outcomes in a brief intervention trial nevertheless went on to use additional services in the community. This may have been because although their outcomes were positive from a research perspective (i.e., in terms of decreased substance use), they continued to have associated problems (e.g., interpersonal) because they felt they needed help maintaining the changes they had accomplished, or for other reasons. In fact, Aasland, Bruusgaard, and Rutle (1987) have suggested that some people enter addiction treatment after they have already changed, with the purpose of treatment being to maintain that change. Whatever the reason, perceptions of the need for treatment by potential consumers may differ markedly from those of professionals. If services are paid for by individuals themselves, this is less of a problem than services that are reimbursed by public programs or insurance providers. Thus, besides having a variety of services available there is also a need to provide triage services to assure that funds are spent wisely to provide necessary care.

Stepped-Care Approach

One way for the addiction field to provide services efficiently would be to embrace a stepped-care model of service provision (Sobell & Sobell, 2000). Such an approach is shown in Figure 7.2 and reflects how services are delivered for many health problems. It suggests guidelines for providers to follow in making treatment recommendations, with the initial recommendations based on both empirically based knowledge and clinical judgment. The guidelines are that the treatment of choice should be (a) individualized, (b) consistent with the contemporary research literature, (c) least restrictive but still likely to work, and (d) acceptable to the consumer. Following the initial treatment disposition, decisions about further interventions are performance-based; that is, they depend on whether the individual shows a good response to treatment. If the response is inadequate, consideration is given to stepping up the intensity of care or to using a different approach. For example, in the treatment of hypertension, typically a family physician

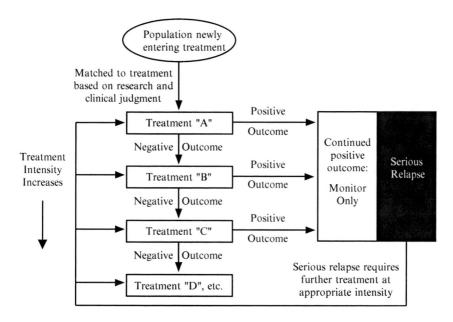

FIGURE 7.2. Stepped-care model of health service delivery.

is likely to recommend various lifestyle changes such as exercise and diet as first treatments of choice, followed by medication, and eventual referral to a specialist if the aforementioned interventions are not effective. Accumulating evidence suggests that individuals who will do well with a brief cognitive–behavioral treatment show substantial change within the first few sessions of treatment (Wilson, 1999). Thus, individuals who do not show early change might be good candidates for stepping up the level of services.

Multiple Functions of Treatment

Finally, in terms of the functions that can be served by treatment, several general themes are evident. Treatment can serve as a forum for people to organize their thoughts about their problems and make informed decisions about priorities. This may be one reason why motivational enhancement treatments incorporate decisional balancing exercises compelling the individual to weigh the pros and cons of changing versus staying the same (Substance Abuse and Mental Health Administration, 1999). Another function of treatment can be to help people understand their predicament and how they got there and to give hope that change is possible. In some cases, when people become aware of the relationship between precipitating factors and consequences and their substance use, this may be sufficient for them to initiate change; however, in other cases, change may be difficult, if not impossible, without the acquisition of necessary skills. Another potential function of treatment is to provide social support and reinforcement for change, especially if clients lack such resources as part of their everyday environment. Lastly, treatment can "buy time" for people. For example, individuals who are under social pressure to change, but not yet ready to change, could enter treatment and attend sessions to satisfy others, but have no intention of changing their substance use.

Summary: Many Ways to Leave Your Lover

It is evident that change in substance use can be accomplished in many ways, with treatment being only one way. This chapter was intended to provide an organizational framework for conceptualizing variables important for precipitating change. Although the multiple components of change were described conceptually rather than reviewed, an important point that this chapter highlighted is that little is known about factors determining (a) how a person decides to try and change, (b) why and when someone seeks help, and (c) how one chooses among alternatives, including treatment. Research on client–treatment matching will be of limited benefit without corresponding research on (a) getting clients to select treatments that are likely to be least restrictive but nevertheless effective, as well as (b) getting service providers to adopt a professional, stepped-care approach to service provision rather than being wed to services developed for severe cases (and therefore too intensive for individuals with less severe problems; Institute of Medicine, 1990; Tucker, 1999).

References

Aasland, O. G., Bruusgaard, D., & Rutle, O. (1987). Alcohol problems in general practice. *British Journal of Addiction, 82*, 197–201.

Aday, L. A., & Andersen, R. M. (1974). A framework for the study of access to medical care. *Health Sciences Research, 9*, 208–220.

Bandura, A. (1997). The anatomy of stages of change. *American Journal of Health Promotion, 12*, 8–10.

Becker, C. H., & Maiman, L. A. (1975). Sociobehavioral determinants of compliance with health and medical care recommendations. *Medical Care, 13*, 10–14.

Carey, K. B., Purnine, D. M., Maisto, S. A., & Carey, M. P. (1999). Assessing readiness to change substance abuse: A critical review of instruments. *Clinical Psychology-Science and Practice, 6*, 245–266.

Davidson, R. (1998). The transtheoretical model: A critical overview. In W. R. Miller & N. Heather (Eds.), *Treating addictive behaviors* (2nd ed., pp. 25–38). New York: Plenum Press.

DiClemente, C. C., Prochaska, J. O., & Gibertini, M. (1985). Self-efficacy and the stages of self-change of smoking. *Cognitive Therapy and Research, 9*, 181–200.

Fagerström, K. O., Kunze, M., Schoberberger, R., Breslau, N., Hughes, J. R., Hurt, R. D., et al. (1996). Nicotine dependence versus smoking prevalence: Comparisons among countries and categories of smokers. *Tobacco Control, 5*, 52–56.

Fiore, M. C., Novotny, T. E., Pierce, J. P., Giovino, E. J., Hatziandreu, P. A., Newcomb, T. S., et al. (1990). Methods used to quit smoking in the United States. Do cessation programs help? *Journal of the American Medical Association, 263*, 2760–2765.

Hasin, D., & Grant, B. (1995). AA and other help seeking for alcohol problems: Former drinkers in the U.S. general population. *Journal of Substance Abuse, 7*, 281–292.

Institute of Medicine. (1990). *Broadening the base of treatment for alcohol problems*. Washington, DC: National Academy Press.

Kavanagh, D. J., Sitharthan, T., Spilsbury, G., & Vignaedra, S. (1999). An evaluation of brief correspondence programs for problem drinkers. *Behavior Therapy, 30*, 641–656.

Klingemann, H., & Hunt, G. (1998). *Drug treatment systems in an international perspective*. Thousand Oaks, CA: Sage.

Marlatt, G. A. (1999). From hindsight to foresight: A commentary on Project MATCH. In J. A. Tucker, D. A. Donovan, & G. A. Marlatt (Eds.), *Changing addictive behavior: Bridging clinical and public health strategies* (pp. 45–66). New York: Guilford Press.

Miller, W. R., Brown, J. M., Simpson, T. L., Handmaker, N. S., Bien, T. H., Luckie, L. F., et al. (1995). What works? A methodological analysis of the alcohol treatment outcome literature. In R. K. Hester & W. R. Miller (Eds.), *Handbook of alcoholism treatment approaches: Effective alternatives* (2nd ed., pp. 12–44). Boston: Allyn & Bacon.

Miller, W. R., & Rollnick, S. (1991). *Motivational interviewing: Preparing people to change addictive behavior*. New York: Guilford Press.

Orleans, C. T., Schoenbach, V. J., Wagner, E. H., Quade, D., Salmon, M. A., Pearson, D. C., et al. (1991). Self-help quit smoking interventions: Effects of self-help materials, social support instructions, and telephone counseling. *Journal of Consulting and Clinical Psychology, 59*, 439–448.

Pescosolido, B. (1991). Illness careers and network ties: A conceptual model of utilization and compliance. *Advances in Medical Sociology, 2*, 161–184.

Prochaska, J. O., & DiClemente, C. C. (Eds.). (1986). *Toward a comprehensive model of change*. New York: Plenum Press.

Project MATCH Research Group. (1997). Matching alcoholism treatments to client heterogeneity: Project MATCH posttreatment drinking outcomes. *Journal of Studies on Alcohol, 58*, 7–29.

Saunders, B., & Allsop, S. (1985). Giving up addictions. In F. N. Watts (Ed.), *New developments in clinical psychology* (pp. 203–220). New York: John Wiley.

Simpson, C. A., & Tucker, J. A. (2002). Temporal sequencing of alcohol-related problems, problem recognition, and help-seeking episodes. *Addictive Behaviors, 27*, 659–674.

Sobell, L. C., Ellingstad, T. P., & Sobell, M. B. (2000). Natural recovery from alcohol and drug problems: Methodological review of the research with suggestions for future directions. *Addiction, 95*, 749–764.

Sobell, L. C., Sobell, M. B., Toneatto, T., & Leo, G. I. (1993). What triggers the resolution of alcohol problems without treatment? *Alcoholism: Clinical and Experimental Research, 17*, 217–224.

Sobell, M. B., & Sobell, L. C. (2000). Stepped care as a heuristic approach to the treatment of alcohol problems. *Journal of Consulting and Clinical Psychology, 68*, 573–579.

Stewart, T. (1987). *The heroin users*. London: Pandora Press.

Substance Abuse and Mental Health Administration. (1999). *Enhancing motivation for change in substance abuse treatment* (Treatment Improvement Protocol Series). Rockville, MD: U.S. Department of Health and Human Services.

Sutton, S. (2001). Back to the drawing board? A review of applications of the transtheoretical model to substance use. *Addiction, 96*, 175–186.

Thom, B. (1986). Sex differences in help-seeking for alcohol problems—1. The barriers to help-seeking. *British Journal of Addiction, 81*, 777–788.

Thom, B., Brown, C., Drummond, C., Edwards, G., & Mullan, M. (1992). The use of services for alcohol problems: General practitioner and specialist alcohol clinic. *British Journal of Addiction, 87*, 613–624.

Tucker, J. A. (1999). Changing addictive behavior: Historical and contemporary perspectives. In J. A. Tucker, D. A. Donovan, & G. A. Marlatt (Eds.), *Changing addictive behavior: Bridging clinical and public health strategies* (pp. 3–44). New York: Guilford Press.

Tucker, J. A., & Davison, J. W. (2000). Waiting to see the doctor: The role of time constraints in the utilization of health and behavioral health services. In W. Bickel & R. Vuchinich (Eds.), *Reframing health behavior change with behavior economics* (pp. 219–264). New York: Lawrence Erlbaum.

Tucker, J. A., & King, M. P. (1999). Resolving alcohol and drug-related problems: Influences on behavior change and help-seeking processes. In J. A. Tucker, D. A. Donovan, & G. A. Marlatt (Eds.), *Changing addictive behavior: Bridging clinical and public health strategies* (pp. 97–126). New York: Guilford Press.

Tucker, J. A., Vuchinich, R. E., & Rippens, P. D. (2002). Environmental contexts surrounding resolution of drinking problems among problem drinkers with different help-seeking experiences. *Journal of Studies on Alcohol, 63*, 334–341.

West, R. (2005). Time for a change: Putting the transtheoretical (stages of change) model to rest. *Addiction, 100*, 1036–1039.

Wilson, G. T. (1999). Rapid response to cognitive behavior therapy. *Clinical Psychology: Science and Practice, 6*, 289–292.

8
Promoting Self-Change: Taking the Treatment to the Community

Linda Carter Sobell and Mark B. Sobell

As discussed in detail in Chapter 1, the vast majority of people with alcohol and drug problems are unlikely to enter traditional substance abuse or addiction treatment programs (Harris & Mckellar, 2003). Several major U.S. surveys have concluded that only a small percentage of individuals with alcohol problems ever seek and enter into treatment (Dawson, Grant, Stinson, et al., 2005; Raimo, Daeppen, Smith, Danko, & Schuckit, 1999). For example, of 4,422 adults 18 years or older classified with prior-to past-year DSM-IV alcohol dependence in the 2001–2 National Epidemiologic Survey on Alcohol and Related Conditions (Dawson, Grant, Stinson, et al., 2005), only 25.5% reported ever receiving treatment (12-Step programs: 3.1%; Formal treatment: 5.4%; both 12-Step and treatment: 17.0%). Another national survey found "only 16% of those with an alcohol use disorder (AUD) had received any treatment in 2001. Similarly, a recent report on utilization of AUD treatment in the Veterans Administration found that only 23% of individuals with an identified disorder received treatment" (Harris & McKellar, 2003, p. 1). Clearly, such figures underscore the need to seriously develop and evaluate alternative, minimally intrusive interventions that will appeal to such individuals.

For close to three decades, treatment for individuals with alcohol and drug problems has been provided almost exclusively at traditional specialty substance abuse agencies. If individuals with substance use and abuse problems are unwilling to come into treatment, the key question is "What can be done to motivate them to change their substance use outside of treatment or as a result of a very brief encounter?" One suggestion has been that we should take the treatment to the people (Sobell, Cunningham, Sobell, et al., 1996; Sobell, Sobell, Leo, et al., 2002). Alternative interventions need to be provided in settings other than traditional substance abuse agencies, such as physicians' offices, primary care settings, or nontraditional ways such as on the Internet or by mail.

Interestingly, effective January 2007, the U.S. Centers for Medicare and Medicaid Services added two new reimbursement codes for use by Medicaid, Medicare, and other third-party payers. These codes allow providers to be reimbursed for alcohol and drug screenings and brief interventions (SBIs) in clinical settings. Bertha Madras (2006), Deputy Director of Demand Reduction from the White House Office of National Drug Control Policy, reported that the "impetus behind the Medicaid decision to reimburse for alcohol and drug screening services was the recognition of the number of people who go unidentified who are in need of an intervention or treatment" (Medscape Medical News, 2006). In addition to the fact that so few substance abusers seek treatment, the other compelling reason behind these two new codes appears to be financial. It is estimated that conducting alcohol and drug SBIs in clinical settings will save the federal Medicaid budget $520 million annually. Given scarce medical resources and health care cost containment, such savings could be used in a stepped-care manner where the first intervention is minimal, of low intensity, least costly, likely to be effective, and has consumer appeal (Sobell & Sobell, 2000). For those where such interventions are successful, their further progress need only be monitored. For those where it was not effective, their care could be stepped up (i.e., more intensive treatment) using some of the savings from the SBIs. Such thinking is consistent with a stepped-care model of treatment (Davison, 2000; Foulds & Jarvis, 1995; Sobell & Sobell, 2000). In summary, successful methods of promoting self–change would allow for widespread impact on substance use problems and at a much lower cost than traditional treatment.

Self–Change Approaches

Self-change approaches have long been part of many brief interventions that help substance abusers evaluate and guide their own behavior change (Apodaca & Miller, 2003; Fleming & Manwell, 1999; Heather, 1994; Heather, Rollnick, Bell, & Richmond, 1996; Sitharthan, Kavanagh, & Sayer, 1996; Sobell & Sobell, 1993, 1999). Factors associated with the development of self-change approaches have included: (a) the need for interventions for individuals whose substance use problems are not severe, particularly those with alcohol problems (Sobell & Sobell, 1993, 1999, 2005), (b) demonstrations that, for many individuals, brief interventions are as beneficial as more intense interventions (Bien, Miller, & Tonigan, 1993; Fleming & Manwell, 1999; Miller et al., 1995; Moyer, Finney, Swearingen, & Vergun, 2002; Project MATCH Research Group, 1998a, b; Saunders, Kypri, Walters, Laforge, & Larimer, 2004; Sobell, Breslin, & Sobell, 1998), and (c) an emphasis on self-control processes in the evolution of cognitive–behavior therapy (e.g., Mahoney & Lyddon, 1988; Thoresen & Mahoney, 1974).

The success of brief self-change treatments for substance abusers suggests that even before entering treatment such individuals possess sufficient skills to function effectively (Sobell & Sobell, 1998). This, in turn, suggests that the major role of these treatments might be motivational; that is, they serve to catalyze people's use of their own resources to bring about behavior change. In a study that provides some support for the idea that self–change approaches and minimal interventions might appeal to adult drinkers, Werch (1990) found that over one-quarter of all drinkers reported an interest in receiving aids to help them drink more moderately. Moreover, drinkers who were interested in receiving one or more self-help aids reported high levels of drinking and a greater motivation to limit their alcohol use. This study suggests that a considerable number of drinkers, especially heavier drinkers, would be receptive to aids to help them drink less.

A nontraditional way of facilitating self-change with regard to excessive drinking has been through the use of very brief interventions by physicians in primary care health settings. These interventions usually consist of a short inquiry followed by brief advice and feedback when warranted. An important characteristic of these interventions is that although typically the patients' reasons for visiting their physician have nothing to do with their alcohol use, as part of the visit doctors can ask an individual about their alcohol use and determine if a patient's drinking exceeds recommended guidelines (Dawson, Grant, & Li, 2005; National Institute on Alcohol Abuse and Alcoholism, 1995, 2007). At this point, physicians can then raise concerns (e.g., "cutting back on your alcohol use might be helpful in lowering your hypertension levels") and suggest that patients reduce their drinking to recommended levels. Such interventions have produced significant decreases in drinking, and they can reach a much broader population than that served by traditional substance abuse programs (Fleming & Manwell, 1999; Fleming et al., 2000, 2002; National Institute on Alcohol Abuse and Alcoholism, 2007; Wutzke, Shiell, Gomel, & Conigrave, 2001). Minimal interventions can also be conducted by correspondence or e-mail for individuals unwilling to come into treatment, in addition to those unable to attend treatment for other reasons such as transportation problems, lack of available child care, or living in rural areas (Breslin, Sobell, Sobell, Buchan, & Kwan, 1996; Jeffery, Hellerstedt, & Schmid, 1990; Lando et al., 1997; Ramelson, Friedman, & Ockene, 1999; Sitharthan et al., 1996; Zhu et al., 1996).

Several studies have reported positive outcomes using media campaigns to reduce the prevalence of smoking (Campion, Owen, Mcneill, & Mcguire, 1994; Giffen, 1991; Hughes, Cummings, & Hyland, 1999; Killen, Fortmann, Newman, & Varady, 1990; Lichtenstein, Lando, & Nothwehr, 1994; Pirie, Rooney, Pechacek, Lando, & Schmid, 1997; Utz, Shuster, Merwin, & Williams, 1994; Warner, 1981, 1989). Typically, these studies involved large-scale ad campaigns that either addressed the health risks of smoking or derided the positive value of smoking behavior (e.g., it's not cool to smoke). Interestingly, large community interventions or mass media campaigns aimed at secondary prevention have almost exclusively targeted smokers. With one exception (Sobell, Cunningham, Sobell, et al., 1996), campaigns for other addictive behaviors (e.g., alcohol or drug problems, gambling) have been noticeably lacking. Finally, another new and promising way of accessing the community on a large scale is through the Internet (Alemi et al., 1996; Wright, Williams, & Partridge, 1999).

In a review of brief interventions, Heather (1989) concluded:

Evidence shows that brief interventions are effective and should be used for individuals who are not actively seeking help at specialist agencies. This justification is, again independent of level of seriousness, although most recipients of community-based interventions will obviously have problems of a less severe variety. (p. 366)

Over a decade later, a meta-analytic review of controlled trials of brief interventions for alcohol problems reached similar conclusions (Moyer et al., 2002).

Tailored Nontraditional Messages

Several studies have shown that the overwhelming reason that people give for either not entering or delaying entering treatment is because of the stigma associated with being labeled (Chiauzzi & Liljegren, 1993; Corrigan, 2004; Cunningham, Sobell, & Chow, 1993; Cunningham, Sobell, Sobell, Agrawal, & Toneatto, 1993; Grant, 1997).

Naturally Recovered Alcohol Abusers Dislike Labels

Respondent 1: "'You are an alcoholic.' People had suggested it to me before but I never really — I had vehemently denied the idea you know or the accusation."

Respondent 2: "So the desire is gone and this is where I part company with Alcoholics Anonymous and people like them, because they operate on a naturalistic bias. A naturalistic way whereas not necessarily Alcoholics Anonymous, because AA started as a Christian organization. But they say you are always an alcoholic."

In the addiction field, if researchers are to develop programs and messages that are perceived as attractive and listened to rather than avoided, then it will be necessary to understand why many individuals even with minimal alcohol and drug problems do not seek treatment. First, studies have demonstrated that

---

Naturally Recovered Individuals Tell Us What Would Attract Them to Treatment

Question: "If an ad were to appear on television or in a newspaper to attract individuals to seek help with their drinking problem, what wording would you suggest?"

Respondent 1: "If you could say something I guess maybe to indicate something like 'You can do it.' 'Help yourself, you can do it.' Something to give them some assurance that all is not lost."

Respondent 2: "Well, that's an interesting question. I would say something that would offer some comfort and dignity to the listener. The words that come to my mind, 'Are you sure?'"

Respondent 3: "People who drink too much are done a disservice by the use of the word 'alcoholic.'"

Respondent 4: "I would say more along the lines of getting people to realize they have a problem. Something like 'Do you drink every day? If you do, you may have a problem.' A nonthreatening thing that would say, that somebody might say 'You know I do drink every day' and then they might make a concerted effort to not drink every day. Something very simple. Not going into the blackouts and all. It's nonthreatening. Just saying 'Do you drink every day?' Not using scare tactics, just using the tactics of be aware."

---

labels such as "alcoholic" and "addict" should be avoided. In fact, negative messages like these are likely to be perceived as inaccurate by high-risk drinkers in the general population. Consistent with the literature, highly effective messages are those that avoid stigmatizing or labeling. Second, the message needs to be proactive. Third, the message should contain information that allows people to make better, more informed decisions about their alcohol consumption.

Because the addiction field has long been dominated by an almost exclusive focus on individuals who are severely dependent on alcohol, the general public, particularly in North America, has developed a stereotypic and stigmatizing impression of anyone who drinks excessively; such individuals are viewed as alcoholics, unable to recover without treatment, and not capable of returning to moderate drinking. In a very recent general population telephone study, respondents ($N = 3006$) were asked about their beliefs concerning drinking problems. It was found that fewer than half (41.5%) felt that someone with an alcohol problem could recover without treatment, and less than one-third (29%) felt such individuals could return to moderate drinking (Cunningham, Blomqvist, & Cordingley, 2007). Several other studies have also reported that the general public does not believe that untreated and moderate drinking outcomes are possible (Cunningham et al., 2007; Cunningham, Sobell, & Chow, 1993; Ferris, 1994; Nadeau, 1997). Furthermore, in two early natural recovery studies (Shaffer & Jones, 1989; Sobell, Sobell, & Toneatto, 1992), researchers reported that several respondents during their interviews asked if they were the only ones who had recovered "this way" (i.e., on their own). Lastly, one study (Cunningham, Sobell, & Sobell, 1998) reported that there was a significantly greater reluctance to self-disclose resolving an alcohol problem compared with quitting smoking cigarettes (23.7% versus 5.1%); the predominant reason (57.1%) for not wanting to talk to others was the stigma or label attached to having an alcohol problem. While self-change is the major pathway to recovery from alcohol problems, most studies suggest that the majority of people are unaware of this fact. In summary, given the beliefs held by the general populace, coupled with those who recover on their own, it is not surprising that trying to persuade someone with an alcohol problem in the general population that they can change on their own might be difficult. The fact that people hold beliefs that are not evidence-based suggests that we need to educate consumers, particularly that not everyone needs to enter treatment and that self-change is a legitimate and predominant pathway to change.

In many ways, attempting to persuade high-risk drinkers to reduce their drinking can be viewed as an exercise in attitude change. Research in cognitive social psychology tells us that when individuals receive a message with which they

---

Naturally Recovered Alcohol Abuser

"Well, as I mentioned previously I had tried to stop on several occasions previously and I would stop maybe for a short or fairly prolonged period of time but then I would fall back into the regular routine. So, at the end in 1960 I just made up my mind very determinedly that this thing wasn't going to beat me, I was going to beat it because it was ruining my relationship with my family. And sooner or later it was going to have an effect on my work."

disagree, they resist it by various means, such as formulating counterarguments (Perloff, 1993). For example, if people who are high-risk drinkers are told, "You are an alcoholic" or "You have an alcohol problem," they are likely to react by generating reasons why they are not. The message does not make sense to them. The way to avoid such counterarguments is to present the message in a nonconfrontational and nonthreatening manner, which is the same strategy used in motivational interviewing in clinical situations (Miller & Rollnick, 2002; Substance Abuse and Mental Health Administration, 2002). When recruiting problem drinkers into treatment or getting individuals to respond to advertisements about changing their drinking on their own, what has been learned is that the "content" of the message is critical.

Over the years, whether in Canada, Australia, the United States, Sweden, or Mexico, studies have recruited alcohol and drug abusers to treatment by using carefully worded statements to attract such individuals. The ads for treatment typically contain phrases such as "Are you concerned about your alcohol or drug use?" or "Are you considering changing your drinking?" (Klingemann, 1991; Miller & Hester, 1980; Miller, Taylor, & West, 1980; Pearlman, Zweben, & Li, 1989; Sobell & Sobell, 1998, 2005).

Many studies have now shown that untreated and naturally recovered substance abusers report several reasons for not seeking treatment or not seeking treatment promptly (Cunningham, Sobell, & Chow, 1993; Cunningham, Sobell, & Freedman, 1994; Cunningham, Sobell, Sobell, et al., 1993; Grant, 1997; Hingson, Mangione, Meyers, & Scotch, 1982; Roizen, 1977; Sobell, Sobell, & Toneatto, 1992; Tuchfeld, 1981). As already mentioned, among the most salient reasons are the stigma associated with the label "alcoholic" or admitting to being an alcoholic (Copeland, 1997; Cunningham et al., 1998; Cunningham, Sobell, Sobell, et al., 1993; Grant, 1997; Roizen, 1977; Sobell et al., 1992; Tuchfeld, 1981). Two other major reasons given for not seeking treatment are of interest. In a general population survey, 96% of respondents who ever had a problem reported they thought they could handle their problem on their own (Hingson et al., 1982). We found similar evidence in our own research (Sobell et al., 1992), in that 38% of naturally recovered alcohol abusers reported that they did not enter treatment because they thought they could solve their problem on their own. In fact, this reason was rated as most influential in their decision not to seek treatment. The second reason that very frequently has been given for not seeking treatment is that problem drinkers have "felt their problem was not serious enough" to seek help (Hingson et al., 1982; Miller, Sovereign, & Krege, 1988; Sobell et al., 1992; Thom, 1986). In the Hingson et al. study, 84% responded in such a manner, as did 46% in our own research. Taken collectively, and combined with the effect of stigma, these studies convincingly demonstrate significant barriers associated with seeking treatment.

In conclusion, a concern articulated in the literature over a decade ago is still salient today: "these barriers must be addressed if we want to encourage the greater proportion of untreated alcohol and drug abusers to seek treatment" (Cunningham, Sobell, Sobell, et al., 1993, p. 353). Changing public perceptions to recognize that self-change is possible and is the predominate pathway to change for many with an addictive behavior is critical, as is the need to provide alternative, nontraditional interventions. Because traditional treatment approaches in the substance abuse field have been hypothesized as deterring problem drinkers—those with less severe problems—from seeking treatment (Sobell & Sobell, 1993), interventions need to be tailored to the needs of different types of drinkers. Finally, it is interesting to note that adults with serious mental illness in a U.S. survey and substance abusers reported similar reasons for not seeking treatment (Substance Abuse and Mental Health Administration, 2003). Besides cost (50.4%), 28.2% of respondents reported that stigma kept them from seeking treatment and 10.4% said they did not feel a need for treatment or that they could handle their problems without treatment.

With respect to prevention and harm reduction, the same reasoning underlying motivational interventions can be used with the general public (Nadeau, 1997; Rehm, 1997). In fact, how messages are presented and what those messages say is probably even more important with substance users in the general population than with self-identified problem users who are considering changing. The reason is that substance abusers in the general public do not perceive themselves as needing to change. Thus, they should be more resistant to messages suggesting change than would be substance abusers who are already ambivalent about their alcohol or drug use. Because many untreated problem drinkers do not view their drinking as serious enough to warrant seeking treatment, one suggestion is to modify drinkers' beliefs about the normality of their drinking. Providing individuals with feedback about their drinking and where it fits in relation to national norms can be viewed as advice feedback that is intended to promote self–change by getting the person to view their heavy drinking from a new perspective. Support for providing this type of feedback also comes from a general population survey where most respondents said they first recognized a problem by recognizing the volume of their intake (Hingson et al., 1982).

For a message to be considered by, and have an impact on, an individual, it is important that the message does not evoke resistance. For example, because a small amount of drinking can have a cardiovascular protective effect (Hanna, Chou, & Grant, 1997; Svärdsudd, 1998), a proactive prevention message could be created describing the beneficial effects of limited drinking, but emphasizing that like so many other aspects of our lives, there needs to be a healthy balance between what you get out of drinking and the risks that are taken. A proactive message is less likely to evoke resistance compared with a critical message. In this regard, several years ago Éduc'alcool, an independent, not-for-profit organization, in Montreal, Quebec, Canada, designed a secondary prevention program, "Alco-Choix" (translated "Drinking Choices") that allowed for moderation goals. To solicit individuals for the program, they designed Ad 1 shown in Figure 8.1. In English the ad says: "You are not an Alcoholic. You just drink a little too much but do not want to completely stop either. P.CRA can help you. Inquire here about the Alcohol Consumption Program." The logo at the bottom says: "Moderation tastes better."

Ad 1

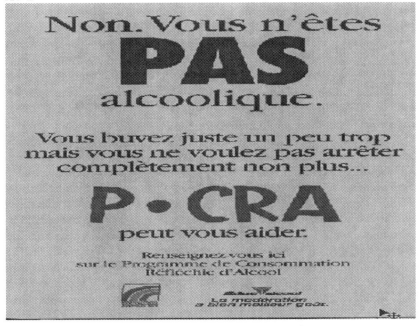

Ad 2

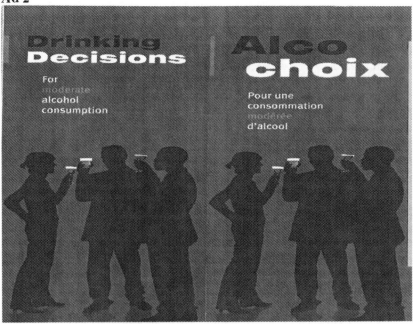

FIGURE 8.1. The tone of an advertisement can make a difference.

After running this ad regularly for slightly more than 2 years, they abandoned it because they had only received 38 registrations. Demonstrating that the tone of a message makes a big difference, they then used Ad 2 in Figure 8.1 and received more than 500 calls over a 5-year period. They concluded the proactive ad was a "huge success" (H. Sacy, Director General, Éduc'alcool, personal communication, October 17, 2003).

In summary, early intervention trials for prevention and harm reduction suggest that it is very important to create a message, and a system for delivering that message, that will be accepted by the intended target audience.

A Community Mail Intervention: Background and Rationale

The Promoting Self-Change (PSC) study, a community based mail intervention funded through the National Institute on Alcohol Abuse and Alcoholism, was conducted in Canada (Sobell, Cunningham, Sobell, et al., 1996). This large-scale community intervention was designed to promote self-change among individuals who were unwilling, not ready, or otherwise unmotivated to access the formal health care system in order to change their drinking. As will be discussed later, while the PSC intervention was designed for problem drinkers, several aspects of the project are relevant to prevention and harm reduction. For example, avenues and procedures that will attract individuals in the general public to consider changing their drinking on their own or with minimal help are likely to be very different from what traditional practices in the alcohol field would suggest. Finally, although the PSC community trial targeted problem drinkers, community interventions have also been successful with cigarette smokers, and therefore, there is every reason to extend and evaluate such trials to individuals with other addictive behaviors.

The PSC intervention represents a convergence of two lines of research. The first involved studies that examined the natural recovery processes with alcohol abusers (Sobell et al., 2001; Sobell, Sobell, Toneatto, & Leo, 1993), and the second involved clinical trials using a Guided Self-Change model of treatment with problem drinkers (Sobell & Sobell, 1993, 1998, 2005). This community-based intervention was designed to take account of three factors found to be associated with heavy drinkers who do not seek treatment or formal help (reviewed in Sobell, Cunningham, Sobell, et al., 1996): (a) stigma or embarrassment of being in treatment for alcohol problems, (b) the desire to change on one's own, and (c) little belief by the general public that self-change is a viable pathway to recovery. The PSC project used several key elements from Guided Self-Change treatment (e.g., Decisional Balance Exercise, Brief Situational Confidence Questionnaire, Timeline Drinking Advice/Feedback; Sobell & Sobell, 1993, 1998) and made them available by mail to individuals in the community who wanted to change their drinking on their own.

The PSC intervention was designed to help problem drinkers analyze their own problems and guide their own change. After the assessment materials were completed and returned by mail, the respondents in the experimental condition were sent a set of personalized feedback materials based on their assessment responses relating to their drinking levels, high-risk situations, and motivation for change (see Appendix A in Sobell, Cunningham, Sobell et al., 1996). Participants assigned to the control group were sent two educational pamphlets available in the community rather than personalized feedback. The sample consists of 825 respondents recruited primarily through newspaper advertisements.

An Empirically Crafted Advertisement

As discussed earlier, when creating a message that will be accepted by the intended target audience (in the present study this was problem drinkers who have never been in treatment and who might be reluctant to seek traditional alcohol treatment services), the message cannot evoke resistance or it will be ignored and thus be ineffective. In this regard, the advertisement for the PSC study contained three messages, all of which were chosen to address issues or concerns we had anticipated in recruiting a group of heavy drinkers who had never accessed the health care system for their drinking. The first line of the ad, "Thinking About Changing Your Drinking?" was chosen because it was felt that this message would not evoke resistance, would prompt people to think about their drinking, and attract the attention of those already thinking about changing. The second line read, "Do you know that 75% of people change their drinking on their own?" This message was chosen because, despite the fact that some Canadian studies (Cunningham, 1999; Sobell, Cunningham, & Sobell, 1996) had shown that over 75% of individuals with an alcohol problem change their drinking without formal treatment or AA (as noted earlier), the general public is still skeptical about the idea that individuals can change on their own (Cunningham et al., 1994, 2007; Cunningham, Sobell, & Chow, 1993; Rush & Allen, 1997). Furthermore, this message clearly puts forth the concept of empowerment (Dickerson, 1998), a message with a proactive approach. The third line, "Call us for free materials you can complete at home" was chosen because, as discussed earlier, one of the major reasons that people have given for not entering treatment was that they wanted to change their drinking on their own (Hingson et al., 1982; Sobell et al., 1993). Thus, the ad made clear that respondents would not need to come to a treatment program. Lastly, the fact that in slightly over a year almost 2,500 people called in response to the ads, suggests that the message was effective in recruiting the target population. A copy of this advertisement appears in Figure 8.2.

Eligible respondents meet the following study criteria: (a) be of legal drinking age (i.e., 19 years old in Ontario, Canada), (b) no prior history of alcohol treatment or self-help such as AA or SMART Recovery (to insure

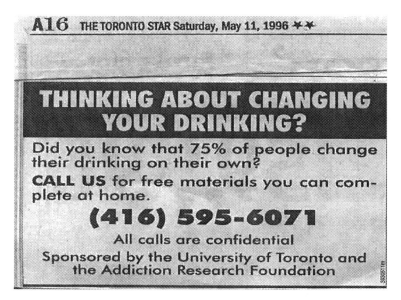

FIGURE 8.2. Promoting self-change study: ad used to recruit participants.

that severely dependent alcohol abusers were not included), and (c) report drinking an average of 12 or more drinks per week or having consumed 5 or more drinks on at least 5 days in the past year. Of the 2,434 individuals who responded to the media solicitations, almost three-quarters (i.e., 72%) met the initial screening criteria and were sent a consent form and assessment materials. The major reasons respondents were ineligible were (a) 90% reported they had previously received some type of treatment or help and (b) 7% were ineligible because of the drinking criteria (i.e., their drinking was not heavy enough to meet the study criteria). Of those meeting the initial screening criteria and mailed the assessment packages, 47% (825) individuals returned their questionnaires and were randomly assigned to one of the two groups. One third of the participants were women and there were no gender differences in terms of the screening criteria.

Eligible participants were randomly assigned to one of two interventions: (a) the Motivational Enhancement/Personalized Feedback (MEPF) condition ($n = 414$), where individuals received personalized advice/feedback based on their assessment of their drinking and related behaviors or (b) the Bibliotherapy/ Drinking Guidelines (BDG) condition ($n = 411$), where participants received two pamphlets on effects of alcohol and guidelines for low-risk drinking and self-monitoring. The experimental intervention (MEPF) was a motivational intervention. Based on the answers from their assessment materials, respondents were sent personalized feedback and a decisional balance exercise, all intended to enhance their motivation to change (Sobell, Cunningham, Sobell, et al., 1996).

Although the control group (BDG) completed the same questionnaires as those in the experimental group, no personalized feedback was provided until their 12-month follow-up interview was completed. Similar to studies in the smoking field (Becoña & Vazquez, 2001; Brandon, Collins, Juliano, & Lazev, 2000; Curry, McBride, Grothaus, Louie, & Wagner, 1995; Ershoff, Quinn, & Mullen, 1995), BDG respondents were given two self-help pamphlets that were freely available in the local community. These pamphlets provided information about the nature of alcohol abuse, about monitoring one's alcohol use, and general advice on how people could deal with their alcohol problem.

PSC Study Results

Of the original 825 participants in the PSC community trial, 79.6% (657; MEPF = 321, BDG = 336) were located for follow-up, a rate similar to that of other large brief intervention and clinical trials (Babor et al., 1996; Edwards & Rollnick, 1997; Fleming et al., 2002; Grant, Arciniega, Tonigan, Miller, & Meyers, 1997; Project MATCH Research Group, 1998c). As reported previously, significant reductions in drinking from 1 year pre- to 1 year postintervention occurred for both groups, but no significant group differences were found for any drinking variables (Sobell et al., 2002). Thus, it appears that the intervention materials for both groups, irrespective of whether they were personalized, facilitated the reduction of drinking.

What Triggered the Change Process?

Although the results in the community trial were unexpected, the question is why both interventions worked equally well. First, it is possible that those who respond to advertisements are ready to change irrespective of the materials used. In this regard, BDG participants were given two informational self-help pamphlets, one of which instructed them only to self-monitor their drinking and provided explicit guidelines for low-risk drinking. Perhaps participants in this group self-monitored their drinking and consequences and recognized that their drinking exceeded recommended guidelines and self-corrected. In contrast, while those in the MEPF group were not given targets for low risk drinking, they received implicit information about the amount of their drinking as compared with national norms and they were asked what changes they wanted to make to their current alcohol use. While several other possible explanations can be posited for changes in participants' drinking, because we used the Timeline Followback (Sobell & Sobell, 1992) to collect drinking data on a continuous calendar from 1 year prior to the intervention through the assessment, to 1 year postintervention, and because we had the dates when all participants originally called in to the ad, completed their assessment, and were sent the intervention materials, we were able to further evaluate when the changes in drinking behavior might have occurred.

Responding to Advertisements: A Critical Event in Promoting Self-Change

Because both participant groups were equally effective in changing drinking behavior, it was concluded that the motivational materials given to the experimental group had no added benefit beyond the two informational pamphlets given to the control group. Therefore, the key question we wanted to address was what caused changes in drinking? To further explore what might be the critical event behind the significant reduction in drinking for this community sample, three testable hypotheses were examined. The first related to evaluating whether completing the detailed assessment materials might have affected all participants equally strongly such that neither intervention would have an appreciable added effect on changing drinking.

For several years now, there has been speculation in the addiction field that lengthy assessments and follow-up interviews might drive or at least start the change process (Bien et al., 1993; Clifford & Maisto, 2000; Clifford, Maisto, Franzke, Longabaugh, & Beattie, 2000). In this regard, for many years it has long been thought that the intensive assessment in Project MATCH contributed to the lack of treatment results (DiClemente, Carroll, Connors, & Kadden, 1994). Unfortunately, the Project MATCH researchers, as with most researchers in the alcohol field, did not collect detailed data that would allow for tracking when change occurred.

Until recently, little attention has been given to possible changes in drinking behavior due to reactivity. While a handful of studies have started to examine reactive effects due to assessments and follow-up interviews, the results have been mixed. Some studies have provided some indirect evidence that assessments and follow-ups may reduce alcohol use (Chang, Wilkins-Haug, Berman, & Goetz, 1999; Clifford et al., 2000; Connors, Tarbox, & Faillace, 1992; Epstein et al., 2005; McCambridge & Strang, 2005), while others have not (Hester & Delaney, 1997; Maisto, Sobell, Sobell, & Sanders; 1985; Ogborne & Annis, 1988; Stephens, Roffman, & Curtin, 2000; Timko, Moos, Finney, Moos, & Kaplowitz, 1999).

The second testable hypothesis related to whether the decision to respond to the ad or the brief screening interview by phone precipitated changes in drinking. The third hypothesis was that changes in the drinking behavior occurred shortly before participants responded to the ad (i.e., a month preceding the call, perhaps owing to a significant life event). As noted earlier, because this study used the Timeline Followback (Sobell & Sobell, 1992, 2003) to collect daily drinking data for long periods of time before, during, and after the interventions, it was possible to evaluate these hypotheses using the data already collected. Lastly, because there were no significant differences between the two groups or for gender, data for all participants were combined for subsequent analyses.

For all drinking variables, it was found that the major reduction occurred between seeing the advertisement and talking to the interviewer during the brief telephone screening, but before the assessment materials were received (Sobell et al., 2003; Sobell, Agrawal, Sobell, & Leo, in preparation). There are two possible reasons for why the change occurred at this time: (a) seeing the ad and then waiting for assessment materials could have facilitated change by increasing participants' motivation to change and (b) the brief telephone eligibility screening in response to the ads may have triggered a process of self-evaluation leading to a decision to change (i.e., first line of the ad "Thinking of Changing Your Drinking?" was chosen because it was felt that this message would get people to think about their drinking). Further, both of the above processes could have jointly contributed to the change as well.

Near the end of the study, we became interested in what was attracting callers to the ads. After being screened for the study, 26.1% (458/1,756) of the remaining eligible callers were asked, "When you saw the ad, what about it attracted you, and led you to call us?" Callers who provided more than one reason were asked, "Which one was most important?" Responses from the 458 callers were coded as follows: (a) 31.7% (n = 145) said it was the title of the ad—"Thinking About Changing Your Drinking?", (b) 28.2% (n = 129) said it was the statement that "Did you know that 75% of people change their drinking on their own?", (c) 12.0% (n = 55) said they wanted to change at home and did not want to come in to treatment, (d) 9.8% (n = 45) said they just "saw the ad and called," (e) 9.2% (n = 42) gave other reasons, (f) 4.4% (n = 20) said it was the "sponsorship by the University of Toronto/Addiction Research Foundation," (g) 1.7% (n = 8) said it was because we offered "free materials," (h) 1.7% (n = 8) said it was because we promised "All calls are confidential," and (i) 1.3% (n = 6) said it was because it was "not AA." Two very distinct statements in the ads (thinking of changing your drinking and learning that the vast majority, 75%, of people with alcohol problems change on their own) were reported by 60% of callers as the reasons they had been attracted to the ad.

Finally, at the end of the 1-year follow-up, each participant was asked to indicate the most helpful parts of the program from a list. A year after the intervention, participants rated the following as the most helpful aspect of the program: (a) Seeing the ad and deciding to call: 45.0% (195/433), (b) Completing the initial questionnaire about my drinking, related consequences, and confidence: 23.1% (100/433), (c) Reading the program materials: 19.0% (82/433), (d) Making the call and talking to the interviewer: 6.9% (30/433), (e) Follow-up reminder letters: 3.5% (15/433), (f) Having the program materials to look over: 1.4% (6/433), and (g) Other: 1.2% (5/433), Thus, 1 year after the intervention, close to one-half of all participants felt that seeing the ad and deciding to call was the most helpful aspect of the program. This is particularly interesting given that 60% of participants after being screened into the study, when asked to name the most important thing that attracted them to the advertisements said that it was one of two statements ("thinking about changing your drinking" or "75% of people change … on their own").

Smoking cessation research may help explain the results of the PSC study. Despite the fact that major organizations like the American Lung Association, American Cancer Society, U.S. Surgeon General, and American Psychiatric Association recommend that smokers set a quit date (American Lung Association, 2007; Fisher, 1998; Hughes et al., 1996; U.S. Department of Health and Human Services, 2000), until recently, little has been known about planned versus unplanned quit attempts (Larabie, 2005). Two very recent studies (Larabie, 2005; West & Sohal, 2006) found that close to one half of smokers' quit attempts were unplanned, and that the unplanned attempts were more successful than the planned attempts (West & Sohal, 2006). To explain how this may have happened, West and Sohal (2006) use catastrophe theory, a branch of mathematics that suggests that tensions develop in systems such that "even small triggers can lead to sudden 'catastrophic' changes" (p. 8). For smokers, West and Sohal propose "that beliefs, past experiences, and the current situation create varying levels of 'motivational tension'" (p. 8), where small triggers can change a motivational state (i.e., smoking cessation that was not planned prior to the trigger). Using such reasoning, one possible explanation for why PSC participants changed their drinking behavior when they saw the ad is that while they had been thinking about changing their drinking (motivational tension), like many people in the general public they did not know or believe that problem drinkers do not have to enter treatment in order to change. Thus, seeing the ad functioned as a catalyst (i.e., trigger) to implement a self-change process.

In conclusion, the findings from the PSC study strongly suggest that the change mechanism that prompted participants to respond to the study, and, according to their reports, may have led them to change their drinking behavior relates to some aspect of the wording of the advertisement. If future research confirms that advertisements motivate people to change their drinking, such low cost, low intensity interventions could have broad public health applicability.

Public Health Implications of Community Interventions

Regardless of how the changes in drinking were achieved, it is clear that a large-scale intervention can produce substantial benefits with little cost. The present community-level mail intervention is consistent with an efficient approach to improving public health where individuals are first provided with an intervention that is minimally intrusive on their lifestyle, yet has a reasonable chance of success (Sobell & Sobell, 2000). The present findings suggest that a low-cost population-level approach has the opportunity of reaching large numbers of individuals who are otherwise unwilling, not ready, or not motivated to access the formal health care system. If such an approach was widely used, it could generate enormous health and related benefits. In this regard, it was estimated recently that the cost savings of screening and brief interventions introduced as part of the new Medicaid codes could result in a net savings of $520 million annually for the federal government (Medscape Medical News, 2006). A population approach to alcohol problems, however, would represent a shift from the alcohol field's longstanding clinical focus to a broader public health perspective.

Given the positive results for both groups, it is reasonable to speculate that the change in participants' behavior occurred earlier than would have happened without the intervention, and therefore the anticipated costs of these participants' alcohol problems to society were reduced. For those for whom the intervention does not work, the level of care can be stepped up (i.e., more treatment or an alternative treatment). In this regard, close to one-quarter of the participants who were located for the 1-year follow-up reported they had their first help-seeking experience during that follow-up year (Sobell et al., 2002). This finding suggests that individuals whose problems were not resolved through the current self-help mail intervention and who felt they needed more help engaged in their own stepped care by seeking help rather than letting their problem worsen. The public health implications of interventions like the one reported here have been succinctly articulated in an article by Humphreys and Tucker (2002) who have called for more responsive and effective intervention systems for alcohol-related problems. In arguing that "[a]lcohol intervention systems are often unresponsive to the full range of problems, resources, treatment preferences, goals, motivations and behavior-change pathways with the affected population" (p. 127), they assert that "systems should enhance the accessibility, appeal and diversity of services" (p. 128). Lastly, they suggest four avenues by which this can be accomplished: (a) not only should interventions be targeted at drinkers with less serious alcohol problems, but they should also be disseminated more broadly, including through nonspecialty health care and community settings, (b) although untested, Telehealth services could reach a large percentage of problem drinkers who have not accessed the formal health care system (American Psychological Association, 2000; Jerome et al., 2000), (c) rather than waiting for individuals to cross the clinical threshold, wider, more active, and novel approaches for getting individuals to consider looking at their alcohol use are needed, and (d) receipt of services should be more rapid, address the person's concerns, be more flexible (e.g., goal choice), and meet people where they are on the readiness-to-change continuum. This radical shift in thinking, viewing alcohol problems as a public health issue, while new to many in the alcohol field, was advocated by the Institute of Medicine over a decade ago (Institute of Medicine, 1990). The findings from the PSC study strongly suggest that such an approach is feasible. Another example of successfully addressing alcohol problems from a public health approach comes from results of the first annual National Alcohol Screening Day in 1999 (Greenfield et al., 2003). At the 1,089 sites, 18,043 were screened, 5,595 were referred for treatment, and of those screened only 13% had reported previous alcohol treatment.

Conclusion and Future Directions

Prevention and early intervention strategies need to be developed that are perceived as attractive and are sought out rather than avoided. Despite the considerable cost to society of substance use and related problems, many individuals whose substance use might place them at risk have not experienced any consequences and do not consider their use as a problem. The Prompting Self-Change intervention described in this chapter was designed to appeal to such individuals. In fact, this intervention is consistent with an efficient approach to public health care where individuals are first provided with an intervention that is least intrusive on their lifestyle yet has a reasonable chance of success (Sobell et al., 2002; Sobell & Sobell, 1999). This and similar approaches have the opportunity of reaching large numbers of individuals who are otherwise unwilling, not ready, or not motivated to access the formal health care system. If such interventions succeed, it is reasonable to speculate that the change in respondents' behavior will have occurred earlier than would otherwise be expected, and therefore that the anticipated costs of these individuals' substance use problems to society will be reduced. If the initial intervention does not work, then the level of care can be stepped up (i.e., more treatment or an alternative treatment). Moreover, if interventions like the one just described are successful, they could then be employed and evaluated in a number of other settings (e.g., health care clinics, high schools and colleges, military bases) and with a variety of addictive behaviors (e.g., drug use, gambling).

Lastly, it is very clear that additional research is critically needed to examine different mechanisms of change beyond treatment effects. Until then, reactivity of any type will confound results and limit the interpretation of findings.

References

Alemi, F., Mosavel, M., Stephens, R. C., Ghadiri, A., Krishnaswamy, J., & Thakkar, H. (1996). Electronic self-help and support groups. *Medical Care, 34*(10 Suppl.), 32–44.

American Lung Association. (2007, January 11). Plan your quit day. Ready to quit? Here are 4 steps to a smoke-free future (Retrieved January 11, 2007, from http://www.cancer.org/docroot/PED/content/PED_10_7_Committing_To_Quit.asp

American Psychological Association. (2000, April). Psychology and the Internet. *Monitor on Psychology, 31*, 1–136.

Apodaca, T. R., & Miller, W. R. (2003). A meta-analysis of the effectiveness of bibliotherapy for alcohol problems. *Journal of Consulting and Clinical Psychology, 59*, 289–304.

Babor, T. F., Acuda, W., Campillo, C., Del Boca, F. K., Grant, M., Hodgson, R., et al. (1996). A cross-national trial of brief interventions with heavy drinkers. *American Journal of Public Health, 86*, 948–955.

Becoña, E., & Vazquez, F. L. (2001). Effectiveness of personalized written feedback through a mail intervention for smoking cessation: A randomized-controlled trial in Spanish smokers. *Journal of Consulting and Clinical Psychology, 69*, 33–40.

Bien, T. H., Miller, W. R., & Tonigan, J. S. (1993). Brief interventions for alcohol problems: A review. *Addiction, 88*, 315–336.

Brandon, T. H., Collins, B. N., Juliano, L. M., & Lazev, A. B. (2000). Preventing relapse among former smokers: A comparison of minimal interventions through telephone and mail. *Journal of Consulting and Clinical Psychology, 68*, 103–113.

Breslin, C., Sobell, L. C., Sobell, M. B., Buchan, G., & Kwan, E. (1996). Aftercare telephone contacts with problem drinkers can serve a clinical and research function. *Addiction, 91*, 1359–1364.

Campion, P., Owen, L., Mcneill, A., & Mcguire, C. (1994). Evaluation of a mass media campaign on smoking and pregnancy. *Addiction, 89*, 1245–1254.

Chang, G., Wilkins-Haug, L., Berman, S., & Goetz, M. A. (1999). Brief intervention for alcohol use in pregnancy: A randomized trial. *Addiction, 94*, 1499–1508.

Chiauzzi, E. J., & Liljegren, S. (1993). Taboo topics in addiction treatment: An empirical review of clinical folklore. *Journal of Substance Abuse Treatment, 10*, 303–316.

Clifford, P. R., & Maisto, S. A. (2000). Subject reactivity effects and alcohol treatment outcome research. *Journal of Studies on Alcohol, 61*, 787–793.

Clifford, P. R., Maisto, S. A., Franzke, L. H., Longabaugh, R., & Beattie, M. C. (2000). Alcohol treatment research follow-up interviews and drinking behaviors. *Journal of Studies on Alcohol, 61*, 736–743.

Connors, G. J., Tarbox, A. R., & Faillace, L. A. (1992). Achieving and maintaining gains among problem drinkers: Process and outcome results. *Behavior Therapy, 23*, 449–474.

Copeland, J. (1997). A qualitative study of barriers to formal treatment among women who self-managed change in addictive behaviours. *Journal of Substance Abuse Treatment, 14*, 183–190.

Corrigan, P. (2004). How stigma interferes with mental health care. *American Psychologist, 59*, 614–625.

Cunningham, J. A. (1999). Resolving alcohol-related problems with and without treatment: The effects of different problem criteria. *Journal of Studies on Alcohol, 60*, 463–466.

Cunningham, J. A., Blomqvist, J., & Cordingley, J. (2007). Beliefs about drinking problems: Results from a general population telephone survey. *Addictive Behaviors, 32*, 166–169.

Cunningham, J. A., Sobell, L. C., & Chow, V. M. C. (1993). What's in a label? The effects of substance types and labels on treatment considerations and stigma. *Journal of Studies on Alcohol, 54*, 693–699.

Cunningham, J. A., Sobell, L. C., & Freedman, J. L. (1994). Beliefs about the cause of substance abuse: A comparison of three drugs. *Journal of Substance Abuse, 6*, 219–226.

Cunningham, J. A., Sobell, L. C., & Sobell, M. B. (1998). Awareness of self-change as a pathway to recovery for alcohol abusers: Results from five different groups. *Addictive Behaviors, 23*, 399–404.

Cunningham, J. A., Sobell, L. C., Sobell, M. B., Agrawal, S., & Toneatto, T. (1993). Barriers to treatment: Why alcohol and drug abusers delay or never seek treatment. *Addictive Behaviors, 18*, 347–353.

Curry, S. J., McBride, C., Grothaus, L. C., Louie, D., & Wagner, E. H. (1995). A randomized trial of self-help materials, personalized feedback, and telephone counseling with nonvolunteer smokers. *Journal of Consulting and Clinical Psychology, 63*, 1005–1014.

Davison, G. C. (2000). Stepped care: Doing more with less? *Journal of Consulting and Clinical Psychology, 68*, 580–585.

Dawson, D. A., Grant, B. F., & Li, T.-K. (2005). Quantifying the risks associated with exceeding recommended drinking limits. *Alcoholism: Clinical and Experimental Research, 29*, 902–908.

Dawson, D. A., Grant, B. F., Stinson, F. S., Chou, P. S., Huang, B., & Ruan, W. J. (2005). Recovery from DSM-IV alcohol dependence: United States, 2001–2002. *Addiction, 100*, 281–292.

Dickerson, F. B. (1998). Strategies that foster empowerment. *Cognitive and Behavioral Practice, 5*, 255–275.

DiClemente, C. C., Carroll, K. M., Connors, G. J., & Kadden, R. M. (1994). Process assessment in treatment matching research. *Journal of Studies on Alcohol, Suppl. 12*, 156–162.

Edwards, A. G. K., & Rollnick, S. (1997). Outcome studies of brief alcohol intervention in general practice: The problem of lost subjects. *Addiction, 92*, 1699–1704.

Epstein, E. E., Drapkin, M. L., Yusko, D. A., Cook, S. M., McCrady, B. S., & Jensen, N. K. (2005). Is alcohol assessment therapeutic? Pretreatment change in drinking among alcohol-dependent women. *Journal of Studies on Alcohol, 66*, 369–378.

Ershoff, D. H., Quinn, V. P., & Mullen, P. D. (1995). Relapse prevention among women who stop smoking early in pregnancy: A randomized clinical trial of a self-help intervention. *American Journal of Preventive Medicine, 11*, 178–184.

Ferris, J. (1994, June). *Comparison of public perceptions of alcohol, drug, and other tobacco addictions—moral vs. disease models.* Paper presented at the 20th Annual Alcohol Epidemiology Symposium, Ruschlikon, Switzerland.

Fisher, E. B. (1998). *American Lung Association 7 steps to a smoke-free life* (Paperback). New York: Wiley.

Fleming, M., & Manwell, L. B. (1999). Brief intervention in primary care settings: A primary treatment method for at-risk, problem, and dependent drinkers. *Alcohol Health & Research World, 23*, 128–137.

Fleming, M. F., Mundt, M. P., French, M. T., Manwell, B., Stauffacher, E. A., & Barry, K. L. (2000). Benefit-cost analysis of brief physician advice with problem drinkers in primary care settings. *Medical Care, 38*, 7–18.

Fleming, M. F., Mundt, M. P., French, M. T., Manwell, L. B., Stauffacher, E. A., & Barry, K. L. (2002). Brief physician advice for problem alcohol drinkers: Long-term efficacy and benefit-cost analysis. *Alcoholism: Clinical and Experimental Research, 26*, 36–43.

Foulds, J., & Jarvis, M. J. (1995). Smoking cessation and prevention. In P. Calverley & N. Pride (Eds.), *Chronic obstructive pulmonary disease* (pp. 373–390). London: Chapman & Hall.

Giffen, C. A. (1991). Community intervention trial for smoking cessation (COMMIT): Summary of design and intervention. *Journal of the National Cancer Institute, 83*, 1620–1628.

Grant, B. F. (1997). Barriers to alcoholism treatment: Reasons for not seeking treatment in a general population sample. *Journal of Studies on Alcohol, 58*, 365–371.

Grant, K. A., Arciniega, L. T., Tonigan, J. S., Miller, W. R., & Meyers, R. J. (1997). Are reconstructed self-reports of drinking reliable? *Addiction, 92*, 601–606.

Greenfield, S. F., Keliher, A., Sugarman, D., Kozloff, R., Reizes, J. M., Kopans, B., et al. (2003). Who comes to voluntary, community-based alcohol screening? Results of the first annual National Alcohol Screening Day, 1999. *American Journal of Psychiatry, 160*, 1677–1683.

Hanna, E. Z., Chou, S. P., & Grant, B. F. (1997). Relationship between drinking and heart disease morbidity in the United States: Results from the National Health Interview Survey. *Alcoholism: Clinical and Experimental Research, 21*, 111–118.

Harris, K. M., & Mckellar, J. D. (2003, June). Demand for alcohol treatment. *Frontlines: Linking Alcohol Services Research and Practices*, 1–8.

Heather, N. (1989). Psychology and brief interventions. *British Journal of Addiction, 84*, 357–370.

Heather, N. (1994). Brief interventions on the world map. *Addiction, 89*, 665–667.

Heather, N., Rollnick, S., Bell, A., & Richmond, R. (1996). Effects of brief counselling among male heavy drinkers identified on general hospital wards. *Drug and Alcohol Review, 15*, 29–38.

Hester, R. K., & Delaney, H. D. (1997). Behavioral self-control program for Windows: Results of a controlled clinical trial. *Journal of Consulting and Clinical Psychology, 65*, 686–693.

Hingson, R., Mangione, T., Meyers, A., & Scotch, N. (1982). Seeking help for drinking problems: A study in the Boston metropolitan area. *Journal of Studies on Alcohol, 43*, 273–288.

Hughes, J. R., Cummings, K. M., & Hyland, A. (1999). Ability of smokers to reduce their smoking and its association with future smoking cessation. *Addiction, 94*, 109–114.

Hughes, J. R., Fiester, S., Goldstein, M., Resnick, M., Rock, N., Ziedonis, D., et al. (1996). Practice guidelines for the treatment of patients with nicotine dependence. *American Journal of Psychiatry, 153*(10 Suppl.), 1–31.

Humphreys, K., & Tucker, J. A. (2002). Toward more responsive and effective intervention systems for alcohol-related problems: Introduction. *Addiction, 97*, 126–132.

Institute of Medicine. (1990). *Broadening the base of treatment for alcohol problems.* Washington, DC: National Academy Press.

Jeffery, R. W., Hellerstedt, W. L., & Schmid, T. L. (1990). Correspondence programs for smoking cessation and weight control: A comparison of two strategies in the Minnesota Heart Health Program. *Health Psychology, 9*, 585–598.

Jerome, L. W., DeLeon, P. H., James, L. C., Folen, R., Earles, J., & Gedney, J. J. (2000). The coming of age of telecommunications in psychological research and practice. *American Psychologist, 55*, 407–421.

Killen, J. D., Fortmann, S. P., Newman, B., & Varady, A. (1990). Evaluation of a treatment approach combining nicotine gum with self-guided behavioral treatments for smoking relapse prevention. *Journal of Consulting and Clinical Psychology, 58*, 85–92.

Klingemann, H. K. H. (1991). The motivation for change from problem alcohol and heroin use. *British Journal of Addiction, 86*, 727–744.

Lando, H. A., Rollnick, S., Klevan, D., Roski, J., Cherney, L., & Lauger, G. (1997). Telephone support as an adjunct to transdermal nicotine in smoking cessation. *American Journal of Public Health, 87*, 1670–1674.

Larabie, L. C. (2005). To what extent do smokers plan quit attempts? *Tobacco Control, 14*, 425–428.

Lichtenstein, E., Lando, H. A., & Nothwehr, F. (1994). Readiness to quit as a predictor of smoking changes in the Minnesota Heart Health Program. *Health Psychology, 13*, 393–396.

Mahoney, M. J., & Lyddon, W. J. (1988). Recent developments in cognitive approaches to counseling and psychotherapy. *The Counseling Psychologist, 16*, 190–234.

Maisto, S. A., Sobell, L. C., Sobell, M. B., & Sanders, B. (1985). Effects of outpatient treatment for problem drinkers. *American Journal of Drug and Alcohol Abuse, 11,* 131–149.

McCambridge, J., & Strang, J. (2005). Deterioration over time in effect of motivational interviewing in reducing drug consumption and related risk among young people. *Addiction, 100,* 470–478.

Medscape Medical News. (2006, September). Medicaid will reimburse for alcohol, drug screening and brief intervention. Retrieved December 17, 2006, from http://www.medscape.com/viewarticle/544548?sssdmh=dm1.217591&src=top10To

Miller, W. R., Brown, J. M., Simpson, T. L., Handmaker, N. S., Bien, T. H., Luckie, L. F., et al. (1995). What works? A methodological analysis of the alcohol treatment outcome literature. In R. K. Hester & W. R. Miller (Eds.), *Handbook of alcoholism treatment approaches: Effective alternatives* (2nd ed., pp. 12–44). Boston: Allyn & Bacon.

Miller, W. R., & Hester, R. K. (1980). Treating the problem drinker: Modern approaches. In W. R. Miller (Ed.), *The addictive behaviors: Treatment of alcoholism, drug abuse, smoking and obesity* (pp. 11–141). New York: Pergamon Press.

Miller, W. R., & Rollnick, S. (2002). *Motivational interviewing: Preparing people to change* (2nd ed.). New York: Guilford Press.

Miller, W. R., Sovereign, R. G., & Krege, B. (1988). Motivational interviewing with problem drinkers: II. The drinker's check-up as a preventive intervention. *Behavioural Psychotherapy, 16,* 251–268.

Miller, W. R., Taylor, C. A., & West, J. C. (1980). Focused versus broad–spectrum behavior therapy for problem drinkers. *Journal of Consulting and Clinical Psychology, 48,* 590–601.

Moyer, A., Finney, J. W., Swearingen, C. E., & Vergun, P. (2002). Brief interventions for alcohol problems: A meta-analytic review of controlled investigations in treatment-seeking and non-treatment-seeking populations. *Addiction, 97,* 279–292.

Nadeau, L. (1997, October). *The promotion of low-risk drinking styles: Sensitizing the public. A critical overview.* Paper presented at the symposium on "The promotion of low-risk drinking patterns in the general public: Strategies and messages," Zurich, Switzerland.

National Institute on Alcohol Abuse and Alcoholism. (1995). *The physician's guide to helping patients with alcohol problems.* Washington, DC: U.S. Government Printing Office.

National Institute on Alcohol Abuse and Alcoholism. (2007). *Helping patients who drink too much: A clinician's guide* (updated 2005 edition). Washington, DC: U.S. Government Printing Office.

Ogborne, A. C., & Annis, H. M. (1988). The reactive effects of follow-up assessment procedures: An experimental study. *Addictive Behaviors, 13,* 123–129.

Pearlman, S., Zweben, A., & Li, S. (1989). The comparability of solicited versus clinic subjects in alcohol treatment research. *British Journal of Addiction, 84,* 523–532.

Perloff, R. M. (1993). *The dynamics of persuasion.* Hillsdale, NJ: Lawrence Erlbaum.

Pirie, P. L., Rooney, B. L., Pechacek, T. F., Lando, H. A., & Schmid, L. A. (1997). Incorporating social support into a community-wide smoking cessation contest. *Addictive Behaviors, 2,* 131–137.

Project MATCH Research Group. (1998a). Matching alcoholism treatments to client heterogeneity: Project MATCH three-year drinking outcomes. *Alcoholism: Clinical and Experimental Research, 22,* 1300–1311.

Project MATCH Research Group. (1998b). Matching alcoholism treatments to client heterogeneity: Treatment main effects and matching effects on drinking during treatment. *Journal of Studies on Alcohol, 59*, 631–639.

Project MATCH Research Group. (1998c). Therapist effects in three treatments for alcohol problems. *Psychotherapy Research, 8*, 455–474.

Raimo, E. B., Daeppen, J. B., Smith, T. L., Danko, G. P., & Schuckit, M. A. (1999). Clinical characteristics of alcoholism in alcohol-dependent subjects with and without a history of alcohol treatment [comment]. *Alcoholism: Clinical & Experimental Research, 23*, 1605–1613.

Ramelson, H. Z., Friedman, R. H., & Ockene, J. K. (1999). An automated telephone-based smoking cessation education and counseling system. *Patient Education and Counseling, 36*, 131–144.

Rehm, J. (1997, October). *Campaigns and core messages: An up-to-date and state of the art from a research perspective?* Paper presented at the symposium on "The promotion of low-risk drinking patterns in the general public: Strategies and messages," Zurich, Switzerland.

Roizen, R. (1977). *Barriers to alcoholism treatment.* Berkeley, CA: Alcohol Research Group.

Rush, B., & Allen, B. A. (1997). Attitudes and beliefs of the general public about treatment for alcohol problems. *Canadian Journal of Public Health, 88*, 41–43.

Saunders, J. B., Kypri, K., Walters, S. T., Laforge, R. G., & Larimer, M. E. (2004). Approaches to brief intervention for hazardous drinking in young people. *Alcoholism: Clinical and Experimental Research, 28*, 322–329.

Shaffer, H. J., & Jones, S. B. (1989). *Quitting cocaine: The struggle against impulse.* Lexington, MA: Lexington Books.

Sitharthan, T., Kavanagh, D. J., & Sayer, G. (1996). Moderating drinking by correspondence: An evaluation of a new method of intervention. *Addiction, 91*, 345–355.

Sobell, L. C., Agrawal, S., Sobell, M. B., and Leo, G. I. (in preparation). *Responding to an advertisement: A critical event in promoting self-change of drinking behavior.*

Sobell, L. C., Agrawal, S., Sobell, M. B., Leo, G. I., Cunningham, J. A., Young, L. J., et al. (2003, November). *Responding to an advertisement: A critical event in promoting self-change of drinking behavior.* Poster presented at the 37th Annual Meeting of the Association for Advancement of Behavior Therapy, Boston.

Sobell, L. C., Cunningham, J. A., & Sobell, M. B. (1996). Recovery from alcohol problems with and without treatment: Prevalence in two population surveys. *American Journal of Public Health, 86*, 966–972.

Sobell, L. C., Cunningham, J. A., Sobell, M. B., Agrawal, S., Gavin, D. R., Leo, G. I., et al. (1996). Fostering self-change among problem drinkers: A proactive community intervention. *Addictive Behaviors, 21*, 817–833.

Sobell, L. C., Klingemann, H., Toneatto, T., Sobell, M. B., Agrawal, S., & Leo, G. I. (2001). Alcohol and drug abusers' perceived reasons for self-change in Canada and Switzerland: Computer-assisted content analysis. *Substance Use and Misuse, 36*, 1467–1500.

Sobell, L. C., & Sobell, M. B. (1992). Timeline Followback: A technique for assessing self-reported alcohol consumption. In R. Z. Litten & J. Allen (Eds.), *Measuring alcohol consumption: Psychosocial and biological methods* (pp. 41–72). Totowa, NJ: Humana Press.

Sobell, L. C., & Sobell, M. B. (2003). Alcohol consumption measures. In J. P. Allen & V. Wilson (Eds.), *Assessing alcohol problems* (2nd ed., pp. 78–99). Rockville, MD: National Institute on Alcohol Abuse and Alcoholism.

Sobell, L. C., Sobell, M. B., Leo, G. I., Agrawal, S., Johnson-Young, L., & Cunningham, J. A. (2002). Promoting self-change with alcohol abusers: A community-level mail intervention based on natural recovery studies. *Alcoholism: Clinical and Experimental Research, 26*, 936–948.

Sobell, L. C., Sobell, M. B., & Toneatto, T. (1992). Recovery from alcohol problems without treatment. In N. Heather, W. R. Miller, & J. Greeley (Eds.), *Self-control and the addictive behaviours* (pp. 198–242). New York: Maxwell MacMillan.

Sobell, L. C., Sobell, M. B., Toneatto, T., & Leo, G. I. (1993). What triggers the resolution of alcohol problems without treatment? *Alcoholism: Clinical and Experimental Research, 17*, 217–224.

Sobell, M. B., Breslin, F. C., & Sobell, L. C. (1998). Project MATCH: The time has come ... to talk of many things. *Journal of Studies on Alcohol, 59*, 124–125.

Sobell, M. B., & Sobell, L. C. (1993). *Problem drinkers: Guided self-change treatment.* New York: Guilford Press.

Sobell, M. B., & Sobell, L. C. (1998). Guiding self-change. In W. R. Miller & N. Heather (Eds.), *Treating addictive behaviors* (2nd ed., pp. 189–202). New York: Plenum Press.

Sobell, M. B., & Sobell, L. C. (1999). Stepped-care for alcohol problems: An efficient method for planning and delivering clinical services. In J. A. Tucker, D. A. Donovan, & G. A. Marlatt (Eds.), *Changing addictive behavior: Bridging clinical and public health strategies* (pp. 331–343). New York: Guilford Press.

Sobell, M. B., & Sobell, L. C. (2000). Stepped-care as a heuristic approach to the treatment of alcohol problems. *Journal of Consulting and Clinical Psychology, 68*, 573–579.

Sobell, M. B., & Sobell, L. C. (2005). Guided self-change treatment for substance abusers. *Journal of Cognitive Psychotherapy, 19*, 199–210.

Stephens, R. S., Roffman, R. A., & Curtin, L. (2000). Comparison of extended versus brief treatments for marijuana use. *Journal of Consulting and Clinical Psychology, 68*, 898–908.

Substance Abuse and Mental Health Administration. (2002). *Enhancing motivation for change in substance abuse treatment* (Treatment Improvement Protocol Series, TIPS #35). Rockville, MD: U.S. Department of Health and Human Services.

Substance Abuse and Mental Health Administration. (2003). *Reasons for not receiving treatment among adults with serious mental illness* (Vol. 2003). Rockville, MD: U.S. Department of Health and Human Services.

Svärdsudd, K. (1998). Moderate alcohol consumption and cardiovascular disease: Is there evidence for a preventive effect? *Alcoholism: Clinical and Experimental Research, 22*, 307S–314S.

Thom, B. (1986). Sex differences in help-seeking for alcohol problems—1. The barriers to help-seeking. *British Journal of Addiction, 81*, 777–788.

Thoresen, C. E., & Mahoney, M. J. (1974). *Behavioral self-control.* New York: Rinehart & Winston.

Timko, C., Moos, R. H., Finney, J. W., Moos, B., & Kaplowitz, M. S. (1999). Long-term treatment careers and outcomes of previously untreated alcoholics. *Journal of Studies on Alcohol, 60*, 437–447.

Tuchfeld, B. S. (1981). Spontaneous remission in alcoholics: Empirical observations and theoretical implications. *Journal of Studies on Alcohol, 42*, 626–641.

U.S. Department of Health and Human Services. (2000, June). You Can Quit Smoking. Consumer Guide. http://www.surgeongeneral.gov/tobacco/consquits.htm

Utz, S. W., Shuster, G. F., Merwin, E., & Williams, B. (1994). A community-based smoking-cessation program: Self-care behaviors and success. *Public Health Nursing, 11*, 291–299.

Warner, K. E. (1981). Cigarette smoking in the 1970's: The impact of the antismoking campaign on consumption. *Science, 211*, 729–730.

Warner, K. E. (1989). Effects of the antismoking campaign: An update. *American Journal of Public Health, 79*, 144–151.

Werch, C. E. (1990). Are drinkers interested in inexpensive approaches to reduce their alcohol use? *Journal of Drug Education, 20*, 67–75.

West, R., & Sohal, T. (2006). "Catastrophic" pathways to smoking cessation: Findings from national survey. *British Medical Journal, 332*, 458–460. Originally published online 27 January 2006; doi:10.1136/bmj.38723.573866.AE.

Wright, B., Williams, C., & Partridge, I. (1999). Management advice for children with chronic fatigue syndrome: A systematic study of information from the Internet. *Irish Journal of Psychological Medicine, 16*, 67–71.

Wutzke, S. E., Shiell, A., Gomel, M. K., & Conigrave, K. M. (2001). Cost effectiveness of brief interventions for reducing alcohol consumption. *Social Science & Medicine, 52*, 863–870.

Zhu, S. H., Stretch, V., Balabanis, M., Rosbrook, B., Sadler, G., & Pierce, J. P. (1996). Telephone counseling for smoking cessation: Effects of single-session and multiple-session interventions. *Journal of Consulting and Clinical Psychology, 64*, 202–211.

9

Hostile and Favorable Societal Climates for Self-Change: Some Lessons for Policymakers

Harald Klingemann and Justyna Klingemann

Introduction

When individuals vote, decide on what to wear or what to eat, they do not do so in a societal vacuum; rather, their actions are influenced and affected by society's values, trends, commercials, and campaigns. From our daily experience, it seems plausible that social and cognitive processes are intertwined. However, in the area of natural recovery research, decisional processes of self-change are often viewed as occurring mainly within the individual or from interactions between individuals. This is not surprising given the importance of clinical psychology and psychiatry in this area as well as the methodological difficulties in measuring society's impact on individual behavior.

From a sociological point of view, the role of primary and secondary groups, organizational settings, societal belief systems, and opportunity structures—all of which may promote or impede self-change—has largely been neglected. Exceptions are the concept of social capital including multilevel resources for change (Granfield & Cloud, 1999) and attempts to apply staging models to understanding health behavior and lifestyle changes within an organizational and environmental framework (Oldenburg, Glanz, & French, 1999). As a result of this restricted point of view, our understanding of the spontaneous recovery process suffers from an individualistic (as compared with a societal) bias. To address such a gap, this chapter intends to highlight links between individual clinical views and social factors such as public images of addiction, treatment systems, the role of the media, and policy measures. These macro-societal aspects are of interest to policymakers.

"Could be about attitudes in the society. Against those who have problems. Even if it is classified as a disease, I don't think that is how it is seen by most people. They rather think it is your own fault, at least kind of. ... So, some better understanding in society for those kind of people who have problems. That would make it easier for them I think. One maybe would dare to make a first step." (shop owner, SINR interview, Stockholm)

Images of Alcohol and Drug Addiction in the General Population: Stigma, Social Support, and Change Optimism

Societal beliefs about social problems and their nature shape individual and collective responses to individual self-change. How visible are these problems? How confident are researchers that people may eventually change their eating disorders, heroin or alcohol use, or pathological gambling on their own? The answers to these questions will depend on the overall concept of addiction or the paradigms that prevail in societies. Are addictive behaviors seen as medical problems, social problems, or as criminal or immoral in nature? Of interest in this context is the informal social response to natural recovery. It can be assumed that the social support or tolerance potential quitters experience in their attempt at self-change will be contingent on the images they see in the general population and more precisely in their reference groups.

A Canadian survey (Cunningham, Sobell, & Sobell, 1998) showed that for potential self-changers who are in the precontemplation phase or weighing strategies for implementing change, the images of the nature of addiction and the public visibility of successful natural recovery were very important. Whereas 53% of the respondents who had overcome their dependence without treatment knew of similar cases, only 14% in a general population group were aware of self-change cases. The other study groups (significant others of self-changers, unsuccessful self-changers, and treatment cases) fell within these two extremes. It seems plausible to assume that societal stigma kept people from telling others about their self-change process; that is, only 5% of self-changers said they did not tell others they had stopped smoking, whereas almost five times more (24%) did not tell others they had stopped drinking. Even though self-changers had a success story to tell, they probably anticipated a negative or ambivalent societal response of varying strength according to the type of addiction.

Although there is a vast literature on the nature of stereotypes and attitudes toward addiction, the perception of self-change processes in the public is clearly underresearched. Only recently have efforts been made to explore attitudinal dimensions of the perception of self-change in the general population. The study on "Societal Images of Natural Recovery from Addictions" (SINR) is an international multicity study conducted thus far in Bern and Fribourg (Switzerland), Frankfurt (Germany), Santa Marta and Bogota (Colombia), Warsaw (Poland), Stockholm (Sweden), Helsinki (Finland), and Toronto (Canada). This collaborative project explored, from a sociological perspective, the social conditions influencing personal change (Zulewska-Sak & Dabrowska, 2004). The aim of the study was to identify dimensions of public attitudes toward self-change using "purposive sampling" in communal settings. In each of the cities, 15 key informants from different social and professional backgrounds (e.g., journalists, law enforcement representatives, health care and mental health treatment professionals, so-called everyday therapists such as barkeepers and taxi drivers) were interviewed regarding the following: (a) their beliefs in chances for self-change, (b) barriers to self-change (Zulewska-Sak, 2004, 2005; Zulewska-Sak & Dabrowska, 2005), and (c) how to promote self-change. Results demonstrate the sophistication of everyday perceptions concerning drug problems. "Without using technical or scientific terms, most respondents appear to be competent barefoot drug policy makers" (Klingemann, 2003, p. 14).

The study results were used as a starting point for the first representative survey study conducted in Switzerland in 2004 which directly measured relevant self-change factors such as "self-change optimism," "social distance," and "self-reported helping behavior." Quotes from the qualitative material from the SINR study mentioned above are used throughout this chapter to illustrate societal conditions pertinent to self-change. It is assumed that disbelief in the possibility of change will discourage potential self-changers. Furthermore, this pessimism will undermine social support by collaterals, which does not seem worth the effort. These assumptions still need to be investigated empirically. Do people believe that addicts can quit on their own? Asked about addiction *in general*, respondents see, on average, a 24% chance for change without professional help which points to a widely held disbelief in natural recovery (see Figure 9.1). More specifically, 26% of the respondents believe there is no chance at all to change.

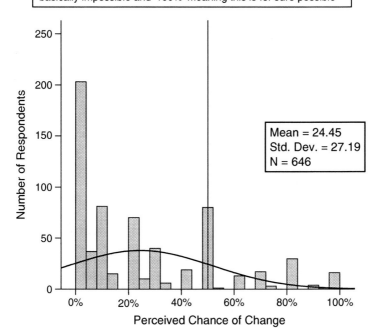

FIGURE 9.1. General optimism for self-change from addictive behaviors.

> "Very difficult. I have met a few people, also friends, who swore they would make it and blah-blah, but it was just talk. It's very difficult, once you fall into it, to get out of that circle. It's totally difficult, from what I've seen. And with therapy, they have really made it, a few of them, and a few are dead, those who haven't done it. There are totally extreme differences." (hairdresser, SINR interview, Frankfurt)

Of the total respondents, 12% believe there is an equal chance to change with or without professional help.

> "Cause I think this is some kind of a lottery. Fifty-fifty, this way or that way." (taxi driver, SINR interview, Warsaw)

A minority (3%; a subgroup which merits a more in-depth analysis) is completely *sure* that addicts can change their lives without paid professionals.

> "In my opinion it's the most important, dominant factor that an addicted person should come to such an inner decision, that he wants to recover from addiction. ... There are addictions easier to recover from... but there are also such addictions where recovery is a long-term process... which doesn't necessarily have to be a success. But I think there are more factors that are easy to deal with than such ones where the help of specialists is required." (lawyer, SINR interview, Warsaw)

As the preceding quotes from the SINR study illustrate nicely, lay theories on addiction are by no means simplistic. The representative survey confirms this by revealing that two-thirds of the population think the chances for self-change depend on the substance to which the person is addicted. This should not come as a surprise if one thinks about the diverging images of licit and illicit drugs in the public arena transmitted by the media. That is, when presented with a list of various addictive behaviors and asked to rate the chances of natural recovery, respondents are more optimistic about self-change from smoking tobacco and cannabis (attributing about a fifty-fifty chance) than about spontaneous remission from hard drugs such as heroin and cocaine (only in approximately 13% of the cases do they see this as a possibility). Men tend to be more optimistic than women, except for the consensus on hard drugs and prescription drugs, in which no significant differences were detected.

Gambling, alcohol, and prescription drugs range in the middle with about a one third perceived chance for natural recovery. This rank order may reflect to some extent the availability of professional treatment (basically none for smoking and cannabis abuse) and may correlate with perceived dangerousness of the substance.

Tobacco and cannabis addiction are set apart from other substances in the public mind, which has implications for policy. That is, with about 70% nonsmokers in the population and increasing pressure from policymakers to pass smoking bans, "change optimism" seems to be most relevant and could possibly be included in campaign concepts. Major conclusions from this study, which still need to be validated through future research in other countries, include the following:

- "Change optimism" proves to be strongly culture-bound and across all types of addictive behaviors is significantly higher in the Francophone minority part of the country, which implements harsher drug policies than in the German-speaking region, which has a higher acceptance of harm reduction policies. In both cases, a gap between the public trust in the ability to make informed choices and the official policymakers discourse can be noted.
- Political views have most impact on the self-change climate when they relate to current debates and high levels of sensitization; a right-wing orientation favors optimism to change from pathological gambling (ongoing debate about casinos and lottery legislation) and proponents of cannabis legalization (a core issue of the debate on the new narcotics law) are significantly optimistic about self-change possibilities from cannabis misuse.
- Personal experience with addiction problems facilitates specific self-change optimism. It significantly increases with self-reported consumption of alcohol and cannabis, respectively. A result which can be interpreted from the general finding is that involuntarily taken risks tend to be underestimated.

Treatment Systems and the Acceptance of Treatment

Self-change or natural recovery is defined as the successful resolution of a behavior perceived as problematic, a process which is primarily driven by the motivation and power of the individual and social forces without relying on treatment or expert help or intervention. The changes that an individual makes through self-change rather than treatment depend to some extent on the availability of treatment resources (Kavanagh, Sitharthan, Spilsbury, & Vignaedra, 1999). This accessibility will vary greatly according to the type of problem at a given time.

> "There is very little treatment for compulsive shopping and gambling. Yes, you can put it that way, that the less help there is out there, the more people have to rely on themselves to heal." (psychologist, SINR interview, Bern)

The treatment of nicotine dependence illustrates this point nicely. Hughes (1999) claims that the statement that 90–95% of smokers who quit do so on their own without treatment is no longer correct. He argues that given the increasing sale of over-the-counter and nonprescription medications as well as bupropion (Wellbutrin) in the United States, 37% of all quits in 1998 could be attributed to medication use. He draws an interesting parallel between the growth of this branch of the treatment industry and the response to some psychiatric disorders. At the turn of the last century, few clinicians thought of depression as a disorder; instead, most believed it could be cured by simple motivation and, thus, few treatment resources were made available. Currently, almost all clinicians agree that clinical depression needs treatment. Perhaps the understanding of nicotine by administrators, clinicians, and the public in the 1990s is where the knowledge of depression was in the early 1900s.

However, the availability of treatment does not only depend on the prevailing concept of a disease or addiction, but also on political parameters. In the last two decades, while expansive growth could be seen in drug treatment systems in most countries, it was at the expense of treatment resources available for alcohol abusers. Taking Switzerland for example, the treatment network for approximately 30,000 drug abusers, compared with the counseling and care services available to more than eight times that number of alcohol abusers, is disproportionately well developed and differentiated (Klingemann, 1998).

The images of addiction and prevailing drug, alcohol, or tobacco policies also largely determine the type of treatment methods and models. Most prominently, harm reduction measures, heroin prescription, and large scale substitution or replacement therapies are available in many countries. Their diffusion and adoption depends on a number of endogenous and exogenous influences such as the moral judgment in the population and the adherence to international drug control (Klingemann & Hunt, 1998; Klingemann & Klingemann, 1999).

> "I do suppose that low-threshold initiatives in the area of drugs, for example when heroin is given for free, or other such programs, they have a certain positive effect on the probability of entering a self-healing process, because people are somehow accepted there." (psychologist, SINR interview, Bern)

Even if equity is assumed in availability of professional help at a given time in a given country, individuals' perception of the accessibility of treatment may still vary and therefore affect the probability that they will look for their own solution and not seek professional assistance.

> "When I have a problem, I don't confide in strangers, rather contact close friends." (hairdresser, SINR interview, Warsaw)

In part, a barrier to treatment is the ability of providers to tailor their services to the needs of potential clients. This is mirrored by statements of the SINR respondents who emphasize that treatment has to be individualized; that is, what works for one person does not necessarily work for another person.

"Important to find treatment which is suited for the specific person. ... You see that people are different and need different kinds of treatment suited for their needs." (journalist, SINR interview, Stockholm)

"So for me that [self-help groups] would be an appropriate possibility, if you are afraid to have your life analyzed with strangers. This is a big fear, even if we think we have quite an easy threshold, but in principle it is very, very high." (head of an outpatient facility for alcohol addicts, SINR interview, Frankfurt)

Natural recovery research provides valuable information on the question of why people do not seek treatment. Lack of information, stigma, and the belief that treatment does not offer what is needed are some of the main reasons (Klingemann, 1991, 1992). Another important reason is culturally supported beliefs. For example, Western values strengthen the idea that individuals have to ideally overcome problems without affecting others (i.e., individual will power and strength) and by downplaying the influence of other circumstances (see Barker and Hunt's chapter in this volume). From a systems perspective, the inability of treatment providers to reach the majority of their target groups points to the increasing importance of lay help, informal referral systems, and therefore also self-change processes. In modern societies, the authority of experts and societal elites, such as scientists and politicians, has been fading in general. The emerging distance between the lay populace and professional treatment also shows the limits of medication and expert help in addiction intervention. This opens an analytical viewpoint that has yet to be discussed—the perspective of the consumer. On both the individual and systems levels, the consumer of treatment services is viewed, according to the sick role definition by Parsons (1951), as a passive, compliant recipient of beneficial treatment by a specialist authority. This is further illustrated by the top-down planning of treatment programs based on scientific paradigms about the nature of addiction, expert knowledge and professional socialization, and the severity of addiction problems.

Yet, addiction treatment is an interaction between the provider and the consumer. Experts are also influenced by their lay counterparts and need their consent to operate and succeed. A better understanding for the dynamics and future changes of treatment systems and the role of natural recovery or assisted self-change will be facilitated by researching the interface between professional and lay cultures and referral systems (Freidson, 1960; Klingemann & Bergmark, 2006). This includes, among others, the following topics:

• The comparison of experts' and lay persons' ideas and concepts of addiction, consequences of addictive behaviors, risk assessment, and the perceived efficiency of formal and informal support
• Individual and organizational strategies to adapt to clients' needs
• Lay strategies to control and check professionals' behavior (e.g., via Internet, second opinion)
• Understanding consumer treatment choices and decisions not to seek professional help

In spite of these underresearched topics, there is at least some evidence that treatment systems have converged in particular areas closer to the target groups they intend to reach. Some indicators for such a development are the following:

• The partial adoption of the *stepped-care* model and brief interventions which acknowledges the everyday life context of clients while using beneficial evidence-based practices
• The long-term trend toward outpatient treatment which brings interventions *closer to the community* and avoids removing clients from daily context, as opposed to inpatient programs
• The inclusion of *affective, spiritual alternative elements* into treatment programs going beyond the "specific symptoms, evidence only" philosophy

To conclude, the current shortcomings in addiction treatment can be viewed from the perspective of self-change research as a lack of trust and confidence. Helping people to change can only be achieved in a self-change friendly society with treatment professionals who are equally legitimized by their professional community and their customers whose needs they are expected to match.

Self-Change in the Global Village: Media Images and Health Information Management as Social Capital

The Portrayal of Alcohol and Drug Users in the Media

The way in which social problems are presented in print, electronic media, and other public arenas can exert considerable influence on stereotypes or the willingness to provide informal support and help.

> "Well, one of the possibilities [to make self-change easier] is certainly information, that you ... I don't know exactly ... show some ways, in newspapers, in books, on the radio, and in TV programs, how people could also quit on their own. Or maybe even in schools, explaining that to people." (journalist, SINR interview, Bern)

Advertising for smoking and alcohol is subject to various restrictions in some countries and it is generally claimed that only brand-specific market shares are at stake (Godfrey, 1995). Although there are no studies showing how advertisement exposure affects recovery, one can speculate that self-change from nicotine and alcohol problems might be more easily accomplished where cues for use are less frequent. The images of smoking, alcohol use, and illicit drug use presented on television, radio, and in print can be understood both as a reflection of and major influence on public opinion about substance use.

Lemmens, Vaeth, and Greenfield (1999) have presented a content analysis of the portrayal of alcohol-related issues in five national newspapers in the United States from 1985 to 1991. Most articles reported alcohol issues neutrally or negatively. Furthermore, a general shift since the 1960s was noted, characterized by emphasizing public health issues, deemphasizing clinical aspects, and stressing external environmental factors more than the biopsychological definition of alcohol-related behavior.

Such changes in media messages may be more conducive to natural recoveries by not glorifying drinking and by stressing the role of environmental factors rather than intrapsychic factors. However, more recent media studies reveal a more differentiated picture by type of drugs. For example, the comprehensive literature review in "Here's Looking at You, Kid': Alcohol, Drugs, and Tobacco in Entertainment Media," prepared for The National Center on Addiction and Substance Abuse at Columbia University by Roberts and Christenson (2000), examined research on the frequency and nature of media portrayals of the use of alcohol, tobacco, and illicit drugs. Results show that for television alcohol remains the substance most likely to be portrayed, with no large past or current changes in frequency; the most recent data indicate that three out of every four episodes of the most popular shows depict alcohol use (Roberts & Christenson, 2000). Drinking has generally been presented as a routine, problem-free activity. If anything, the overall message is largely positive, in that those who drink on television are more likely to be central characters, more attractive, and of higher status then those who do not drink (Mathios, Avery, Bisogni, & Shanahan, 1998). Older studies, such as the analysis of 48 German and American soap operas and crime series shown on German television, also highlight the reinforcement of positive, beverage-specific social stereotypes such as the association between beer and friendship (Weiderer, 1997).

Portrayal of tobacco use decreased markedly on TV from the 1950s through the 1980s, but rose during the 1990s, with the most recent data indicating that 22% of episodes of the most popular shows depict tobacco use (Roberts & Christenson, 2000). Christenson, Henriksen, and Roberts (2000) found that negative statements were made about smoking in 23% of the shows in which smoking occurred, yet explicit refusals occurred in none of 31 episodes that showed tobacco use.

According to Roberts and Christenson (2000), illicit drug use portrayals appear to be more frequent now than in the 1970s; currently about one in five episodes of top television shows portray illicit drug use. In their own study, Christenson et al. (2000) found that when drug use appears on television it is often portrayed negatively; that is, 67% of episodes that portrayed illicit drug use also depicted negative consequences, while only 3% contained statements that could be interpreted as pro-use.

Although the impact of television on viewers and potential risk groups is difficult to assess, one can assume that modeling influences people, especially in later stages of change (Rogers, Vaughan, & Shefner-Rogers, 1995; Slater, 1997). Such modeling approaches, based on social learning theory, proved to be quite efficient by using, for instance, melodrama. The more positive portrayal of alcohol and tobacco use in the media, compared with illicit drugs, is consistent with the attitudes in the population about the possibility of self-change from various types of addiction reviewed earlier.

Active Information Retrieval and Media Use as a Tool for Self-Change

Individuals involved in self-change and their collaterals are not only passively exposed to addiction-related messages in the media, but once they have reached the contemplation/action stage of change they may also extend their human capital by actively seeking information useful to gain control of their habit. The concept of human capital, as a part of the social capital for successful self-change, refers to knowledge, understanding, skills, and other personal attributes that can be used to achieve one's desired goals and successfully negotiate personal difficulties (Granfield & Cloud, 1999).

Using "How to..." Books

Written material can assist people in the recovery process. Most bookstores have a "Self-help" section. People trying to gather information about what they can do concerning their eating, sex, drinking, or work stress problems can turn to some type of bibliotherapy. Self-help material may (a) be based explicitly on the principles of self-change and stages of change theory, (b) help to monitor and structure personal observations (e.g., drinking occasions and quantities consumed), and (c) provide general information with no stepwise or didactic program. Self-help manuals are available for both problem drinkers and their partners (Barber & Gilbertson, 1998). The appeal of the "how to improve your life" literature on the book market is probably due to the choice it leaves readers, its time flexibility, and its confidentiality (e.g., Carlson's 1998 book on simple ways to minimize job stress was a national bestseller in the United States). Self-help material has a middle position between manuals requiring minimal contact with a therapist (Heather, 2001) and personal diaries that help monitor personal changes including addiction problems.

> "Thursday 3 August: 8 st. 11, thigh circumstance 18 inches (honestly what is the bloody point), alcohol units 0, cigarettes 25 (excellent considering), negative thoughts: approx. 445 per hour, positive thoughts 0." ("Bridget Jones's Diary," by Helen Fielding, 1999, p. 184)

Using the Internet, Cyber Hugs, and Telephone Helplines

Health information and related discussions lists, chat rooms, and cyber self-help groups on the Internet are becoming increasingly popular and are a standard item for many providers (Maxwell, 1998). Examples include McCartney's (1999) resources on perinatal nursing and Moran's (1999) information on geriatric rehabilitation.

These sources can also be tapped by individuals trying to come to terms with their addiction problem on their own. Major advantages for many self-quitters are anonymity and the opportunity to compare advice. Young people and individuals living in remote areas are probably most inclined to use the Internet to improve their health status and possibly to handle problems with addictive behaviors. There are numerous websites for addiction information and counseling such as Smart Recovery, Web of Addiction, Moderation Management, and NHS Direct Online ("Advice On-line," 2000). Behavioral self-control training has also been made available via the computer and could produce substantial reductions in the consumption of heavy drinkers. The Drinker's Check-Up is a brief motivational intervention designed to assist clients achieving moderation or abstinence (Saladin & Santa Ana, 2004).

Lastly, the use of popular self-help books is most likely skewed by social strata. This is probably even more the case with Internet usage because it varies with age, income, gender, and educational level (Korgaonkar & Wolin, 1999). The possibility to easily retrieve health-related information from the Internet is by no means equally distributed among societal groups or countries. In North America, which represents only 5.1% of the world population, the Internet penetration rate amounts to 69.1% compared with Europe with a rate of 31.2% (12.4% of the world population), Asia with a rate of 10.8% (56.4% of the world population), and Africa with a rate of 3.6% (14.1% of the world population; "Internet World Stats," 2006). This distribution of access to self-change-related information on the Internet appears to be in reverse proportion to the needs and development of treatment systems in these regions.

Compared with Internet use, many more people have access to telephone helplines. A rationale for helplines is that, given the stigma of addiction, receiving initial help from an anonymous therapist might be more acceptable than face-to-face contact. Helplines can provide immediate motivational material, brief counseling, and information on what kind of treatment is available and how to seek it. Lichtenstein, Glasgow, Lando, Ossip-Klein, and Boles (1996) conducted a meta-analysis of 13 studies of helplines for smoking cessation. Such helplines appear to be efficient and useful as a public intervention for large populations. Meta-analysis confirmed a significant increase in long-term abstinence rates.

An American study (Hughes, Riggs, & Carpenter, 2001) of a convenience sample of 30 helplines for alcohol- cocaine- heroin- marijuana- or tobacco-dependent individuals seeking treatment analyzed the quality of the service by making "undercover" client calls. Responses were categorized as helpful (sending useful mailings, referrals to self-help programs or a drug dependence treatment center), neutral (referrals to another national helpline), or unhelpful (incorrect information such as "nicotine is not really addicting," or inadequate responses, for instance, unfulfilled promises to return a call or declining competence with respect to the caller's problem). Almost none of the U.S. helplines attempted to give concrete therapeutic advice over the phone (which seems to be the case in Europe); instead they served almost exclusively as referral agencies or mailed written information. The percentage of helplines for illicit drugs described by the evaluators as helpful was relatively low (25% for marijuana) in comparison with alcohol telephone counseling, which was coded as 41% helpful.

To conclude, specific features of the various forms of low-threshold help possibly influence their usefulness for various subgroups of potential self-changers. That is, easy access and personal voice contact by telephone may be attractive for some groups, whereas more neutral contact with Internet websites may be more valuable for others. The former allows for a more passive and guided approach, while the latter provides a more active role, critically comparing information on the web. The use of various types of media may depend not only on group characteristics, but also on the individual's specific stage of change.

Media Campaigns Setting the Stage for Change?

Drug, alcohol, and smoking campaigns are launched to sensitize the public and to influence attitudes and behavior patterns of risk groups. Similar to the question of "How does the amount of advertising influence consumption?", one may also ask, "How are the motivation for and chances of self-change affected by national sensitization campaigns?" Wilde's (1991) conclusion from a decade ago asserted that mass communication prevention programs for health were hardly ever evaluated systematically, a criticism that is still valid today.

Conceptual shortcomings and a lack of theoretical underpinnings are seldom identified as reasons for failure. Slater (1999) has suggested that the stages of change model could in fact provide a framework for integrating theories of media effects on self and others and prove to be useful for the planning of communication campaigns to change health behaviors. More specifically, relevant theories for the transition from precontemplation to contemplation are agenda setting, situational theory, and multistep flow which lead to interpersonal discussion of the problem behavior. Initial awareness can be built by using simple sources and dramatic messages. Moving from contemplation to preparation assumes the acceptance of the campaign messages and the perception of models and skills illustrated in engaging narrative or entertainment programming (i.e., social learning theory). Finally, the iterative process from preparation to action may require continued messages which help maintain the motivation and keep the behavior change goal salient. Providing more persuasive evidence and using more directive messages have been useful for probing behavior change. At the same time, this may cause reactance among potential self-changers (Slater, 1999). The stage specific definition of campaign objectives seems to be a promising avenue to promote natural recovery. However, using the stages of change model to integrate theories that address health communication campaigns in general and facilitate self-change of problem behaviors has rarely been done in the addiction field.

The following three Swiss campaigns, where ideas and findings from natural recovery research have been used as conceptual foundations, will be briefly described: (a) the 1997 drug campaign "A Sober Look at Drugs" concentrated on self-efficacy, (b) the 1999 alcohol campaign "Handle With Care" used a stages of change approach, and (c) the 1999/2000 tobacco campaign "Milestone" focused on significant life events as agents of self-change. As part of an experimental approach to drug policies (Klingemann & Hunt, 1998), the prevention debate in Switzerland has moved from a traditional, substance-specific informational approach toward an orientation concerning health promotion and empowerment of the individual to successfully cope with life's challenges. The focus has shifted to protective factors (e.g., individuals' beliefs in having control over their life, having confidence in other people, trusting in one's ability to overcome setbacks, seeing difficulties as a positive challenge, finding meaningful objectives in life). From this approach, prevention is viewed as a concern of society as a whole. Key elements and ideas from natural recovery research can be used for campaigns based on this mode of thinking.

"A Sober Look at Drugs"

The Federal Drug Sensitizing Campaigns, which started in 1991, set out to promote a better understanding of drug issues among the public at large and included, among others, the following studies: (a) a 7-year follow-up of heroin users conducted by the Zurich Institute for Addiction Research (Dobler-Mikola, Zimmer-Höfler, Uchtenhagen, & Korbel , 1991), (b) natural recovery studies on alcohol and heroin remitters by the Swiss Institute for the Prevention of Alcohol and Drug Problems (Klingemann, 1992), and (c) an epidemiological survey among heroin and cocaine users done by the University of Bern (Estermann, Herrmann, Hügi, & Nydegger, 1996). These three studies provided empirical data which were used by the campaign organizers to illustrate their point. The national poster campaign, launched in 1997 under the theme of "A Sober Look at Drugs," tried to change the attitude "once an addict always an addict," by giving information about the chances of stopping drug use and trying to strengthen hope and optimism with the slogan "Getting into drugs does not mean to stay with them—Most drug users succeed in quitting their habit" (see Figure 9.2).

Even though annual campaign budgets for these studies (about $2 million U.S.) were low compared with commercial advertising, the objectives were reached. A representative survey conducted in 1997 showed a positive reaction and a good recall rate of 31% for that year's campaign. The (stigma relevant) perceived rate of drug users quitting rose from 18% in 1996 to 29% in 1997 (Moeri, 1997). Those directly concerned with the problem preferred the more direct and specific message, "Coercion is no help most of the time but with our support most drug users will manage to quit." This is consistent with Slater's (1999) stage-specific recommendations for media

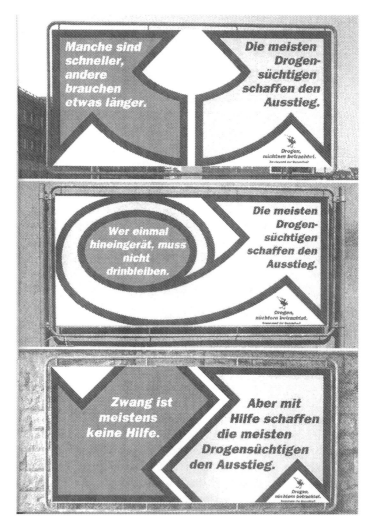

FIGURE 9.2. Poster campaign for "A Sober Look at Drugs."

campaigns mentioned earlier. Taken together, self-efficacy and mobilizing social support for self-change was at the center of this campaign.

"Handle With Care"

The campaign "Handle With Care" was the first-ever, large-scale alcohol prevention program in Switzerland. It was sponsored by the Swiss Alcohol Board and launched by the Swiss Office for Public Health and the Swiss Institute for the Prevention of Alcohol and Other Drug Problems as part of the National Alcohol Program 1998–2002. The "Handle With Care" logo was a bottle opener which was repeated in all messages and incorporated in billboard poster campaigns that started in July 1999 with ads in the print media published simultaneously. This campaign went a step further than "A Sober Look at Drugs" by adopting the theoretical underpinnings of a simple stages of change model. The objectives of this campaign were to gently push at-risk consumers who were in the precontemplation stage forward to the contemplation stage and to influence motivated at-risk consumers to move toward the action phase. The campaign was based on the results of a representative survey conducted in November 1998. The distribution across consumption patterns and stages showed that 84% of all respondents were in the precontemplation stage, 6.5% were in the contemplation stage, and a remarkable 9.5% were in the action stage. Males thought about their drinking more than women while age and linguistic region were not related to stage progression.

Five 18-second TV spots labeled "minor mishaps" were shown on all Swiss TV channels and non-Swiss channels with Swiss advertising slots starting in March 1999. These spots featured everyday scenarios showing self-confident individuals consuming alcohol and ending up with minor mishaps such as the following:
A man starting to pour a glass of wine but misses the glass (wet socks clip), a woman burping at a ladies tea party (burp clip), a man dropping ashes from a cigar into the glass of another guest (ashes clip), a man falling off his chair (falling clip), and a woman almost going to the men's restroom (wrong door clip). All situations are in leisure-time settings and meant to be nondramatic. The spots end with the on-screen question "Everything under control?," prompting viewers to evaluate if their alcohol consumption is maybe a bit problematic and should be given more thought ("Spectra," 1999a,b).

"Handle With Care" was targeted at the population segment progressing to the action stage and promoted self-monitoring material consistent with the principles of assisted self-change and minimal intervention. To monitor one's own alcohol consumption, a handy alcohol slide ruler was distributed in physicians' waiting rooms and at counseling agencies (see Figure 9.3).

The program was still operating in 2006, although with a lower budget, combined with a community prevention program and new elements such as an information table in credit card form to monitor one's Blood Alcohol Concentration level and an Internet game ("Space Bar," 2006). The current content of messages has shifted to a more traditional emphasis on alcohol-related negative consequences. It remains to be seen to what extent the new Swiss National Alcohol Program 2007–2011, which is still being planned, will draw on the ideas and results of self-change research.

"Milestone"

"A lifestyle is born. Milestone—the most pleasurable non-smoking campaign since we know cigarettes!" This was the opening slogan when the campaign was launched in October 1999 by the Swiss Cancer League and

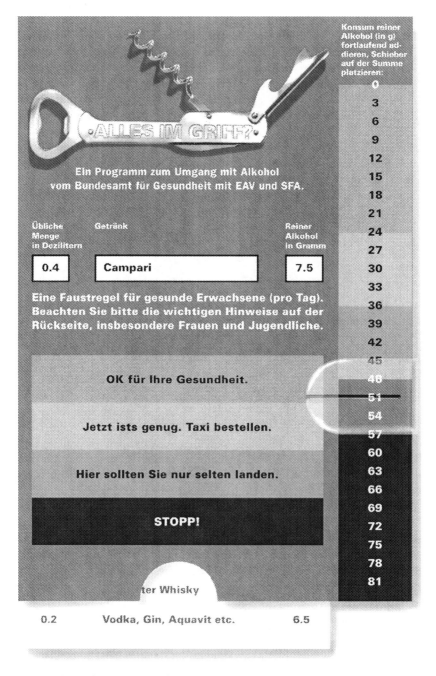

FIGURE 9.3. Tools to assist self-change: Alcohol slide ruler distributed during the "Handle With Care" campaign.

the Swiss Office of Public Health. The concept of "Milestone" is explicitly based on significant life events that trigger spontaneous remission, a classic theme of natural recovery. Key elements are the special moments which make life worthwhile and break through the daily routine such as "the first child, the sumptuous wedding, the new sports car, the trip around the world, the dream job, the successful exam, the important birthday, the new apartment with a view on the lake. ... 'Milestone' symbolizes the end of a phase in your life and a new beginning" (see Figure 9.4; "Swiss Cancer League," 1999).

The campaign was aiming specifically at dissonant smokers in the contemplation phase and wanted to provide chronic smokers with the motivation necessary to quit. It was the first largely Internet-based campaign in Switzerland, although it also used a telephone helpline and printed informational material. First, smokers signed up on the website and defined their personal milestone—a date and event marking the start of their attempt to quit smoking. This was part of a public data base including portraits of all the participants. Second, they received an e-mail on their quit date reminding them of their intention. After 3 months participants

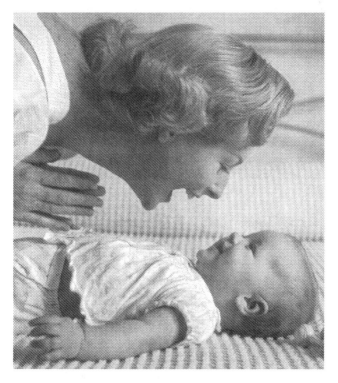

Figure 9.4. Life events as personal milestones for change when quitting smoking.

received another e-mail asking them to report their success or failure. Finally, reported successes were filed under the category "congratulations" and the participants received a gift. Those reporting failures were encouraged to resubscribe by choosing another milestone (i.e., another quit date). During the phase of remission, the website offered tools for assisted self-change such as information on nicotine replacement, self-help groups, and self-monitoring devices. After 100 days of the campaign, about 300 people had signed up and indicated a personal milestone. During the first 3 months the website had 25,000 visitors and 18,000 of them downloaded the nonsmoking questionnaire ("Swiss Cancer League," 2000; see also Siegenthaler, 2000). More recent campaigns have not used the idea of individual turning points. For example, the poster used as part of the Swiss National Program on Tobacco Prevention (2001–2005) emphasized negative consequences of tobacco, with a focus on passive smoking (www.rauchenschadet.ch). Which approach will influence dissonant smokers more and facilitate self-change remains to be seen.

Structural Prevention and Chances of Change: How Far Is It to the Next Pub and Where Am I Still Allowed to Smoke?

Availability of alcohol and drugs is subject to change and varies greatly between societies, groups, and regions. Taxation policies and various degrees of competition on drug markets will influence prices and consumption patterns (e.g., Klingemann, 1994; Öesterberg, 1992). Most of the discussion in the natural recovery field has focused on general consumption levels and has not been concerned with addiction and effects on individual behavior. How sensitive are drug consumers in various stages of change to price changes? Are substitution processes (i.e., one drug for another) affected by differential prices, health policies, or income fluctuations? In this context Godfrey (1995) highlights interesting implications of Becker and Murphy's (1988) economic model of rational addiction for self-change processes by stating the following:

Permanent changes in prices may have small short-run effects, but the long run demand for addictive goods is predicted to be more elastic than the demand for non-addictive goods. Some addictive behavior patterns such as "binges," abrupt discontinuity of consumption, and repeated quitting behavior are also consistent with this model of "rational behavior." (p. 180)

Self-reward schemes of quitters (i.e., spending the money I saved for something else I like) and the pressure to quit because of the increasing financial burden of keeping up the habit could serve as examples of how these environmental conditions can affect individual behavior.

"This is difficult, we have to change the structure of society and that is not made just like that. I think it's really difficult." (hairdresser, SINR interview, Stockholm)

The definition of alcohol-related social harm and ideas regarding what should be done about it vary across time and within the same country, as demonstrated by trend studies in the Netherlands. For example, Bongers, Goor, and Garretsen (1998) define the social climate on alcohol as the blend of different views on drinking, conceptions of alcohol-related problems, and appropriate measures for dealing with them. The study dealt with, among other things, tolerance toward drinking behavior of close relatives and drinking behavior at a party, and found that tolerance increased between 1958 and 1994. Furthermore, it was found that support for advertisement restrictions and higher prices for alcoholic beverages in the Dutch population is fading.

Taking an example from Switzerland, the liberalization of the markets has allowed for longer hours of operation, the abolishment of the so-called need clause (limiting the number of outlets as a function of the population), and the introduction of unified tax rates for distilled spirits after a ruling of the World Trade Organization in July 1999. The British government has also reformed the licensing laws and changed opening hours since 2000, even though national opinion polls do not necessarily show public support for such a policy ("Alcohol Policy," 2000; "Minister Lays Down the Law," 2000; "White Paper," 2000).

However, contextual conditions for change are by no means stable across time and countries. For example, conditions for self-change have been altered in the Nordic countries with the erosion of their alcohol monopolies after they joined the European Union (Holder et al., 1998). In 2000, the European Commission refused to extend exemption clauses to Sweden which limited alcohol imports.

Comparing the United States and Canada in 1989/1990, Giesbrecht and Greenfield (1999) found a greater polarization of opinion within both countries for policy items relating to promotion of alcohol or control of physical, demographic, or economic access, and virtually no polarization with regard to curtailing services to drunken customers or providing information on treatment.

In a recent study, Giesbrecht, Anglin, and Ialomiteanu (2005) presented survey respondents with a list of evidence-rated policy measures according to a World Health Organization-sponsored project. The respondents consisted of Ontarians drawn from cross-sectional surveys conducted with representative samples of adults between 1993 and 2003. Results showed that lay people indicated support for a wide range of policies, including both evidence-based measures (e.g., introducing a monopoly retailing system, raising the minimum legal drinking age) and less effective strategies (e.g., banning alcohol- and smoking-related advertisements on shows popular with young viewers, using warning labels). In some cases, support for effective policies (e.g., raising taxes on alcohol, restricting outlet density) was modest. This shows that the attitudes toward policy measures which would improve structural conditions for self-change are not necessarily viewed by the public as negative and should be taken into account. Not only in treatment, but also in policy, acceptance of citizens and consumers is pivotal for the implementation of change.

Finally, the most recent and impressive example of environmental changes potentially relevant to self-change is the partial or complete ban on smoking, not only in the United States (Clean Indoor Air Act, 2003) and Ireland (Public Health Tobacco Act, 2003), but also in Italy (2005), Norway (1996), Spain (2006), Scotland (2006), New Zealand, Australia, South Africa, Tanzania, Canada, and Bhutan. In Switzerland, preliminary steps have been taken to curb tobacco consumption, such as the smoking ban on public transportation in December 2005 and discussions of smoking restrictions in restaurants and bars in various cantons (see Figure 9.5).

Research on the impact of smoking bans on smoking behavior and self-change processes is scarce so far. Indirect measures include reductions in cigarette sales, the air quality in public indoor places, and smoking-related health problems (e.g., respiratory problems; see Allwright et al., 2005). Direct measures focus on the effects of reduced access to smoking at the workplace on smokers as well as nonsmoking employees and finally on customers and smokers in general. It remains to be seen if reported declines in cigarette sales, for instance an 11.3% reduction in Ireland by the market leader Gallaher (www.rauchenschadet.ch), will continue into the future. As to the effect of workplace smoking bans, older studies demonstrated that heavier smokers benefit most and that "the imposition of environmental restrictions may make long-term controlled smoking more viable in itself, and a useful way station for those who would eventually like to stop smoking completely" (Borland, Chapman, Owen, & Hill, 1990, p. 180). The comprehensive systematic review of 26 studies on the effect of smoke-free workplaces on smoking behavior by Fichtenberg and Glantz (2002) comes to the conclusion that "while producing benefits for non-smokers ... smoke-free work places make it easier for smokers to reduce or stop smoking" (p. 190). More specifically, a consumption reduction of 29% can be assumed. Also, smoking bans seem to have some effects on smoking cessation in general, at least in the short term. The Tobacco Control study has shown that the smoking ban in Ireland helped people quit smoking and 83% of Irish smokers responded positively to the ban (Eaton, 2005). Italy's smoking ban in public places has led to an 8% drop in cigarette consumption (23% among 15- to 24-year-olds; Dobson, 2005) and the study by Fichtenberg and Glantz (2002) mentioned above shows that a smoking ban at all workplaces would lead to a 4.5% drop in per capita consumption in the United States.

Although the causality is unclear, one can assume that these restrictions will support self-change processes. The Australian study by Trotter, Wakefield, and Borland (2002) on the perceived effects of smoking bans in bars, nightclubs, and gaming venues on smoking behavior focused on socially cued smoking

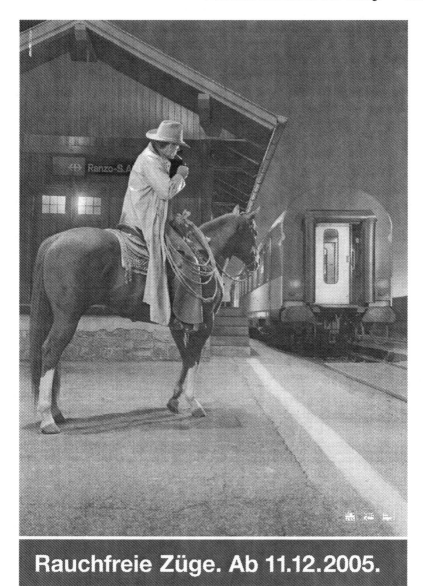

FIGURE 9.5. Poster campaign for the introduction of a smoking ban on public transportation in Switzerland.

and readiness to quit. Of the smokers frequently going to those places, 70% reported smoking more in these settings and 25% said they would be more likely to quit if bans were imposed. From a self-change perspective an interesting finding is that, compared with smokers not likely to quit after a ban, smokers who reported they would quit tended to be younger and indicated socially cued consumption. They were also in favor of bans and 2.22 times more likely to be in the contemplation or preparation stages of change. So far there are no studies which directly address the effect of smoking bans on self-change from smoking (and possibly gambling and problem alcohol use), but it could be speculated that at least dissonant smokers who are already contemplating changing might benefit considerably from these environmental changes.

Motivation of Change and References to Society and Politics of Self-Change

Most likely, individuals interviewed about why they recovered will not make reference to society, outlet density, or similar macro-concepts. Most of the contextual references (i.e., environmental features) discussed in this chapter are not often revealed in narrative accounts presented in natural recovery research. This could be an artifact and consequence of the individualistic bias described in the introduction. However, this does not mean that the macro-societal factors outlined in this chapter do not have an effect on the change process at the individual level. Identity transformation processes do become visible when people talk about religious and spiritual experiences as the causes of their remission and when they assume professional roles as helpers to foster their change and make productive use of their past deviant experiences for current respectable roles (Klingemann, 1999).

The promotion of a "self-change friendly society" might include efforts to influence social interactions between addicts and the general population, which may reduce social distance and encourage social support. Such a policy would also take into consideration societal images of various addictions and present counterarguments to addiction-related attributions of dangerousness and blame.

> "Addiction [should] be more accepted in this society here, [should be] talked about more openly, so that addicts don't necessarily feel rejection from public life.... Prejudices are so big, that people who are addicted can't work, they are not in a position to be independent." (social worker, SINR interview, Frankfurt)

Interactions between the various self-change context parameters and the empirical study of the link between context and individual change could be studied best in limited communal settings similar to community prevention programs under the following slogan: "Creating our self-change friendly town—steps to a communal self-change laboratory."

> "It could be that the environment should pay more attention to it and be more supportive ... but it depends on what stage you are in and if you listen to others. You cannot clear the country from drugs or alcohol. It seems unrealistic that all the narcotics would disappear." (social worker, SINR interview, Stockholm)

Future research is also needed to expand the range of indicators for self-change friendly societies. These concepts need to be empirically validated and tested on a cross-national level. Their relevance for the prevalence of self-change rates and the evolution of self-change processes over time should be subject to closer investigation. Aggregate data analysis and connecting context variables with individual behavior, such as the stages of change approach, will be methodological challenges for self-change research to come closer to answering the old question "why do (or don't) people change?"

References

Advice on-line. (2000). *Alcohol Alert*, *1*, 8–9.

Alcohol policy: What the public thinks. (2000). *Alcohol Alert*, *1*, 2–4.

Allwright, S., Paul, G., Greiner, B., Mullally, B. J., Pursell, L., & Kelly, A. (2005). Legislation for smoke-free workplaces and health of bar workers in Ireland: Before and after study. *British Medical Journal*, *331*, 1117.

Barber, J. G., & Gilbertson, R. (1998). Evaluation of a self-help manual for the female partners of heavy drinkers. *Research on Social Work Practice*, *8*, 141–151.

Becker, G. S., & Murphy, K. M. (1988). A theory of rational addiction. *Journal of Political Economy*, *96*, 675–700.

Bongers, I. M., Goor, I. A., & Garretsen, H. F. (1998). Social climate on alcohol in Rotterdam, the Netherlands: Public opinion on drinking behavior and alcohol measures. *Alcohol and Alcoholism*, *33*, 141–150.

Borland, R., Chapman, S., Owen, N., & Hill, D. (1990). Effects of workplace smoking bans on cigarette consumption. *American Journal of Public Health*, *80*, 178–180.

Carlson, R. (1998). *Don't sweat the small stuff at work*. New York: Hyperion.

Christenson, P. G., Henriksen, L., & Roberts, D. F. (2000). *Substance use in popular prime-time television*. Washington, DC: Office of National Drug Control Policy and Mediascope Macro International, Inc.

Cunningham, J. A., Sobell, L. C., & Sobell, M. B. (1998). Awareness of self-change as a pathway to recovery for alcohol abusers: Results from five different groups. *Addictive Behaviors*, *23*, 399–404.

Dobler-Mikola, A., Zimmer-Höfler, D., Uchtenhagen, U., & Korbel, R. (1991). *Soziale Integration und Desintegration in der 7-Jahreskatamnese bei (ehemals) Heroinabhängigen*. Forschungsinformation aus dem Sozialpsychiatrischen Dienst: Zürich, Report No. 38.

Dobson, R. (2005). Italy's smoking ban has led to an 8% drop in tobacco consumption. *British Medical Journal*, *331*, 1159.

Eaton, L. (2005). Northern Ireland will introduce a smoking ban. *British Medical Journal*, *331*, 922.

Estermann, J., Herrmann, U., Hügi, D., & Nydegger, B. (1996). Zusammenfassung der wichtigsten Ergebnisse: Empfehlungen. In J. Estermann (Ed.), *Sozialepidemiologie des drogenkonsums* (pp. 155–162). Berlin: Verlag für Wissenschaft und Bildung.

Fichtenberg, C. M., & Glantz S. A. (2002). Effect of smoke-free work places on smoking behaviour: Systematic review. *British Medical Journal*, *325*, 188–191.

Fielding, H. (1999). *Bridget Jones's diary*. New York: Penguin.

Freidson, E. (1960). Client control in medical practice. *American Journal of Sociology*, *65*, 374–382.

Giesbrecht, N., Anglin, L., & Ialomiteanu, A. (2005, May). *Alcohol policy effectiveness and public opinion: Is there support for effective policies in Ontario?* Paper presented at the 31st Annual Alcohol Epidemiology Symposium of the Kettil Bruun Society for Social and Epidemiological Research on Alcohol, Riverside, CA.

Giesbrecht, N., & Greenfield, T. K. (1999). Public opinion on alcohol policy issues: A comparison of American and Canadian surveys. *Addiction, 94,* 521–531.

Godfrey, C. (1995). Economic influences on change in population and personal substance behavior. In G. Edwards & M. Lader (Eds.), *Addiction: Processes of change* (pp. 163–187). Oxford: Oxford University Press.

Granfield, R., & Cloud, W. (1999). *Coming clean: Overcoming addiction without treatment.* New York: New York University Press.

Heather, N. (2001). Brief interventions. In N. Heather, J. P. Timothy, & T. Stockwell (Eds.), *Alcohol dependence and problems* (pp. 605–626). New York: John Wiley & Sons.

Holder, H. D., Kuhlhorn, E., Nordlund, S., Osterberg, E., Romelsjo, A., & Ugland, T. (1998). *European integration and Nordic alcohol policies: Changes in alcohol controls and consequences in Finland, Norway, and Sweden 1980–1997.* Aldershot, UK: Ashgate.

Hughes, J. R. (1999). Four beliefs that may impede progress in the treatment of smoking. *Tobacco Control, 8,* 323–326.

Hughes, J. R., Riggs, R. L., & Carpenter, M. J. (2001). How helpful are drug abuse helplines? *Drug and Alcohol Dependence, 62,* 191–194.

Internet World Stats, Usage, and Population Statistics. (n.d.). Retrieved November 22, 2006, from http://www.internetworldstats.com

Kavanagh, D. J., Sitharthan, T., Spilsbury, G., & Vignaedra, S. (1999). An evaluation of brief correspondence programs for problem drinkers. *Behaviour Therapy, 30,* 641–656.

Klingemann, H. (1991). The motivation for change from problem alcohol and heroin use. *British Journal of Addiction, 86,* 727–744.

Klingemann, H. (1992). Coping and maintenance strategies of spontaneous remitters from problem use of alcohol and heroin in Switzerland. *The International Journal of the Addictions, 27,* 1359–1388.

Klingemann, H. (1994). Environmental influences which support or impede change in substance behavior. In G. Edwards & M. Lader (Eds.), *Addiction: Multiple processes of change* (pp. 131–161). Oxford: Oxford University Press.

Klingemann, H. (1998). Harm reduction and abstinence: Swiss drug policy at a time of transition. In H. Klingemann & G. Hunt (Eds.), *Drug treatment systems in an international perspective: Drugs, demons, and delinquents* (pp. 94–111). Thousand Oaks, CA: Sage.

Klingemann, H. (1999). Addiction careers and careers in addiction. *Substance Use and Misuse, 34,* 1505–1526.

Klingemann, H. (2003, August). *How optimistic are the hairdresser and the lawyer about addicts "kicking their habit" on their own?: Public images on "natural" recovery from addiction in Switzerland, Colombia, and Germany: International collaborate study on "Societal Images of Natural Recovery from Addictions."* Paper presented at the Summer Academy "Social Work and Society," St. Petersburg, Russia.

Klingemann, H., & Bergmark A. (2006). The legitimacy of addiction treatment in a world of smart people. *Addiction, 101,* 1230–1237.

Klingemann, H., & Hunt, G. (Eds.). (1998). *Drug treatment systems in an international perspective: Drugs, demons, and delinquents.* Thousand Oaks, CA: Sage.

Klingemann, H., & Klingemann, H.-D. (1999). National treatment systems in global perspective. *European Addiction Research, 5*, 109–117.

Korgaonkar, P. K., & Wolin, L. D. (1999). A multivariate analysis of web usage. *Journal of Advertising Research, 39*, 53–68.

Lemmens, P. H., Vaeth, P. A., & Greenfield, T. K. (1999). Coverage of beverage alcohol issues in the print media in the United States, 1985–1991. *American Journal of Public Health, 89*, 1555–1560.

Lichtenstein, E., Glasgow, R. E., Lando, H. A., Ossip-Klein, D. J., & Boles, S. M. (1996). Telephone counseling for smoking cessation: Rationales and meta-analytic review of evidence. *Health Education Research, 11*, 243–257.

Mathios, A., Avery, R., Bisogni, C., & Shanahan, J. (1998). Alcohol portrayal on prime-time television: Manifest and latent messages. *Journal of Studies on Alcohol, 59*, 305–310.

Maxwell, B. (1998). *How to find health information on the Internet.* Washington, DC: Congressional Quarterly.

McCartney, P. R. (1999). Internet communication and discussion lists for perinatal nurses. *Journal of Perinatal and Neonatal Nursing, 12*, 26–40.

Minister lays down the law. (2000). *Alcohol Alert, 1*, 6.

Moeri, R. (1997). *Auswertung der Kurzevaluation zur Kampagne ,Drogen, nüchtern betrachtet' – eine Mehrheit beurteilt die Kampagne positiv.* BAG Bulletin, 42.

Moran, M. L. (1999). Dissemination of geriatric rehabilitation information via the Internet. *Topics in Geriatric Rehabilitation, 14*, 80–85.

Oldenburg, B., Glanz, K., & French, M. (1999). The application of staging models to the understanding of health behavior change and the promotion of health. *Psychological Health, 14*, 503–516.

Österberg, E. (1992). Effects of alcohol control measures on alcohol consumption. *International Journal of the Addictions, 27*, 209–225.

Parsons, T. (1951). *The social system.* New York: The Free Press.

Roberts, D. F., & Christenson, P. G. (2000). *"Here's looking at you, kid": Alcohol, drugs, and tobacco in entertainment media. A literature review prepared for The National Center on Addiction and Substance Abuse at Columbia University.* Menlo Park, CA: Kaiser Family Foundation.

Rogers, E. M., Vaughan, P., & Shefner-Rogers, C. L. (1995, May). *Evaluating the effects of an entertainment-education radio soap opera in Tanzania: A field experiment with multi-method measurement.* Paper presented at the Annual Conference of the International Communication Association, Albuquerque, NM.

Saladin, M. E., & Santa Ana, E. J. (2004). Controlled drinking more than just a controversy. *Current Opinion in Psychiatry, 17*, 175–187.

Siegenthaler, U. (2000). Jedem Projekt seine eigene website? Der erfolg der Milestone-website weckt neue Gelüste. *Krebsliga Intern, 1*, 11–12.

Slater, M. D. (1997). Persuasion processes across receiver goals and message genres. *Communication Theory, 7*, 125–148.

Slater, M. D. (1999). Integrating application of media effects, persuasion, and behavior change theories to communication campaigns: A stages-of-change framework. *Health Communication, 11*, 335–354.

Space Bar. (n.d.). Retrieved November 22, 2006, from http://www.alles-im-griff.ch

Spectra. (1999a). Petits malheurs. *Spectra, 15*, 8.

Spectra. (1999b). Un million de personnes ont un comportement risqué avec l'alcool. *Spectra, 16*, 7.

Swiss Cancer League. (1999, October). Press release for October 21, 1999. Bern: Federal Office of Public Health.

Swiss Cancer League. (2000, February). Press release fact sheet for February 29, 2000. Bern: Federal Office of Public Health.

Trotter, L., Wakefield, M., & Borland, R. (2002). Socially-cued smoking in bars, nightclubs, and gaming venues: A case for introducing smoke-free policies. *Tobacco Control*, *11*, 300–304.

Weiderer, M. (1997). Aspects of alcohol drinking and alcohol abuse in soap-operas and crime series of German television. *Sucht*, *43*, 254–263.

White paper. (2000). *Alcohol Alert*, *1*, 7.

Wilde, G. J. (1991). Effects of mass media communications upon health and safety habits of individuals: An overview of issues and evidence. *Addiction*, *88*, 983–996.

Zulewska-Sak, J. (2004, May). *"I'm gonna try with a little help from my friends": Social perception of factors improving or impeding chances of the natural recovery from addiction*. Paper presented at the 30th Annual Alcohol Epidemiology Symposium of the Kettil Bruun Society for Social and Epidemiological Research on Alcohol, Helsinki, Finland.

Zulewska-Sak, J. (2005, May). *Social perception of factors impeding chances for natural recovery from addiction: A cross-cultural qualitative perspective*. Paper presented at the 31st Annual Alcohol Epidemiology Symposium of the Kettil Bruun Society for Social and Epidemiological Research on Alcohol, Riverside, CA.

Zulewska-Sak, J., & Dabrowska, K. (2004). *Comparative analysis of qualitative data from Warsaw (Poland), Bern (Switzerland), Stockholm (Sweden), Frankfurt (Germany) within International Collaborative Study on Societal Images of Natural Recovery from Addictions (SINR; Final report)*. Warsaw: National Bureau for Drug Prevention.

Zulewska-Sak, J., & Dabrowska, K. (2005). Percepcja spoleczna czynnikow udaremnia-jacych samodzielne przezwyciezenie uzaleznienia: Jakosciowa analiza porownawcza. *Alkoholizm i Narkomania*, *18*, 63–77.

10
Natural Recovery: A Cross-Cultural Perspective

Judith C. Barker and Geoffrey Hunt

As has already been seen, the idea of "natural recovery" or "self-change" from addictions is a poorly understood and much contested concept. Some commentators in the field of alcohol and drug studies accept that this phenomenon exists, while others remain skeptical. Given the nature of this debate occurring within Anglo-European societies, it is not surprising to find that the idea of natural recovery becomes even more problematic and unclear when considering other non-Western societies. Unfortunately at this juncture, little cross-cultural research has been done on these issues. In fact, as a recent review (Sobell, Ellingstad, & Sobell, 2000) has demonstrated, the majority of the investigations have been conducted in North America (of 40 studies 59.1% were in the United States, 16.2% in Canada, 18.9% in Europe). In an earlier review, Klingemann (1994), found similar results; that is, of 80 studies reviewed on environmental influences impeding or promoting change in substance use, 7 came from outside the United States and only 1 from a non-Anglophone country.

In this chapter, information will be presented about alcohol and drug use and abuse from a broad range of cultural settings to bring relevant questions to the forefront. This is done to sensitize therapists, researchers, and other health care practitioners to the range and depth of issues underlying work with substance abusers from different cultural backgrounds. Attention to cross-cultural issues is important because it allows practitioners dealing with refugee or migrant populations from non-Western nations to understand how they might differ from dominant Anglo-European populations in attitude or response to problem substance use or addiction (Galanti, 1991). Such a focus also allows a more refined understanding of underlying concepts and assumptions central to promoting self-change or "natural recovery" from problem substance use, for example, concepts and issues such as disease, addiction, treatment, drug abuse, dependency, and control.

> **Recovered Heroin Addict**
>
> "I made a decision in favor of her, in favor of life, that gave me the strength for that decision which was definite for me. Where I grew up in the countryside, you keep what you promise, this is how I was raised which is of course an important background."

Cross-Cultural Variation in Beliefs and Normative Behaviors

Underlying the ideas of "recovery" and "treatment" are notions of disease or unacceptably disordered behavior versus well-being or normatively proper behavior. Such notions intrinsically influence opportunities and means for self-change or natural recovery.

Ideas such as these vary widely, not just by culture, but also by historical era, population demographics, prevailing theories of medicine, the degree of socially approved latitude in behavior, and modes of social control (Good, 1986). For example, it is common for highland Peruvian peasants to chew coca leaves and ingest the juice as a necessary adjunct or stimulant to work whereas in the West, cocaine, the refined substance extracted from coca leaves, has not been generally accepted as a beneficial substance (Allen, 1988). In early nineteenth century Europe, absinthe was a fashionable drink among the urban middle class until it was banned decades later because of its deleterious, even deadly, effects on physical well-being and social life. Cigarette smoking by adults, especially males, is tolerated in most societies, whereas smoking by children or females is frequently punished (Marshall, 1987). Whether excessive consumption of alcohol is a disease, an addiction, or a symptom of a disordered life has been hotly debated in the literature. What comprises "excessive" or "moderate" consumption can be equally disputed. In many non-Western societies alcohol abuse, even when resulting in domestic violence or public displays of lewd or enraged behavior, is viewed as a regrettable but intrinsic characteristic of an individual for which he or she is not responsible, a characteristic made visible by but not caused by drinking.

> **Recovered Alcohol Abuser**
>
> "Anything, shooting guns in town, or running your car through people's yards, or just anything. I never set out to do that, but I was always, I was with them. Me and my brother ... he's died of cirrhosis of the liver....He didn't quit. Just—used to have a saying that they don't even have anymore. But when we'd go to court, the lawyer would always plead your case, you know, just good ole boys, didn't mean no harm."

Among Cook Islanders in the Pacific, drunken brawls are not just mechanisms for release of aggression, but also a culturally approved means to point up and punish in public infractions of family and community morals

(Banwell, 1989). Strict distinctions may be drawn by gender. For example, drunkenness by women, whether due to ingestion of alcohol or kava, a local brew from *Piper methysticum*, is not tolerated in most Western Pacific societies (Marshall, 1987). Chewing of betel (*Areca catechu*) is a widespread custom throughout Asia and the Pacific, yet this stimulant is barely recognized in the West nor is there much research on its pharmacological properties let alone its social uses (Marshall, 1987).

What is normal, natural, and proper in one society seems strange, disturbing, and repulsive in another. Understood in context, however, each society's assumptions and behaviors become comprehensible and rational. For example, in certain South American Indian groups, male shamans (specialist healers and seers) deliberately ingest hallucinogens in order to invoke communication with the gods, especially about important and socially central activities such as warfare or hunting expeditions. Moreover, they will often blow the same substances into the nostrils of their hunting dogs to enhance the animals' abilities to detect game which is so essential to survival. In contrast, most Western cultures view very negatively any but the most mildly altered state of consciousness or cognitive ability, including any loss of control, especially when these states are induced deliberately or chemically. Pharmacologically active substances, however, such as alcohol, kava, betel, tobacco, ginger, mushrooms and other fungi, bark of various trees, and exudates from insects, amphibians, or plants, are all widely used to stimulate altered physiological or cognitive states and to induce or enhance out-of-body or out-of-mind experiences. The boundary between food, medicine, cosmetic, religious material, and drugs is a blurry one, particularly outside American or European settings (Dobkin De Rios, 1984; Etkin, 1996; Schivelbusch, 1992).

Cultural Types: Broadly Drawn

No social or cultural group is homogeneous. Within every group, some people know more about or are more interested in health issues than are other people. Often these people are recognized within their society as health professionals (e.g., shamans, acupuncturists, chiropractors, homeopathic practitioners, midwives, dentists, surgeons) with an elaborate medical knowledge and recognized set of beliefs and practices. Generally, people are pragmatic about treatment, seeking and using anything that provides relief, and people will change behavior around illness far more readily than they will change their underlying beliefs about the cause of the disorder. The more similar a patient and healer, in terms of age, sex, ethnicity, religion, education, occupational status, geographic location (e.g., rural versus urban setting), and socioeconomic class, the more likely they are to hold the same health beliefs and engage in mutually comprehensible behaviors (Galanti, 1991).

Health beliefs alone do not explain why people act, react, or think the way they do. Basic cultural values and assumptions about the nature of life (e.g., proper ways of relating to various categories of people, animals, and objects) and behavioral norms and expectations—in short, worldview or general orientation to life—all help form individuals' health beliefs or explanatory models (Kleinman, 1980).

Recovered Alcohol Abuser

"Being a nice person, being in control, being healthy, being intelligent. Those [are] all good things. I guess those are all values, like you said earlier, and those are things that I strive for. That I work towards. And it's one, it's not greater than anything else. Being healthy is not greater than being intelligent or being in control ... [it's being] the good kind of person."

To understand how worldviews can affect therapeutic endeavors, two different cultural "styles," first outlined by Hall (1956, 1959), will be discussed. These variants, or styles, have a long tradition especially in Western social psychological thought that contrasts forms of group organization and values. These variants are often described as "individualist" or "collectivist" in orientation (Oyserman, Coon, & Kemmelmeier, 2002). Such terms are heuristic devices rather than real, immutable degrees of absolute difference. They represent the ends of a continuum, the extremes. Presenting them as distinguishable and nonoverlapping permits each style and its main features to be identified and conceptualized. However, every group contains aspects of both forms, flexibly melded together and manifest differently in different circumstances. This chapter deliberately highlights the differences, the extremes, so the impact of these orientations or propensities for action becomes clear (Barker, 1994). Most cultural groups, however, hold more nuanced, less strident, more middle-of-the-range views that nevertheless can be illuminated and informed by the ideas presented here.

Specialist Cultures

The first cultural style is that associated with Western, Anglo-Europeans. This "individualist" cultural framework has been characterized as "specialist" in orientation (Hall, 1956, 1959). A core element of individualism is the assumption that individuals in a group act independently from one another. "From the core, a number of plausible consequences or implications of individualism can be discerned" (Oyserman, Coon, & Kemmelmeier, 2002, p. 4).

Basic mottoes of life in specialist cultures seem to be: "Every person for him- or herself" and "Keep your eyes on the prize." Such cultures are future oriented, actively seeking to prevent problems. Time is a commodity that can be spent, wasted, donated, or saved. Specialist cultures are also technologically innovative, deliberately seeking to devise and use new therapies and healing devices. They are egalitarian, secular, and heavily focused on the individual and independence. A model of the proper life course is a "shooting star"—a steep, straight upward trajectory ending in a blaze of glory. In other words, through education and accumulation of personal wealth, anyone can and should achieve, and should rise rapidly in individual esteem, renown, capability, and wealth; in short, such individuals should quickly fulfill their potential.

Specialist cultures prize health, for educational and financial successes depend on it. They tend to distinguish physical from mental/emotional health. Physical health is "correctable" through appropriate diagnosis and technological treatment with medications or surgery, whereas mental or emotional disorders are seen as fundamentally disruptive to the social fabric and results in marginalization of the sufferer. In such an individualistic society, one must have a strong and stable sense of self that is able to act independently in and on the world because no one else can help one achieve one's own personal responsibilities or goals for life. Addiction to alcohol or drugs is extremely disruptive to achieving one's full potential.

Anglo-European cultures represent particular variations on this idea of specialist culture. Despite being so fundamentally similar, they can differ markedly in their attitudes toward use and abuse of alcohol and drugs. So-called "wet" cultures, such as France and Spain, for example, are liberal in permitting access to alcohol, and tolerant in their treatment of problems arising from abuse. In contrast, Scandinavian countries, so-called "dry" cultures, strictly control access to addictive substances such as alcohol and tend to be more punitive in their responses to alcohol and drug abuse (Klingemann & Hunt, 1998; Klingemann, Takala, & Hunt, 1992). Moreover, the premium choice of alcoholic beverage varies widely between Southern and Northern European regions (i.e., wine versus vodka), a difference due partly to agriculture, economics, and trade, partly to historical precedent, and partly to complex cultural symbolism and ideology. Intranational differences can be as profound as international ones; for example, the drinking rate for the German-speaking cultural population in Switzerland has decreased since 1981, unlike the alcohol consumption rate for the general Swiss population that has remained steady (Klingemann, 1994). Just as differences within specialist cultures can sometimes be crucial in terms of attitude and practice, so too can they be relatively mute. Sobell and colleagues (Sobell et al., 2001), for example, found that people in Switzerland and Canada used very similar processes of cognitive evaluation and assessment to spur natural remission from alcohol and drug abuse.

Generalist Cultures

In contrast to Anglo-European cultures, many non-Western cultures can be described as "generalist" cultures (Hall, 1956, 1959), with a collectivist orientation or an "up-and-down, roller coaster" model of life. "The core element of collectivism is the assumption that groups bind and mutually obligate individuals" (Oyserman, Coon, & Kemmelmeier, 2002, p. 5).

Such cultures are portrayed as present-oriented and motivated more by immediate need to accomplish a task than by future planning or prevention of problems (Barker, 1994). These are hierarchical, sacred/religious, traditional cultures with a strong focus on family and group interconnections or interdependence. Basic, guiding mottoes seem to be: "Go with the flow" and "Enjoy the ride." Individual achievement, through education or wealth accumulation, is good as long as the outcomes can be and are redistributed to benefit everyone in the family. Health is valued but sometimes an individual has to forego or wait for treatment if some other family member's need is seen as more urgent. Illness is often accepted with a degree of stoicism or fatalism, and mental and physical health is often not separated. A person suffering from mental and emotional distress remains a valued member able to contribute something, however meager, to the family. To survive in a group with this basic life trajectory, one needs a mobile, flexible sense of self that is able to adapt to various contingencies and to sublimate individual desires for the collective good. Time is not a commodity so much as a flexible medium in which one lives in the here-and-now, and so one worries not about things over which one has no control, such as the future. Indeed, individual ability to control life is not a major concern and is often deliberately eschewed in order to achieve other culturally desirable ends. In these societies, an addicted individual is likely to be less disruptive of personal, familial, or community life.

As among specialist cultures, there is variation among and within generalist cultures in attitude and practice around alcohol, drugs, and other substances or addictive habits. Marshall (1979, 1987) presents examples of this variability among Pacific Island nations.

Variability is also well documented in the comparative literature on alcohol and drug treatment. The Latin-influenced nations of Argentina, Peru, and Colombia, for example, deal with drug addiction largely through voluntary treatment in nongovernmental organizations whereas the East Asian nations of China and Japan resort to compulsory detoxification in formal government controlled units (Klingemman & Hunt, 1998; Klingemann et al., 1992).

Ethnic Minorities and Mainstream Populations

Today it is common to find populations from generalist cultures within the context of mainstream Anglo-European specialist cultures. Over the past 2 decades there has been massive migration of non-Western peoples to: (a) European countries (e.g., Turks in Germany, Indonesians in Holland, Algerians in France, West Africans and West Indians in Britain), (b) various Anglo-affiliated countries (e.g., East Indians in Canada, Pacific Islanders in New Zealand and Australia), and (c) the United States (e.g., Asians, Latinos, Afghanis, Ethiopians, Haitians). These migrant groups bring attitudes toward knowledge and practices with respect to alcohol and drugs that vary from the mainstream Anglo-European populations. Such differences often, but not always, become muted over time, with second- or third-generation ethnic minorities adopting the mainstream pattern of consumption and beliefs. For example, Kitano and colleagues (1988, 1992) report that Japanese men in Japan were far less accepting of drinking by women, and were heavier consumers of alcohol than were Japanese-American men born and raised in Hawaii. Religious Jews, however, tend to be abstemious consumers of alcohol, regardless of where in the world they live or how long they have been there.

> "How I started with my drinking was with the European, when I was only young then I get involved with European ways of living. In that time I got deeper and deeper involved in alcoholism. At the end I was stupid, I didn't know what was going on. I was blindfold by the alcoholic spirit. It's poison to us, mainly the Aboriginal people because we can't handle it, because it's not our culture in other words." (Brady, 1993a, p. 96)

Despite the presence of multiple, distinct, non-Western, generalist populations in most major Anglo-European cities worldwide, a paucity of literature addresses normative practices of substance use or abuse by these minority or ethnic groups. Stereotypes about such groups often substitute for careful empirically based knowledge, and unresolved conceptual issues abound. These shortcomings are not only underacknowledged by researchers and clinicians, but also seriously diminish the utility of the extant literature. Here, the case of Asian Americans is considered in more detail, not because they are unique or special in the degree to which they represent conceptual and methodological problems, but rather because they illustrate so well issues common in understanding minority/ethnic populations everywhere. Asian Americans are also selected for study because they, along with other allegedly collectivist, nonindustrial cultures, are so often contrasted with Euro-American, industrial, Western nations and the individualism that is presumed to be characteristic of these groups. This contrast or separation is rarely neat and often incomplete (Kitayama, Markus, Matsumoto, & Norasakkunkit, 1997; Yamaguchi, 1994).

Individuals presently fleeing into various European nations may be Croatian or Serbian, Muslim or Christian, wealthy or poor, but as long as researchers, clinicians, social workers, and government agents identify them as "refugees from Kosovo," knowledge about their attitudes toward and use of addictive substances will be no more adequate than is the information on Asian Americans.

> "Well, at the time, when I got a taste of it I thought it was good for me, I didn't know, I was blindfold—no-one ever taught Aboriginal people all the wide world, no-one ever taught us what alcohol could do to our people. We just got in, just like cattle in a trough, just like Jack and few other people saying, we just go straight into the trough and have as much as we can drink." (Brady, 1993a, p. 97)

Asian Americans

The U.S. Census Bureau officially aggregates all people of Asian origin into a single category "Asian Pacific Islander," a term encompassing at least 60 distinct, named ethnic groups from more than 20 different nations

(Kim, McLeod, & Shantzis, 1992). Some of these Asian ethnic groups (e.g., Chinese, Japanese) have been in the United States since the 1850s and have large, generationally complex, well-established communities in metropolitan areas. Other Asian groups have been in the United States for only the past 2 decades (e.g., Cambodians or Laotians, recent refugees from Southeast Asia) and comprise smaller, economically struggling enclaves of shallow generational depth. To further separate this heterogeneous group, national origin is often used as a descriptor (e.g., Chinese, Vietnamese, Guamanian). While more fine-grained than the census term, national origin does not eliminate problems arising from important social, cultural, historical, and linguistic differences. The Hmong and the Iu-Mien, for example, are two distinct ethnic groups from the highlands of Southeast Asia, a region overlapping the national borders of Laos, Cambodia, Vietnam, and Thailand. Until 30 years ago, opium was a major cash crop in this region, especially for the Iu-Mien, and older members of these groups often still regard this drug as a useful home remedy for many everyday maladies. Further, "Vietnamese" as a descriptor makes no distinction between a person with origins in a Vietnamese cultural group and a person with origins in a migrant, ethnic Chinese group residing in Vietnam. While "China" might be an unambiguous descriptor of geographic or national origin, it makes no allowance for differences due to language or dialect (e.g., Cantonese versus Mandarin), nor does it indicate if a person comes from the dominant Han ethnic group or from the Dai or Hakka (to name but a few) minority ethnic groups in China. Recording and reporting the specific name of the ethnic group as recognized and used, its members, as well as their nation of origin, would go a long way toward overcoming some present inadequacies in available data.

For many years, a common stereotype of Asians in the United States has been that they constitute a "model minority," a quiet, law abiding, hard-working, family-oriented group that excels educationally and is economically successful (Furuto, Biswas, Chung, Murase, & Ross-Sheriff, 1992). When data about Asians in the United States are disaggregated, however, a severe challenge is issued to this stereotype. Instead of "model minority," a more complex picture emerges, one of different histories, of a broad range of distinctive settlement and demographic patterns, and of widespread variations in wealth, health, and longevity (Kim et al., 1992; Tanjasiri, Wallace, & Shibata, 1995; Uehara, Takeuchi, & Smukler, 1994). Also evident are distinct patterns of practice and belief about substance use and abuse, especially concerning alcohol and smoking. For example, well-established Asian communities tend to have smoking rates similar to U.S. rates, between 25% and 30%, depending on gender and age. However, newer Asian immigrant groups, such as those from Cambodia or Vietnam, are distinctly different. Fewer women in these populations smoke (usually less than 20%, even as low as 5% for some age groups) but many more men smoke (between 50% and 65%, depending on age groups; Jenkins et al., 1997; McPhee et al., 1995; Surgeon General, 1998). There is evidence, too, that alcohol and drug prevalence rates also vary by specific Asian ethnicity, as well as age and gender (Chi, Lubben, & Kitano, 1989; Kim et al., 1992; Kitano & Chi, 1988; Wong, Klingle, & Price, 2004).

The stereotype of "model minority" has prevented social welfare and health officials from recognizing diversity within the Asian community and from dealing with both short- and long-term consequences of migration stress, especially among refugees. These underrecognized stresses are often due to role reversals between (a) children and parents when only the children speak English or understand the American way of life or bureaucratic system and (b) spouses especially when only the wife can obtain a job. Intergenerational tensions also exist, when grandparents are no longer given respect or obedience or can no longer communicate with their monolingual English-speaking grandchildren, or when children shed allegiance to animistic, Taoist, Confucian, Buddhist, Shinto, Hinduism, or other non-Abrahamic religions and adopt Christianity but their parents and grandparents do not. Life events, such as death of a parent or spouse, divorce, severe illness or trauma, or the uprooting act of migration itself, have been associated with prompting or exacerbating substance use. However, intrapersonal evaluation of the meaning of such life events and their multiple, long-term consequences seems to have as much, if not greater, potential for negatively affecting self-esteem and increasing substance use (Klingemann, 1994). While the specific mechanisms remain unclear, the stresses and tensions outlined above have led some Asians, youths in particular, to increasingly poor educational performance, increasing alienation from family and community, increasing gang membership, increasing violence and criminal activity, and increasing substance use and abuse (Furuto et al., 1992).

Some Central Domains for Self-Change

Cross-cultural differences with respect to addiction and recovery will be vividly displayed around the following five domains: (a) definition and trajectory of the problem behavior from onset to recovery, (b) concepts and use of time, (c) management and display of emotions and cognition, (d) sense of identity, and (e) access to and use of experts. There is, of course, a great deal of overlap between the domains, which serves to reinforce the point that these comprise heuristic distinctions rather than intrinsically separate arenas. This overlap also serves to reinforce the idea that addiction and recovery are complex notions, inextricably intertwined with cultural values, social behaviors, and environmental (treatment/recovery) contexts. Within each domain, central questions are posed about its influence on the nature of self-improvement or self-change, thus providing brief commentaries and pertinent illustrations.

Problem Definition and Trajectory

• How, when, and by whom do substances come to be classed as "dangerous" or "addictive"?

- What is the definition and progression of the illness or addicted state and the trajectory of recovery?
- How, when, and where can this trajectory be interrupted, through self-change or professional treatment?
- For or from what is recovery or treatment sought? What is being treated, behavior or pathophysiology?
- From what kinds of (ingested) substances or nonnormative behaviors is recovery sought—excess alcohol consumption, food, cigarettes, illegal drugs, legal drugs, other behaviors?
- Who gets addicted and who needs to recover?

Definitions of substances as legal or illegal, beneficial or harmful, controlled or commercially available, often produce the "problem" being "treated" and the need for "recovery." Moreover, there is wide variation in what different nations, populations, or cultural groups deem to be a "drug," not to mention the differences between the lay public and professional definitions.

> "The publican asked me if I had a permit and I said 'what the hell's a permit?' and he said 'are you an Aboriginal?' I said 'yeah.' In no uncertain terms he called me a black so-and-so and to get out of there. So I hopped the bar and clobbered him and I was arrested and I said 'why are you arresting me, why don't you arrest the barman?' and they said 'because you're an Aboriginal.' I said 'what that's got to do with it?' and they said 'you're not allowed to drink alcohol.'" (Brady, 1993a, p. 162)

Khat (variously known also as *qat, gat, or chat*) is a plant-derived substance (*Catha edulis*) widely used by Somali, Yemeni, or Ethiopian populations (Cassanelli, 1986). In Europe and North America, physicians or counselors unfamiliar with these migrant communities often have not heard of this plant, let alone know its psychoactive properties. There could well be a sizable proportion of people in such ethnic groups who resort to this particular drug. Precisely because the majority of research is focused heavily on substances better known and more commonly used in Western societies, examining "natural recovery" in these groups will almost certainly miss important cultural underpinnings unless researchers are open to and active in discovering new information. Furthermore, recovery from such "exotic" substances, if it occurs at all, might involve the input or intervention of other individuals in societies (e.g., healers from the local community, family members, or even friends) in ways that are markedly different from those more familiar to mainstream professionals.

Even within dominant populations in Western societies, different groups vary in their categorizations of and response to addiction, be they government officials, healing practitioners, or ordinary citizens. Among professional treatment providers (e.g., physicians, social workers, counselors) concerned with managing or monitoring the effects of psychoactive substances, definitions of addiction change over time. For example, beneficial legal drugs are officially listed and controlled by legislation and prescription by certain licensed professionals. The addictive qualities of many of these drugs (e.g., Valium®) was not recognized initially, in part at least due to the fact that it was mainly prescribed to middle-class, white housewives in urban areas. Unlike other segments of the population (e.g., ethnic minorities, adolescents, blue collar workers), the above-mentioned demographic group is not usually viewed as having a drug problem, or constituting a "dangerous class" in society (see Hunt & Barker, 1999). Even when recognized, the addictive qualities did not force these therapeutic products from the market, in large part because these "addicts" were not societally disruptive. Rather, it remains legal for a physician to prescribe such compounds without regulated follow-up or monitoring of outcome, although general awareness has become heightened about the potential for problematic outcomes. With a few notable exceptions, ceasing to use these licit addictive drugs is not categorized as "recovery." Currently, one might need to stop using marijuana as a recreational pursuit in Anglo-European society, but would one need to stop if it was being used as a medicine, a reclassification that many groups of patients with specific conditions (e.g., glaucoma) would likely advocate? Not all substances alleged (or known) to have psychoactive properties are yet officially recognized or regulated as drugs in Anglo-European contexts. For example, herbal preparations (e.g., St. John's wort and compounds now called nutriceuticals, "foods" containing some substance, such as vitamins and minerals or similar products) are alleged to have some vital pharmacological or therapeutic properties. Until recently, the possibility of addiction to or need to cease the use of these types of substances had not been raised. Gammahydroxybutyrate (GHB) is a case in point. Until 2000, it was a widely used legal substance in the United States, available via Internet sales and in nutrition stores as a dietary supplement. As its use as a psychoactive substance increased, mainly by youths attending dance-music events at clubs and raves, and as the incidence of adverse events increased (up to and including death), the substance was recategorized as a controlled substance by the Drug Enforcement Agency (Anderson, Kim, & Dyer, 2006; Snead & Gibson, 2005).

Throughout the twentieth century, in Western societies tobacco was a legal substance that was readily available to all adults. Moreover, it is a highly addictive substance from which the majority of former smokers "recovered" spontaneously. For at least one migrant Asian group in the United States, Vietnamese men who generally have very high rates of smoking, a formal cessation program resulted in fewer people among the intervention group quitting compared with the control group (Jenkins et al., 1997; McPhee et al., 1995). In other words, spontaneous recovery worked as well as, if not better than, clinical intervention. Therapeutic endeavors developed in and effective for one cultural group cannot always easily or successfully generalize into a different context.

Estimates suggest that as many as 80% to 90% or more former smokers quit without any form of professional help other than public education campaigns

(Fiore et al., 1990; Orleans et al., 1991). Despite the enormous scale of this example of natural recovery, researchers know extraordinarily little about it. These later examples highlight the sociopolitical-economic nature of many decisions around the classification of drugs, and hence, around the need for or possibility of natural recovery from their use.

Given these potential differences in problem definition, steps taken to "cure" the malady will differ across cultures. For example, the notion of addiction as a long-lasting disease, especially one that cannot be cured but only held in remission, may not exist in non-Western societies. An illness which persists is viewed either as having been improperly cured (i.e., once a good cure from a good healer is administered the illness will disappear) or as having originated through sorcery, witchcraft, or evil directed toward the sufferer, the removal of which is necessary before a cure can be successful (Fabrega & Manning, 1972).

Recovered Alcohol Abuser

"So the desire is gone and this is where I part company with Alcoholics Anonymous and people like them, because they operate on a naturalistic bias. A naturalistic way whereas not necessarily Alcoholics Anonymous, because AA started as a Christian organization. But they say you are always an alcoholic. And I say 'No, I am no longer an alcoholic because I have been totally cured.' And in second Corinthians, v.17, it says that if any man is in Christ, he is a new creation. All things have passed away before all things have become new. And I have just taken that verse, it may be out of context, but I have taken that verse as my particular inspiration that I am no longer an alcoholic."

Time

- When in the context of a person's life is addiction likely to occur and recovery generally expected to take place (e.g., at what age or social stage, such as youth, marriage, birth of first child, or widowhood)? In what life context(s) do specific "triggers" for addiction or recovery operate (e.g., death of a parent, birth of a grandchild)?
- What is the trajectory or sequence of expected change(s) that mark recovery?
- What is the expected endpoint of recovery? Is recovery expected to be permanent and robust or a persistently fragile accomplishment?
- What temporal patterns in daily or ceremonial life facilitate or hinder recovery?

In every culture, one's occupation or productive economic/subsistence activity is probably the single most important mechanism for structuring everyday life. Work permits the development of a regular temporal sequence of events and behavioral opportunities, (e.g., when to eat, sleep, take one's leisure, participate in family or community ceremonies or rituals). These are reflected, too, in diurnal patterns of officially permitted access to legal substances, such as, the hours during which pharmacies, pubs, or liquor stores are open. It is not just the timing of consumption that matters, but also the place.

"I think with ... my experiences it just seemed like ... Asians ... when we do drugs it's like at a very specific place. Like raves. And a very specific context. Like in the privacy of your own home. Um ... it's not something that you necessarily want to ... show that you're using.... I think it's just very hard for people to, one, to admit that they're using ... and, two, to bring that into a public space, that's ... I would think that people will look down on that. You know. I know I would, if I saw someone walk in ... into a club and ... was totally high off speed or ... I wouldn't ... I wouldn't ... appreciate that at all."

Temporal sequencing of daily life is highly cross-culturally diverse. To take just one small example, the number of meals per day, the time they are taken, the amount and composition of food consumed, when the main meal is taken, and how meals interface with other activities, all vary widely from group to group (Counihan & Van Esterik, 1997). Many American tourists in Italy and other (Southern) European countries, for example, have remarked at the "extreme lateness" of the hour at which people typically eat their evening meal. Similarly, in these and other nations, such as Mexico, the midday meal is often a rather leisurely affair that permits time to relax or take a nap. In Anglo-American hotels, it is common to see a menu in which a "continental breakfast" of grains, pastries, and coffee is offered as an alternative to a "full English breakfast" consisting of hot items such as eggs and meats, as well as grains, pastries, fruits, and cheeses.

Hours for work or leisure not only vary by the nature of the job but also by socially expected and approved patterns of interaction. In many Middle Eastern societies, for example, a man is expected to meet regularly at local coffee bars to exchange news and gossip with kin, friends, and clients. In Lebanon, consumption of *arak*, a powerful alcoholic aperitif, is an important social lubricant, often accompanying a lengthy meal during which men conduct business. Many refugees in Anglo-European cities work as janitors or watchmen, who usually work at night, and therefore have different rhythms for eating and sleeping, and thus different access to alcohol or cigarettes.

Brady (1993b) points to a pattern in drunkenness among rural Australian Aborigines, noting weekday "dry spells" versus weekend "binges." Seasonality is often evident in the consequences of drunkenness, too. In Papua New Guinea, for example, there are a greater number of fatal drunk-driving crashes on weekends than on weekdays (Sinha & Sengupta, 1989). How do family, friends, and professionals (be they licensed or local healing experts) assist in maintaining normative patterns of daily or seasonal behavior? When and how are addictive substances incorporated into the temporal sequences of life? How does work act to increase, reduce, or ameliorate addictive behaviors?

"Well I suppose around about that time I was growing up, pub was like an [employment agency]. To go in and get a job, just by going to the pub. You'd walk into a pub and someone will speak to you on Cairns area, whether it's guinea grass, or up on Tablelands picking spuds. They're the places [the pubs] that some farmers used to go, and especially when the cane season's just about to start." (Brady, 1993a, p. 23)

Addicts, especially those unable to maintain employment, find it extraordinarily difficult to uphold the structure of everyday life. Indeed, their temporal sequencing often comes to revolve entirely around finding the next "hit" or drink in order to stay high or inebriated (Ames, Grube, & Moore, 1997). Further, their activities become increasingly clandestine, especially if they are addicted to an illegal substance. Recovery, or at least being on the way to recovery, is often indicated by once more engaging in the same temporal pattern of activities as the nonaddicted. Professional programs aimed at assisting recovery can sometimes unwittingly be counterproductive. For example, methadone maintenance clinics in the United States frequently disrupt an addict's attempt to maintain full-time employment through having limited, daytime and weekday only hours that coincide, and thus clash with most job schedules (Hunt & Rosenbaum, 1998).

Sudden conversion experiences have been recorded, such as when a person renounces alcohol or finds God. Indeed, religious conversion was a major reason reported by some Australian Aborigines for "giving away the grog" (Brady, 1993a,b).

Example 1: Recovered Alcohol Abuser

"Yeah, I was drunk. So I walked inside that night. I sit down and listen to the music. So next morning went back in again and this preacher was preaching about alcohol, how God works and alcohol is speaking against that, especially for our people the alcohol had a grip on our people. Same with me, I had nothing, I never owned nothing because of that poison. But I really thank God now for that brother, that really supported me. Supported me and teached me how to live a life without alcohol." (Brady, 1993a, p. 88)

Example 2: Recovered Alcohol Abuser

"I was reading a Christian book, I was drinking a drink, I put it down on the counter, I went into my parents bedroom, they were not there, and I got on my knees ... And I admitted in prayer to the Lord the fact that I was an alcoholic and that I was now asking for his help to heal me and to cure me of alcoholism.... I prayed that would happen, and I thanked the Lord and I claimed it and I believed. And I got up, poured out the drink that I was drinking, and I never even finished it.... Got on the airplane because I knew from the minute that I got off my knees that I was healed."

While complete cessation of problem consumption is the accepted endpoint in many Anglo-European settings, significant moderation of use of the addictive substance is an acceptable endpoint or state of recovery in many other cultures (Everett, Waddell, & Heath, 1976). It might be easier to cut down to acceptable levels or refrain from substance use entirely in a context where temporary abstinence from prized activities is culturally appropriate (e.g., during Lent for active Christians). In the Anglo-American world, however, total abstinence is frequently touted as the only acceptable state, as the mark of complete recovery.

Emotion

• What is the range of emotions normally permitted and what is the form and circumstances proper for doing so? By whom and when are particular kinds of emotional displays improper?

- What cognitive states are permitted? Which ones make people uncomfortable?
- What is the role of social or community forces outside the individual (e.g., family, professionals in law-and-order, medicine, spirituality) in mediating and ameliorating troublesome behaviors, especially those due to alcohol or drug use?
- How is display of emotion affected by addiction, and how is it supposed to change in recovery?

Interviewer: "How do you think that other [East] Indians would perceive you and your [drug] use?"

Respondent: "As a heathen. I feel like they'd judge me. I mean ... in the same way that they judge me for not knowing Hindi ... and that ... represents my assimilation into American culture, I feel like they would also judge me for ... assimilating into hip-hop culture or assimilating into drug culture. And so ... my use of drugs ... or former use of drugs, or my partying habits ... that's not the way they do it. They're more risk-averse, they're more like ... I don't know ... old school. Like way old school."

Most cultures generally do not approve the unfettered expression of all emotional states, but mask some states while allowing others to rein free. In specialist Anglo-European societies, for example, joy, pleasure, amusement, and cheerfulness are states that are positively valued and can be overtly manifest in most circumstances without needing to be muted or explained. Sadness, puzzlement, shyness, irritation, distress, fright, worry, and grief can also be expressed but not for too long or too forcefully, for these are less approved emotions. Strong, negative emotions (e.g., anger, rage, terror) are rarely permitted, and are expected to be quickly squelched. Thus, from a European drunkard, singing and loud maudlin sentimentality is more acceptable than vituperative rage or physically aggressive anger. Noisy, shambling drunken behavior might still make others uneasy or wary, but it is far more acceptable than bursts of profanity or violence.

Years ago, MacAndrew and Edgerton (1969) coined the phrase "drunken comportment" to describe how alcoholics learn to behave in a culturally approved fashion when inebriated. In Western societies, it is common for others to withdraw from the presence of a drugged/drunken/enraged person, to leave him "to cool off" by himself. Such a tactic acknowledges the centrality of the individual, his essential independence from others, and the need for him to regain control of himself by himself. Withdrawal does not work well in generalist cultures, in groups where interdependence is key. For example, among Polynesians it is important that trusted friends or family remain present to ameliorate and contain a person's (drunken) rage. This ensures that group norms of acceptable emotions and displays of behavior are modeled, and that the person is drawn back into the circle of relationships, not excluded from it. The drunk is placated precisely because his rage is legitimated through public acknowledgment.

Different cultures have different standards for comportment when "under the influence" of alcohol or drugs or when in emotional pain. This is easily overlooked in the heat of the moment when police, social services, or health care workers have to confront intoxicated members of different cultural groups. Consider Ethiopians, for example, a soft-spoken, mild-mannered people not given to loud or public displays of emotion. For these individuals the proper emotional and behavioral response on hearing of the death of a loved one is immediate, loud uncontrolled wailing and screaming, the flailing of limbs, and the literal tearing of clothes and hair, especially as family and friends gather in response to the news (Beyene, 1992). Neighbors often seriously misinterpret such sudden, dramatic, and unaccustomed changes in demeanor, ascribing these outbursts of "wild" behavior to drunkenness or drug use and calling in the police to restore order. This has led to considerable misunderstanding and anger between civil authorities trying to "keep the peace," and Ethiopians trying to mourn properly the death of their loved one, especially when the behaviors are accompanied by incompletely understood explanations in unfamiliar languages.

Western cultures are highly rationalist and focus on a rather concrete, empirical reality. Generally, in these cultures, people are very uneasy around those who hallucinate or have cognitive patterns different from the norm. Those who are actively dementing, delirious, or hallucinating, whether for organic or chemical reasons, make others nervous and uneasy, thus are often shunned (Leibing & Cohen, 2006). Conversely, in many other cultures, talking to long-dead ancestors, or seeing or hearing people, noises, or activities that is not apparent to others, is not a suspect activity, even if stimulated by plant or chemical ingestion. Rather, hallucinatory or alternate cognitive states are often highly regarded, as signs of an important ability to establish direct contact with spirits or a parallel world.

Identity

- Is the addicted person's "deviant status" privately or publicly acknowledged?
- What is considered to be the possibility of "change" in identity? That is, is a person seen as having a "career" as an alcoholic or drug addict as, say, in the West versus having a persona or personality characteristic as a bully or argumentative person that is exacerbated by alcohol or drugs, as in many non-Western cultures?
- How does the role of outside forces (e.g., family, healing expert) articulate with ideas of independence, control, and self/identity?
- What is the link between identity and social position (e.g., developmental/ life trajectory/age/chronology issues and gender, ethnic, and within-group socioeconomic class differences)?
- Who is thought to be "at risk" for need of recovery, and how and when should they be treated?

The acceptability of nonnormative behavior varies significantly by age, gender, ethnicity, socioeconomic class, and geographic location (Marsella & White, 1982). For example, among low-income adults over age 65 in rural settings in the United States, it has been found that a much smaller proportion of women than men smoke. Not only do such women currently smoke far fewer cigarettes than their male counterparts, but they also smoke less than younger females and women of the same age but have higher incomes or live in urban locations. Social expectations and rules around inappropriate behavior, both now and when these women were younger, helped shape this finding. When these women were young adults, smoking (especially in a public setting) was not only a declaration of rebellion but also acceptance, albeit often reluctantly, of a reputation as an "easy" or "loose" woman. In general, far fewer older women than older men willingly quit smoking (Colsher et al., 1990).

> "There was a time there for ... two or three years where I ... I didn't think about my ethnic identity at all. I was just thinking about like ... who I was as a person ... as a gay woman, you know. But I ... I noticed ... I remember thinking ... you know, looking around and seeing ... the straight Filipinos on campus, and I remember thinking 'God, I wonder if they're using [drugs] too or ... ?' And ... I remember ... wanting to be a part of that community again. You know, after ... using ... Ecstasy for as much as I did and ... I remember thinking 'I wonder if this is something that's acceptable? Do other Filipino kids do this?' And ... I later learned from my other Filipino friends, straight friends, that, yeah, they had tried drugs too. And so ... so ... but I remember thinking ... 'Am I being less Filipino because I'm hanging out with some white people and ... and Vietnamese people and ... a lotta white people [laughs], you know, and doing drugs with them, or ... ?' You know, I ... I kinda had a hard time with that, like I ... didn't know if I wasn't being true to my people."

A major difference between Western, Anglo-European cultures and non-Western cultures is the degree to which stigmatization of the addicted person occurs, or the degree to which the addict is viewed as deviant (Lemert, 1958; Partanen, 1991). In Western cultures, whether deviancy is due to criminal activity (e.g., stealing to support a drug habit), personal inadequacy (e.g., drinking to excess), or functional rather than organic illness (e.g., mental or emotional conditions), alienation of the deviant from family and the wider society commonly occurs. Should remission from the problem take place whether it is due to natural recovery or through professional therapeutic encounters, the person is reintegrated into mainstream society, though usually still with a "suspect" label as a "recovering" addict. Sometimes, the deviant label is so indelible, the extrusion so permanent, that people who share a particular outcast status band together to form subcultural groups, each with its own values and norms of behavior (e.g., homeless mentally ill, injection drug users).

Consistent with the values of generalist cultures, in non-Western settings mental or emotional illness or addiction frequently does not result in extreme social marginalization (Lemert, 1958; Partanen, 1991). While the family or community might condemn the behavior, they rarely carry over that condemnation to include the actual person. Rather, the individual remains within the family circle and receives public support for his or her efforts to deal with addiction. Possession cults in some West African societies, for example, are organizations that sufferers join in order to express collectively through dance, trance, and chant their mental or emotional anguish, and to display their affliction and nonnormative behavior in a public place to a mainstream audience of nonmembers. Their addiction/illness is not shameful nor is it kept secret from mainstream society. This approach is juxtaposed by the therapeutic self-help groups in the West such as Alcoholics Anonymous. Here, meetings are held out of sight of the general public and, while each member is supported on an individual journey to recovery, there is not the same kind of collective celebration or acceptance of the disease or addiction that unites group members.

Expertise

- Who properly can treat various states of altered consciousness?
- Does recovery involve "experts"? If so, an expert in what?
- Does the "recovered" person pay? Whom? How? What?
- Where does recovery take place (home versus community setting versus other special location)?
- What procedures or means are used to treat altered states of consciousness (e.g., fasting, sweat lodges, herbal medicines)? How could these be used to facilitate self-change or natural recovery?

Professionals can have a profound influence on an addict's desire and resolve to quit, depending on when in the addict's career this intervention occurs. Health was the primary reason Australian Aborigines gave for spontaneously quitting drinking, after some physician, nurse, or other respected expert told them "knock it off or die" (Brady, 1993b).

> "Then she took me up and I went in the hospital here. The doctor said 'you're sick from drinking too much.' And they had a plastic bag that shifted through my nose and a plastic bag down here and they drained it out, a bottle of Moselle and beer, I think that was what I was drinking. They flew me up in Darwin Hospital and I still had that tube and thing through my nose and I had that operation. My liver and kidney was really bad, and I was told from doctor not to be drinking anymore because I sick. You see, doctor told me, 'if you drink again you should have been dead.'" (Brady, 1993a, p. 32)

What this also means, however, is that the alcoholic or drug user has to have been consuming for a long enough period of time or heavily enough that some deleterious physical effect is evident. And that he or she has reached a life stage where no longer drinking, smoking, snorting, sniffing, or injecting is acceptable. A young adult, especially male, in the prime of life might be teased or tormented by peers for not drinking alcohol, whereas an older adult might be excused. Both Australian Aborigines (Brady, 1993b) and urban American Indians (Barker & Kramer, 1996) have commented on how drunkenness is unacceptable at older ages, especially as a person adopts, willingly or otherwise, certain highly valued social roles (e.g., becoming a grandparent).

If the client and the expert come from the same cultural backgrounds, then it is likely that they will share the same cultural assumptions both about the origins of the addiction and the possible need for treatment (Galanti, 1991).

However, if the client and treatment practitioner do not come from the same background, then there may be cultural misunderstandings. For example, in Western societies, the precise procedures adopted during treatment are generally perceived as a somewhat private affair, even if group methods are adopted. In contrast, in many non-Western societies, treatment processes may be seen primarily as a social event, not solely for the purpose of the patient but also for the community as well, a process Kleinman (1980) calls "cultural healing." Put another way, in such societies the healing process acts as an integrative process, restoring both group cohesion and individual integration. Once the client's disruptive behavior has been resolved, the healing process works to repay obligations incurred while the individual was ill.

Although developed within a specific cultural system, treatment modalities are often "imported" or "exported" across national boundaries, depending on the political and policy climate with respect to substance use and treatment (Klingemann & Klingemann, 1999; MacGregor, 1999). While Anglo-European countries frequently take the lead in devising and exporting/importing treatment methods (e.g., Liverpool experiments in England, Swiss heroin trials, various 12-step programs from the United States), the development and export of treatments is not limited to Western settings. For example, *naikan* therapy, a group-oriented personal insight therapeutic approach that originated in Japan, is now used in a number of other countries, including those in Europe (Konuma, Shimizu, & Koyanagi, 1998). As already noted with the smoking cessation program among Vietnamese men, the success of exported treatment modalities is variable, especially among population groups for which the therapy was not originally designed (Klingemann & Klingemann, 1999).

The role the family is expected to play in treatment varies widely, even within European countries (MacGregor, 1999). In some societies, "illnesses" and "problem behaviors" may be solved within the family, rather than going to outside "professionals" (Chin, 1992). Reasons for this may involve politics and socioeconomic status within the community. In Western societies, discussing one's problems, either with friends or professionals, may be viewed as a way of gaining a solution to the problems, while keeping them hidden is seen as "dangerous." However, in other societies, openly discussing problems outside the close-knit extended family group may be seen as dangerous, and the best way forward is to keep them private. When treatment is sought outside the family, it frequently involves a trusted individual with whom family members have longstanding complex relations, such as a business patron or a spiritual guide (e.g., priest, shaman). For example, in Hispanic/Latino societies, *co-madres* are key resources to which people turn in times of stress, trouble, and need for practical day-to-day assistance, especially if there is trouble (e.g., illness, sudden small financial shortfalls, pressing need for urgent childcare) within the family unit.

Furthermore, if the individual's illness is perceived as the result of some malevolent behavior on the part of others in the community, then part of the healing process may entail reparation from those who are suspected of causing the misfortune. Frequently, reparation involves not only the afflicted transgressing individual but also his or her wider family or clan. Only after reparation has taken place can the community become integrated again. Joining with other family or community members to make reparation could be a major way in which self-change takes place. This process is fundamentally different from the process of healing in Western societies. There, once an individual has become labeled as an alcoholic or drug addict, he or she becomes separated or alienated from the rest of society, even after treatment. Unlike other illnesses, the alcoholic or drug addict remains in a permanent state of being in recovery. Consequently, compared to many non-Western societies, the societal process of labeling erects barriers around the individual and separates him or her from the social groups of which they are part.

In examining the role of the expert in non-Western societies, the shaman is particularly important. In nations with few resources for the treatment of problem substance use, such as Peru (Lara-Ponce, 1998), shamans can be key, especially in rural areas. In cases of possession (a state similar to that of the dependent substance abuser), the shaman may adopt practices which allow him to become possessed by the same spirits as those possessing the afflicted in order to return that individual to a prior state. However, as Lewis (1971) notes, whereas the state of possession for the shaman is controlled, the possession for the client is not. In this state of "controlled abnormality" the shaman is able to master or neutralize the spirits, not just those afflicting him but also those affecting his client (Hellman, 1984). Shamanic control occurs in two realms, that of symbolic ritual and that of physiological/psychological process. What comforts the mind and soul, heals and cures the body.

Conclusion: Implications for Research and Clinical Practice

This chapter has shown how the idea of "self-change" or "natural recovery" becomes exceptionally problematic but also extremely instructive when considered cross-culturally. Therapists, counselors, researchers, and others working with people from minority cultures who are undergoing recovery from an addiction, need to be acutely aware of the impact of cross-cultural differences. They need to appreciate the crucial role played by the social location of the problem substance user and how social forces work in both the mainstream and minority cultures.

Within all cultural groups, social location and social forces affect definitions, values, and behaviors around addictive substances, especially alcohol and drugs. The social location of the addict or person in recovery (i.e., age, gender, ethnicity, socioeconomic class, geographic and historical cohort) affects access to and use of particular substances. Wider social forces impinging on the individual (e.g., laws and regulations, resources such as treatment clinics or social services, social policies) directly impact an individual's access to and success with treatment. Practitioners need to be alert to cues that "problems" with and recovery from alcohol and drug use may be manifested in quite distinct ways in different cultural groups.

While it is desirable that counselors and therapists not only speak the language of their minority clients but also be aware of key cultural values and behavioral norms, this is usually exceptionally difficult to achieve when dealing with multiple distinct minority groups. In the absence of such detailed knowledge, it is imperative that treatment professionals learn to recognize central issues around which many miscommunications occur (Barker, 1994). These are most likely to include the following:

- Ideas about basic trajectory of life and its goals
- Range of allowable expression of emotions
- Time patterning of everyday behaviors, especially work
- Beliefs and behaviors about addictive substances, about the course of illnesses in general and substance abuse in particular, the trajectory of recovery, and evidence for success in treatment
- Issues of identity, stigma, and independence
- Notions of family as a source of decision-making, as having authority over individual members, and as a caregiving unit. Awareness of generational differences, especially in migrant groups
- Appropriate time to consult an expert to assist in an individual's recovery

Differences in the impact of social location and social forces become even more marked and complex when assisting a client from a minority group as opposed to the mainstream. Such differences, especially between "specialist" (e.g., Western, Anglo-European) and "generalist" (e.g., non-Western) groups, carry important implications for the global "import/export" of addiction treatments, including the concept of "natural recovery" or "self-change." The more specific the information one knows about their clients and their cultural affiliation, the more helpful it will be in interventions (Barker, 1994). Providers should seek to know the name, geographic origin, and historical background of a minority group, as well as its demographic and health profile. They should also be wary of lumping groups that are distinct into unitary categories, thus eschew stereotypes. Moreover, one must remember that difficulties and miscommunications are not caused by minority clients or mainstream therapists, but rather are the results of two different cultural systems interacting. Whenever unexpected occurrences happen or difficulties arise in treating a client from a different cultural group, practitioners are encouraged to consult an expert (i.e., a bilingual, bicultural individual knowledgeable of both minority and mainstream populations) who can help resolve the impasse stemming from different backgrounds, expectations, and experiences through a culturally appropriate and sensitive translation.

References

Allen, C. J. (1988). *The hold life has: Coca and cultural identity in an Andean community.* Washington, DC: Smithsonian Institution Press.

Ames, G. M., Grube, J. W., & Moore, R. S. (1997). The relationship of drinking and hangovers to workplace problems: An empirical study. *Journal of Studies on Alcohol, 58*(1), 37–47.

Anderson, I. B., Kim, S. Y., & Dyer, J. E. (2006). Trends in gamma-hydroxybutyrate (GHB) and related drug intoxication: 1999 to 2003. *Annals of Emergency Medicine, 47*, 177–183.

Banwell, C. (1989). *The place of alcohol in the lives of Cook Islands women living in Auckland (Report No. 2).* The Place of Alcohol in the Lives of New Zealand Women Project. Department of Anthropology, University of Auckland.

Barker, J. C. (1994). Recognizing cultural differences: Health-care providers and elderly patients. *Gerontology & Geriatrics Education, 15*, 9–21.

Barker, J. C., & Kramer, B. J. (1996). Alcohol consumption among older urban American Indians. *Journal of Studies on Alcohol, 57*, 119–124.

Beyene, Y. (1992). Medical disclosure and refugees: Telling bad news to Ethiopian patients. *Western Journal of Medicine, 157*, 328–332.

Brady, M. (1993a). *Giving away the grog: Aboriginal accounts of drinking and not drinking.* Canberra: Australian Government Printing Service.

Brady, M. (1993b). Giving away the grog: An ethnography of Aboriginal drinkers who quit without help. *Drug and Alcohol Review, 12*, 401–411.

Cassanelli, L. V. (1986). Qat: Changes in the production and consumption of a quasi-legal commodity in Northeast Africa. In A. Appadurai (Ed.), *The social life of things: Commodities in cultural perspective* (pp. 236–257). New York: Cambridge University Press.

Chi, I., Lubben, J. E., & Kitano, H. H. L. (1989). Differences in drinking behavior among three Asian-American groups. *Journal of Studies on Alcohol, 50*, 15–23.

Chin, S.-Y. (1992). This, that, and the other: Mental illness in a Korean family. *Western Journal of Medicine, 157*, 257–293.

Colsher, P. L., Wallace, R. B., Pomrehn, P. R., LaCroix, A. Z., Cornoni-Huntley, J., Blazer, D., et al. (1990). Demographic and health characteristics of elderly smokers. *American Journal of Preventive Medicine, 6*, 61–70.

Counihan, C., & Van Esterik, P. (Eds.). (1997). *Food and culture: A reader.* New York: Routledge.

Dobkin De Rios, M. (1984). *Hallucinogens: Cross-cultural perspectives.* Albuquerque: University of New Mexico Press.

Etkin, N. L. (1996). Ethnopharmacology. In C. F. Sargent & T. M. Johnson (Eds.), *Medical anthropology: Contemporary theory and methods* (rev. ed.). Westport, CT: Praeger.

Everett, M. W., Waddell, J. O., & Heath, D. B., (Eds.). (1976). *Cross-cultural approaches to the study of alcohol: An interdisciplinary perspective.* The Hague: Mouton.

Fabrega, H., & Manning, P. K. (1972). Disease, illness, and deviant careers. In R. A. Scott & J. D. Douglas (Eds.), *Theoretical perspectives on deviance.* New York: Basic Books.

Fiore, M. C., Novotny, T. E., Pierce, J. P., Giovino, G. A., Hatziandreu, E. J., Newcomb, P. A., et al. (1990). Methods used to quit smoking in the United States. *Journal of the American Medical Association, 263*, 2760–2765.

Furuto, S. M., Biswas, R., Chung, D. K., Murase, K., & Ross-Sheriff, F. (Eds.). (1992). *Social work practice with Asian Americans.* Thousand Oaks, CA: Sage.

Galanti, G. A. (1991). *Caring for patients from different cultures.* Philadelphia: University of Pennsylvania Press.

Good, B. (1986). Explanatory models and care-seeking: A critical account. In S. McHugh & T. M. Vallis (Eds.), *Illness behavior: A multidisciplinary model.* New York: Plenum Press.

Hall, E. T. (1956). *The hidden dimension.* Garden City, NY: Doubleday.

Hall, E. T. (1959). *The silent language.* Garden City, NY: Doubleday.

Hellman, C. (1984). *Culture, health, and illness.* Bristol: Wright.

Hunt, G., & Barker, J. C. (1999). Drug treatment in contemporary anthropology and sociology. *European Addiction Research, 5,* 126–132.

Hunt, G., & Rosenbaum, M. (1998). "Hustling" within the clinic: Consumer perspectives on methadone maintenance treatment. In J. A. Inciardi & L. D. Harrison (Eds.), *Heroin in the age of crack cocaine.* Thousand Oaks, CA: Sage.

Jenkins, C. N., McPhee, S. J., Le, A., Pham, G. Q., Ha, N. T., & Stewart, S. (1997). The effectiveness of a media-led intervention to reduce smoking among Vietnamese-American men. *American Journal of Public Health, 87,* 1031–1034.

Kim, S., McLeod, J. H., & Shantzis, C. (1992). Cultural competence for evaluators working with Asian-American communities: Some practical considerations. In M. A. Orlandi, R. Weston, & L. G. Epstein (Eds.), *Cultural competence for evaluators: A guide for alcohol and other drug abuse prevention practitioners working with ethnic/racial communities* (pp. 203–260). Rockville, MD: U.S. Department of Health & Human Services, Office for Substance Abuse Prevention.

Kitano, H. H. L., & Chi, I. (1988). *Asian Americans and alcohol: The Chinese, Japanese, Koreans, and Filipinos in Los Angeles.* In D. Speigler, D. Tate, S. Aitken, & C. Christian (Eds.), *Alcohol use among U.S. ethnic minorities.* Rockville, MD: National Institute on Alcohol and Alcohol Abuse.

Kitano, H. H. I., Chi, I., Rhee, S., & Lubben, J. E. (1992). Norms and alcohol consumption: Japanese in Japan, Hawaii, and California. *Journal of Studies on Alcohol, 53,* 33–39.

Kitano, H. H. I., Chi, I., Law, C. K., Lubben, J. E., & Rhee, S. (1988). Alcohol consumption of Japanese in Japan, Hawaii, and California. In L. H. Towle & T. C. Hartford (Eds.), *Cultural influences and drinking patterns.* Washington, DC: U.S. Government Printing Office.

Kitayama, S., Markus, H. R., Matsumoto, H., & Norasakkunkit, V. (1997). Individual and collective process in the construction of the self: Self enhancement in the United States and self-criticism in Japan. *Journal of Personality and Social Psychology, 72,* 1245–1267.

Kleinman, A. (1980). *Patients and healers in the context of culture: An exploration of the borderland between anthropology, medicine, and psychiatry.* Berkeley: University of California Press.

Klingemann, H. K. H. (1994). Environmental influences which promote or impede change in substance behavior. In G. Edwards & M. Lader (Eds.), *Addiction: Processes of change* (pp. 131–161). New York: Oxford University Press.

Klingemann, H., & Hunt, G. (Eds.). (1998). *Drug treatment systems in an international perspective: Drugs, demons, and delinquents.* Thousand Oaks, CA: Sage.

Klingemann, H., & Klingemann, H.-D. (1999). National treatment systems in global perspective. *European Addiction Research, 5,* 109–117.

Klingemann, H., Takala, J. P., & Hunt, G. (Eds.). (1992). *Cure, care, or control: Alcoholism treatment in sixteen countries.* Albany: State University of New York Press.

Konuma, K., Shimizu, S., & Koyanagi, T. (1998). Social control and the model of legal drug treatment: A Japanese success story? In H. Klingemann & G. Hunt (Eds.), *Drug treatment systems in an international perspective: Drugs, demons, and delinquents.* Thousand Oaks, CA: Sage.

Lara-Ponce, A. (1998). Who is to blame? The discovery of domestic drug problems and the quest for recognition of therapeutic communities in Peru. In H. Klingemann & G. Hunt (Eds.), *Drug treatment systems in an international perspective: Drugs, demons, and delinquents.* Thousand Oaks, CA: Sage.

Leibing, A., & Cohen, L. (Eds.). (2006). *Thinking about dementia: Culture, loss, and the anthropology of senility.* New Brunswick, NJ: Rutgers University Press.

Lemert, E. M. (1958). The use of alcohol in three Salish tribes. *Quarterly Journal of Studies on Alcohol, 19,* 90–107.

Lewis, I. M. (1971). *Ecstatic religion: An anthropological study of spirit possession and shamanism.* New York: Penguin.

MacAndrew, C., & Edgerton, R. (1969). *Drunken comportment: A social explanation.* Chicago: Aldine.

MacGregor, S. (1999). Drug treatment systems and policy frameworks: A comparative social perspective. *European Addiction Research, 5,* 119–125.

Marsella, A. J., & White, G. M. (Eds.). (1982). *Cultural conceptions of mental health and therapy.* New York: Reidel.

Marshall, M. (Ed.). (1979). *Beliefs, behaviors, and alcoholic beverages: A cross-cultural survey.* Ann Arbor: The University of Michigan Press.

Marshall, M. (1987). An overview of drugs in Oceania. In L. Lindstrom (Ed.), *Drugs in Western Pacific societies: Relations of substance* (pp. 13–49). New York: University Press of America.

McPhee, S. J., Jenkins, C. N. H., Wong, C., Fordham, D., Lau, D. Q., Bird, J. A., et al. (1995). Smoking cessation intervention among Vietnamese Americans: A controlled trial. *Tobacco Control, 4*(Suppl. 1), S16–S24.

Orleans, C. T., Schoenbach, V. J., Wagner, E. H., Quade, D., Salmon, M. A., Pearson, D. C., Fielder, J., Porter, C. Q., & Kaplan, B. H. (1991). Self-help quit smoking interventions: Effects of self-help materials, social support instructions, and telephone counseling. *Journal of Consulting and Clinical Psychology, 59,* 439–448.

Oyserman, D., Coon, H. M., & Kemmelmeier, M. (2002). Rethinking individualism and collectivism: Evaluation of theoretical assumptions and meta-analyses. *Psychological Bulletin, 128,* 3–72.

Partanen, P. (1991). *Sociability and intoxication: Alcohol and drinking in Kenya, Africa, and the modern world.* Helsinki: The Finnish Foundation for Alcohol Studies.

Schivelbusch, W. (1992). *Tastes of paradise: A social history of spices, stimulants, and intoxicants.* New York: Pantheon Books.

Sinha, S. N., & Sengupta, S. K. (1989). Road traffic fatalities in Port Morseby: A ten year survey. *Accident Analysis and Prevention, 21,* 297–301.

Snead, O. C., III, & Gibson, K. M. (2005). Gamma-hydroxybutyric acid. *New England Journal of Medicine, 352,* 2721–2732.

Sobell, L. C., Ellingstad, T. P., & Sobell, M. B. (2000). Natural recovery from alcohol and drug problems: Methodological review of the research with suggestions for future directions. *Addiction, 95,* 749–764.

Sobell, L. C., Klingemann, H., Toneatto, T., Sobell, M. B., Agrawal, S., & Leo, G. I. (2001). Alcohol and drug abusers' perceived reasons for self-change in Canada and Switzerland: Computer-assisted content analysis. *Substance Use and Misuse, 36,* 1467–1500.

Surgeon General. (1998). *Tobacco use among U.S. racial/ethnic minority groups.* Rockville, MD: U.S. Department of Health & Human Services, Centers for Disease Control and Prevention.

Tanjasiri, S. P., Wallace, S. P., & Shibata, K. (1995). Picture imperfect: Hidden problems among Asian Pacific Islander elderly. *The Gerontologist, 35,* 753–760.

Uehara, E. S., Takeuchi, D. T., & Smukler, M. (1994). Effects of combining disparate groups in the analysis of ethnic differences: Variations among Asian American mental health consumers in level of functioning. *American Journal of Community Psychology, 22*, 83–99.

Wong, M. M., Klingle, R. S., & Price, R. K. (2004). Alcohol, tobacco, and other drug use among Asian American and other Pacific Islander adolescents in California and Hawaii. *Addictive Behaviors, 29*, 127–141.

Yamaguchi, S. (1994). Collectivism among the Japanese: A perspective from the self. In U. Kim, H. C. Triandis, C. Kagitcibasi, S. Choi, & G. Yoon (Eds.), *Individualism and collectivism: Theory, method, and applications* (pp. 175–188). Thousand Oaks, CA: Sage.

11
Self-Change Toolbox: Tools, Tips, Websites, and Other Informational Resources for Assessing and Promoting Self-Change

Andrew Voluse, Joachim Körkel, and Linda Carter Sobell

Introduction

This chapter is intended to provide tools, tips, and resource information (e.g., websites, manuals, other materials) to assess, assist, and promote the self-change process. Included in this toolbox are brief assessment instruments, a listing of addictive behavior websites categorized by country, and various resources that can be requested online.

It is not the intention of the authors to provide an all-encompassing list of self-change tools, tips, and resources. Rather, the selection reflects the experiences and preferences of the authors.

Assessment Instruments to Promote Self-Change

There exists no shortage of instruments for assessing addictive behaviors (Allen & Wilson, 2003; American Psychiatric Association, 2000; López Viets & Miller, 1997; Rounsaville, Tims, Horton, & Sowder, 1993; Sobell, Toneatto, & Sobell, 1994; Substance Abuse and Mental Health Administration, 1993, 1995, 2002). This toolbox lists and describes, in most instances briefly, selected instruments that can be used to facilitate and evaluate the self-change process. The criteria used for choosing the measures were that they had to be (a) brief, (b) require minimal time and resources, (c) readily accessible, and (d) free. When selecting an instrument for use in facilitating self-change, it should, whenever possible, provide meaningful advice and feedback which can then enhance or strengthen individuals' motivation for change (Substance Abuse and Mental Health Administration, 2002).

The use of brief measures (Breslin, Sobell, Sobell, & Agrawal, 2000; Cherpitel, 1997; Rollnick, Morgan, & Heather, 1996; Samet, Rollnick, & Barnes, 1996; Sklar & Turner, 1999; Sobell & Sobell, 2000, 2005) has increased dramatically over the past decade, spurred by the growing interest in the fields of self-change and brief interventions (Fleming & Manwell, 1999; Fleming, Manwell, Barry, Adams, & Stauffacher, 1999; Heather, 1990, 1994; Rollnick, Butler, & Stott, 1997). For example, while an instrument such as the Addiction Severity Index (ASI) has excellent psychometric characteristics and has been used in many drug programs (McLellan et al., 1992), it is a structured interview with 147 questions (assessing problems in seven different areas) that must be administered by a trained interviewer and takes approximately 30 to 45 minutes to complete. Consequently, instruments such as the ASI are too labor-intensive and resource-demanding for use in brief self-change interventions, where the process can be as short as one session.

Tools for Assessing Problem Severity or Adverse Consequences of Addictive Behaviors

Alcohol Use Disorders Identification Test (AUDIT): This 10-item self-administered questionnaire takes approximately 3–5 minutes to complete. It addresses both past and recent alcohol consumption patterns and alcohol-related problems. Moreover, it identifies individuals drinking at high-risk levels as well as those already experiencing consequences (Allen, Litten, Fertig, & Babor, 1997; Allen & Wilson, 2003; Saunders, Aasland, Babor, De La Fuente, & Grant, 1993). The AUDIT is available in English, French, German, Portuguese, and Spanish.

AUDIT Alcohol Consumption Questions (AUDIT-C): This 3-item questionnaire is a shortened version of the 10-item AUDIT measure. The AUDIT-C uses the first three questions from the full AUDIT, which concentrates on levels of alcohol consumption rather than negative consequences that clients have experienced due to heavy drinking. This scale was developed, partially, as a quick screening tool for general medical practitioners to identify at-risk, heavy drinkers (Gual, Segura, Contel, Heather, & Colom, 2002). In addition, it was created because physicians reported that clients appeared to start responding to the full AUDIT defensively after the third question (i.e., once the items began to probe negative consequences experienced from alcohol use). Although relatively new, the AUDIT-C has demonstrated that it is at least equally effective in screening risky drinking as the full AUDIT and is even superior in identifying heavy drinkers (Bush, Kivlahan, McDonell, Fihn, & Bradley, 1998).

Lübeck Alcohol Dependence and Abuse Screening Test (LAST): This 7-item questionnaire takes approximately 1–2 minutes to complete. It screens for alcohol dependence and abuse and is especially suited for use in health care settings (Rumpf, Hapke, Hill, & John, 1997).

Drug Abuse Screening Test (DAST): This 10-item self–administered questionnaire takes roughly 3–5 minutes to finish. It measures the consequences of drug use that have occurred in the previous year (American Psychiatric Association, 2000; Skinner, 1982; Sobell, Toneatto, & Sobell, 1994). The form is available in English, Portuguese, and Spanish.

Drug Use Disorders Identification Test (DUDIT): This 11-item questionnaire addresses past and recent drug consumption and identifies various drug-related problems. The categories of questions on the survey are almost identical to those on the AUDIT. That is, while both probe frequency and amount of use, they also inquire about consequences and negative effects due to drug use. As with the AUDIT, this survey identifies at-risk individuals and those who have already experienced consequences from drug use. While still in its infancy, the DUDIT has demonstrated that it could predict drug dependence with a sensitivity of 90% in a drug user sample (Berman, Bergman, Palmstierna, & Schlyter, 2005).

Fagerström Tolerance Questionnaire (FTQ): This well-established 8-item questionnaire is a self-report instrument that measures individuals' dependency on nicotine. The instrument has shown high correlations with physiological measures such as carbon monoxide, nicotine, and cotinine levels (Fagerström & Schneider, 1989). Two revisions of the FTQ have also been developed: (a) the 6-item Fagerström Test for Nicotine Dependence (Heatherton, Kozlowski, Frecker, & Fagerström, 1991) and (b) the 10-item Revised Tolerance Questionnaire (Tate & Schmitz, 1993).

Time to the First Cigarette: While a nicotine dependence score is useful for research purposes, the following single question is clinically valuable: "How many minutes upon waking until the first cigarette is smoked?" The latency of smoking the first cigarette after waking is strongly predictive of nicotine dependence (Pomerleau, Pomerleau, Majchrzak, Kloska, & Malakuti, 1990). This question is part of the Fagerström scale for assessing nicotine dependence (Fagerström & Schneider, 1989).

South Oaks Gambling Screen (SOGS): This 20-item self-administered questionnaire takes roughly 3–5 minutes to complete. It assesses gambling-related consequences that have occurred over an individual's lifetime (Lesieur & Blume, 1993).

Eating Disorders Inventory (EDI): This self-report questionnaire measures eating behaviors, attitudes regarding body satisfaction, and psychological traits and symptoms (e.g., perfectionism, interpersonal distrust; Garner, Olmsted, & Polivy, 1983). The instrument takes approximately 15 minutes to complete and is designed to be used throughout treatment to assess progress.

Assessing Addictive Behaviors

Drug History Questionnaire (DHQ): The DHQ uses a card-sort technique and takes roughly 5–10 minutes to finish. It captures both lifetime and recent information (e.g., years used, route of administration, year last used, frequency of use) regarding the use of various drugs (Sobell, Kwan, & Sobell, 1995; Sobell & Sobell, 2000).

One Alcohol Question: Three studies have found that a single question such as "Have you ever had a drinking problem?" results in more individuals being successfully identified as having an alcohol problem as opposed to more time-consuming screening tests such as the Michigan Alcohol Screening Test (Cyr & Wartman, 1988; Taj, Devera-Sales, & Vinson, 1998; Woodruff, Clayton, Cloninger, & Guze, 1976).

Self–Monitoring: This technique requires clients to record specific aspects (e.g., amount, frequency, mood, urges) of their addictive behaviors (e.g., alcohol, drug, smoking, gambling) throughout treatment. Self-monitoring has the following clinical uses: (a) helps clients to continually be aware of their substance use or other addictive behaviors and thus safeguards against distorted perceptions of use, (b) presents a detailed description of clients' addictive behaviors during treatment, (c) identifies potential high-risk use and relapse situations, (d) provides a basis for evaluating whether a change in the target behavior is occurring, and (e) allows clients opportunities to discuss their addictive behaviors with their therapist without awkwardness (Korotitsch & Nelson-Gray, 1999; Sobell & Sobell, 2000, 2005).

Assessing High-Risk Triggers to Addictive Behaviors

Brief SCQ-8 (BSCQ-8): Given that addictive behaviors have a high rate of relapse, it is essential that high-risk triggers to use be evaluated during an intervention (Marlatt & Gordon, 1985). The BSCQ-8, a variant of the Situational Confidence Questionnaire (SCQ; Allen & Wilson, 2003; Annis & Graham, 1988), probes eight major categories of situations related to alcohol or drug use (Breslin, Sobell, Sobell, & Agrawal, 2000). Unlike the original SCQ, the BSCQ-8 is easy to score, can be used to provide immediate feedback to clients concerning high-risk trigger situations concerning their alcohol or drug use, and is free (Breslin, Sobell, Sobell, & Agrawal, 2000; Substance Abuse and Mental Health Administration, 2002). A similar brief instrument has recently been developed for gamblers (May, Whelan, Steenbergh, & Meyers, 1998). The BSCQ-8 can be freely accessed through <http://www.nova.edu/gsc> and then by clicking on the link to "online forms."

Assessing Motivation and Readiness to Change

There has been an increasing recognition of the importance of assessing the extent to which individuals with addictive behaviors believe change is necessary (Substance Abuse and Mental Health Administration, 2002). Motivation can be conceptualized as a state of readiness to change that may fluctuate over time and can be influenced by several factors, including the role of the health care practitioner (Substance Abuse and Mental Health Administration, 2002). The important issue for mental health providers is that interventions for individuals who are not strongly committed to changing their addictive behavior should initially focus on increasing motivation, rather than on methods for changing.

Decisional Balance Exercise (DBE): This task asks clients to evaluate the perceived costs and benefits of continuing to engage in their addictive behaviors versus changing. The exercise is intended to make more salient the pros and cons of changing their current behaviors, which then will allow them to identify obstacles to change (Sobell & Sobell, 1998; Sobell, Sobell, Leo, Agrawal, Johnson-Young, & Cunningham, 2002; Sobell, Sobell, Toneatto, & Leo, 1993). Copies of the Decisional Balance Exercise can be found in a recent publication on motivational interviewing (Substance Abuse and Mental Health Administration, 2002) and can be freely accessed through <http://www.nova.edu/gsc> and then by clicking on the link to "Online forms."

Readiness to Change Ruler: This tool is designed to ultimately build clients' self-efficacy. By using a scaling technique, it allows individuals to give voice to their current motivation level and, more importantly, enables them to explore how to gain more of it. Clients are asked to rate their readiness to change their targeted behavior on a scale from 1 (not ready at all) to 5 (very ready to change) at the present time and also 6 months ago. By deploying discrepancies between the two numbers at the different time points, clients are able to give voice to changes they have made in their life, thus building greater self-efficacy and motivation.

Interviewing Style: Interviewing style is extremely important for obtaining accurate and useful information about individuals' substance use. The way in which questions are phrased can affect clients' answers. An important component of motivational interviewing is avoiding the use of labels. Individuals with substance use problems, particularly those whose problems are not severe, generally are reluctant to be labeled as "alcoholics" or "drug addicts." Not only does labeling serve no therapeutic advantages, it should also be avoided because it has been associated with substance abusers delaying or even avoiding entry into treatment (Cunningham, Sobell, Sobell, Agrawal, & Toneatto, 1993; Sobell, Ellingstad, & Sobell, 2000; Sobell, Sobell, & Toneatto, 1992). Asking individuals with an alcohol or drug problem to "Tell me about your use in the past year" is more likely to elicit an open, candid dialogue about their use compared with asking, "How long have you been an alcoholic (or drug addict)?" The following two references provide examples of how to ask nonjudgmental (i.e., avoiding labeling) yet clinically useful questions: Miller and Rollnick (2003) and Substance Abuse and Mental Health Administration (2002).

Motivational Strategies and Procedures to Increase Motivation: The major strategies and techniques that promote self-change in addictive behaviors are as follows: (a) help individuals identify discrepancies between their current behavior and their future goals, (b) allow individuals to identify reasons for changing, (c) enhance individuals' reasons for change by providing feedback on the risks and consequences of their behaviors, and (d) assist people in developing and evaluating plans for changing.

Addiction Self-Change Websites by Country

North America

Brown University Center for Alcohol and Addiction Studies: <http://www.caas. brown.edu>. This website offers curriculum and training materials for health care professionals. Brown University, Box G-BH, Providence, RI 02912. Tel.: (401) 863–1000.

Canadian Centre on Substance Abuse: <http://www.ccsa.ca>.

Canadian Foundation on Compulsive Gambling: <http://www.responsiblegambling. org>.

Cancer Prevention Research Center at the University of Rhode Island: <http:// www.uri.edu/research/cprc>. Provides information on the Transtheoretical Model of Change. Specifically, the website offers instruments to assess stages and processes of change for alcohol and smoking as well as related constructs (e.g., decisional balancing, self-efficacy).

Center for Online Addiction: <http://www.netaddiction.com>. This website gives information regarding Internet addiction, book presentations and press reviews, addiction tests, and online counseling.

Center on Alcoholism, Substance Abuse, and Addictions (CASAA): <http:// www.casaa.unm.edu>. This organization's mission is "to generate, convey, and apply knowledge to reduce suffering related to addictions and improve the quality of life for those affected by addiction." The website has a vast amount of downloadable materials. Tel.: (505) 925–2300.

Centre for Addiction and Mental Health: <http://www.camh.net>. 33 Russell St., Toronto, Ontario, M5S 2S1, Canada.

Free self-help material and self-monitoring software: <http://www.behavior-therapy.com>.

Guided Self-Change Clinic: <http://www.nova.edu/gsc>. This website provides free forms, calendars, instructions, and materials both in English and in Spanish for the (a) Promoting Self-change Community-based Mail Intervention, (b) Timeline Followback, (c) Family Tree Questionnaire, and (d) Brief Situational Confidence Questionnaire (BSCQ). At the bottom, click on the link to "Online forms," then go to the relevant files to download for free. L. C. Sobell, Center for Psychological Studies, Nova Southeastern University, 3301 College Ave., Ft. Lauderdale, FL 33314. sobelll@nova.edu.

Higher Education Center for Alcohol and Other Drug Prevention: <http:// www.edc.org/hec>. This website offers access to databases as well as other information about effective substance abuse prevention programs; public policy options; publications; and substance abuse educational opportunities for parents, students, and community leaders.

National Clearinghouse for Alcohol and Drug Information: <http://www.health.org>, <telnet.ncadi.health.org>, <ftp.health.org>, <info@prevline.health.org>. This organization is the Information Service division of the Center for Substance Abuse Prevention of the U.S. Department of Health and Human Services. It serves as the central point in the federal government for information about alcohol and other drug problems. Many of the publications can be obtained free of charge by calling the toll free number ([800] 729–6686) and providing one's name and address. Items are also available online for downloading. P.O. Box 2345, Rockville, MD 20852. Tel.: (301) 468–2600.

National Institute on Alcohol Abuse and Alcoholism: <http://www.niaaa.nih.gov>, <http://www.etoh.niaaa.nih.gov>. This website, among other features, provides literature searches on alcohol-related topics. 6000 Executive Blvd. Rockville, MD 20892–7003.

National Institute on Drug Abuse: <http://www.nida.nih.gov>. NIDA infofax gives empirically-based information on drug abuse and addiction. Fact sheets can be obtained by calling (888) 644–6432.

Rutgers University Center of Alcohol Studies: <http://www.alcoholstudies.rutgers.edu> This website contains a large collection of alcohol information. Smithers Hall, Busch Campus, Piscataway, NJ 08855-0969. Tel.: (908) 445–2190.

Smoking Websites:

<http://www.ahcpr.gov> (smoking cessation clinical practice guideline; published free by the Agency for Healthcare Research and Quality. Tel.: [800] 358-9295)

<http://patient.education.upmc.com/S.htm#Smoking> (smoking cessation behavior modification)

<http://www.kickbutt.org> (smoking cessation facts)

<http://www.lungusa.org> (American Lung Association)

<http://www.tobacco.org>

<http://www.tobacco.org/History/Tobacco_History.html>

<http://www.wonder.cdc.gov> (Centers for Disease Control and Prevention's smoking guidelines)

Great Britain

Advisory Council on Alcohol and Drug Education: <http://www.tacade.com>. The aim of this website is to provide support for professionals working with young people by supplying a range of publications and training products. 1 Hulme Place, Salford, Manchester, M5 4QA. Tel.: 0161-745-8925.

Alcohol Concern: <http://www.alcoholconcern.org.uk>. This website, created by a national agency on alcohol use, contains a vast amount of information about the effects of drinking and includes a page of local contact points and links to other alcohol-related sites. 32–36 Loman Street, London, SE1 0EE. Tel.: 020-7928-7377.

Alcohol Problem Advisory Service: <http://www.apas.org.uk>. This website offers information, training, and advice on alcohol misuse. 26 Park Row, Nottingham, NG1 6GR. Tel.: 0115-948-5570.

Centre for Health Economics: <http://www.york.ac.uk/inst/che>. University of York, Heslington, York, YO10 5DD. Tel.: 01904-433-646.

Department of Health: <http://www.doh.gov.uk>. This website offers statistics and information on alcohol use and misuse. In addition, government reports and official documents can be obtained via the website. Richmond House, 79 Whitehall, London, SW1A 2NL. Tel.: 020- 7210-4850.

Free drinking evaluation: <http://www.camh.net/About_Addiction_Mental_Health/Drug_and_Addiction_Information/evaluate_your_drinking.html>.

Institute of Alcohol Studies: <http://www.ias.org.uk>. This website aims at increasing knowledge of alcohol misuse and has a range of fact sheets and publications related to alcohol issues. Alliance House, 12 Caxton Street, London, SW1H 0QS. Tel.: 020-7222-4001.

Medical Council on Alcoholism: <http://www.medicouncilalcol.demon. co.uk>. This organization has an education and advisory role within the medical profession and produces handbooks and newsletters related to alcohol misuse. The website contains links to further resources. 3 St. Andrew's Place, London, NW1 4LB. Tel.: 020-7487-4445.

National Health Service Direct: <http://www.nhsdirect.nhs.uk>. This website provides information, advice, and details on support groups for health issues such as alcohol and smoking. Tel.: 0845 4647.

National Institute for Health and Clinical Excellence: <http://www.nice.org. uk>. This website contains information on behavioral changes and the benefits of motivational interviewing as well as support for doctors, nurses, and other health professionals. MidCity Place, 71 High Holborn, London, WC1V 6NA. Tel.: 020-7067-5800.

Smoking Websites:
   <http://www.ash.org.uk>
   <http://www.cancernet.co.uk/smoking.htm>
   <http://www.givingupsmoking.co.uk> (offers free publication materials)
   <http://www.healthnet.org.uk/quit/guide.htm>
   <http://www.recovery.org.uk>

Training by Distance Learning: e-mail: <training@lau.org.uk>. This online course offers extensive teaching materials, weekly telephone tutorials with an experienced practitioner, and video-linked supervised practice. Leeds Addiction Unit, 19 Springfield Mount, Leeds, LS2 9NG. Tel.: 0113-295-1330.

Wrecked: Think about drink: <http://www.wrecked.co.uk>.

Austria, Germany, and Switzerland

Controlled Consumption of Illegal Drugs: <http://www.kiss-heidelberg.de>. This website is targeted at individuals with drug problems as well as drug treatment professionals. It provides information especially about the "KISS" program, a 12-session individual and group treatment approach for controlled consumption of illegal drugs. Also, free downloads of power point slides and articles as well as addresses of therapists offering "KISS" treatments are available.

Controlled Drinking (CD): <http://www.kontrolliertes-trinken.de>, <http://www.kontrolliertes-trinken.ch>. This website is intended for people with alcohol problems, health professionals, and the media. It contains the following: basic information about CD, three German-speaking behavioral self-control programs for CD (bibliotherapy, individual treatment, and group treatment), diverse self-tests (e.g., AUDIT, online Blood Alcohol Concentration calculation, drinking diary), a 15-item questionnaire for deciding on direction of change (i.e., abstinence or controlled drinking), and the addresses of therapists and self-help groups offering CD treatment.

Controlled Smoking Websites: <http://www.kontrolliert-rauchen.de>. This website offers a scientific overview of studies addressing the possibility and effects of controlled/reduced smoking and uses smoking diaries to help individuals self-register the number of cigarettes smoked weekly.

<http://www.rauchfrei.de/rauchen>. This website gives 10 tips to help individuals reduce their smoking.

Eating Disorders Websites: <http://www.bundesfachverbandessstoerungen.de>. This is an association of different counseling centers and treatment facilities offering help for people with eating disorders.

<http://www.bzga-essstoerungen.de>. This website, produced by the Federal Center for Health Education (BZgA), contains a large amount of information about eating disorders (including addresses of treatment providers, literature, and counseling by phone), brochures, and many Austrian and Swiss links pertaining to this topic.

<http://www.hungrig-online.de>. This nonprofit website addresses two forms of eating disorders. The first, <http://www.bulimie-online.de>, is for individuals with bulimia nervosa, their relatives, and professionals. It provides basic information about the disorder, self-tests, addresses of professionals and self-help groups, online chats, discussion groups, and relevant literature. The second website, <http://www.magersucht-online.de>, focuses on anorexia nervosa and is structured the same as the one for bulimia nervosa.

Federal Center for Health Education ("Bundeszentrale für gesundheitliche Aufklärung" [BZgA]): <http://www.bzga.de>. This official website of the German Federal Center for Health Education offers various tools for changing one's consumption of alcohol, cigarettes, or drugs. The following is a list of websites from this organization which focus on various aspects of addiction: <http://www.bist-du-staerker-als-alkohol.de> (targeted for adolescents and offers a self-test and information regarding alcohol), <http://www.kinder-starkmachen.de> (concentrates on prevention of addictive behaviors in the areas of leisure-time and sports activities), <http://www.rauchfrei-info.de> (information about smoking and a program to quit, assisted by a 21-day mail support system), <http://www.rauch-frei.info> (aimed at adolescents and provides facts about smoking and an individualized program for quitting), <http://www.drugcom.de> (provides adolescents with comprehensive information about legal and especially illegal psychoactive substances ["druglex"], professional counseling via the Internet and chat rooms ["drug help," "drug talk"], self-tests of one's knowledge regarding drugs, self-tests about one's alcohol and cannabis consumption patterns, and a program called "Quit the Shit" for youths willing to reduce or stop their cannabis use).

Federal Ministry of Health ("Deutsches Bundesministerium für Gesundheit"): <http://www.bmg.bund.de>. This website, which is part of the commissary for drugs and addiction, informs visitors of federal policies on drugs and addiction.

German Cancer Research Center ("Deutsches Krebsforschungszentrum Heidelberg" [DKFZ]): <http://www.tabakkontrolle.de>. This website is one of the World Health Organization's focal points for tobacco control. Specifically, the center plans political activities against smoking, publishes materials advocating for a smoke-free environment, maintains a stop-smoking telephone helpline, provides personal support for individuals trying to quit smoking (e.g., by using motivation, action plans, relapse prevention), and gives a list of therapists and treatment centers.

German Center for Addiction ("Deutsche Hauptstelle für Suchtfragen"): <http://www.dhs.de>. This federally funded association is composed of all organizations, mostly nonprofit, operating in the addiction field. The website contains basic information about addictions (through brochures, links, and relevant literature) and addresses of treatment agencies and self-help groups. Moreover, the association organizes an annual addiction conference and publishes the addiction journal *Jahrbuch Sucht* which has up-to-date epidemiology data and discusses select addiction topics.

German Protestant Council for Helping People with Addiction Problems ("Gesamtverband für Suchtkrankenhilfe im Diakonischen Werk der Evangelischen Kirche in Deutschland" [GVS]): <http://www.sucht.org>. This website informs individuals about substance use and addiction, addresses legal questions, and offers specialized, continuing education for addiction professionals.

German Society for Addiction Medicine ("Deutsche Gesellschaft für Suchtmedizin"): <http://www.dgsuchtmedizin.de>. This website was created by an association of physicians researching or working in the field of addiction, with their ultimate objective being to bridge the gap between addiction research and practice. The organization also publishes the scientific journal *Suchttherapie* (*Addiction Therapy*).

Illegal Drugs: The following websites contain diverse information and guidance to change drug use: <http://www.cannabis-archiv.de>, <http://www. drogen-und-du.de>, <http://www.eve-rave.net>, <http://www.suchtknacker. ch>, and <http://www. xtc.mesh.de>.

Institute for Addiction Research ("Institut für Therapieforschung" [IFT]): <http://www.ift.de>. The IFT is a research institute in Munich, Germany, with a primary focus on substance use disorders (e.g., alcohol, illicit drugs, pharmaceuticals, tobacco), pathological gambling, and eating disorders. The organization empathizes epidemiology, prevention, and treatment research of addictive behaviors.

Internet Addiction ("Onlinesucht"): <http://www.onlinesucht.de>. This website offers assessment and support for individuals with Internet addiction, with field reports by Internet addicts, self-tests, and relevant literature.

Ludwig-Boltzmann-Institute for Addiction Research at the Anton-Proksch-Institute ("Ludwig-Boltzmann-Institut für Suchtforschung am Anton-Proksch-Institut"): <http://www.api.or.at>. This Austrian research group on alcohol and illicit drugs focuses its research on epidemiology, alcohol- and drug-related problems, alcohol and drug policies, social history, treatment and prevention, and evaluation of prevention as well as methodological issues.

Self-Help Association of Drug Addicts, Recovering Addicts, and Substituted Heroin Addicts ("JES - das bundesweite Netzwerk von Junkies, Ehemaligen und Substituierten"): <http://www.jes.aidshilfe.de>. This self-help association of individuals currently using drugs or recovering from drug consumption advocates for the rights of these people (e.g., legalization of drugs, acceptance of nonabstinence goals, support of safe injection rooms).

Self-Testing for Addiction Problems Websites (with or without online feedback): alcohol: <http://www.kontrolliertes-trinken.de/kontrolliertes-trinken/web/1_ selbsttest>, <http://www.alkohol-selbsttest.de>, <http://www.expertentest-alkohol.de>, <http://www.sfa-ispa.ch/Extranet/publication/PublicationUpload/ Parkscheibe.pdf>, <http://www.fazit-verlag.de/downloads/MPU-brochure.pdf> (for DUI drivers).

drugs: <http://www.drogen-und-du.de>, <http://www.suchtknacker.ch/ html/04/ quiz2.php>, <http://www.drugcom.de>, <http://www.forump.it/kms/ test_cannabis/ cannabis_konsum.php>.

eating disorders: <http://www.anad-pathways.de/11/bin_ich_essges-toert.html>, <http://www.anad.de/20/mein_persoenliches_ess_protokoll.html>, <http://www. psychotherapiepraxis.at/e_survey.phtml>, <http://www.netzwerk-essstoerungen.ch>.

gambling: <http://www.caritas.erzbistumkoeln.de/neuss_cv/sucht_hilfe/gluecksspiel/ selbsttest.html>, <http://www.beges.ch/glueck-im-unglueck/index1.shtml#zitrone>.

Internet addiction: <http://www.kstw.de>, <http://www.dr-walser.ch>, <http:// www. stangl-taller.at/arbeitsblaetter/sucht/InternetsuchtTest.shtml>, <http:// www.firstsurf.com/piuform.htm>, <http://www.psychotherapiepraxis.at>.

shopping   addiction: <http://www.suchtberatung-rostock.de/kauf.htm#2>, <http://www.stangl-taller.at/arbeitsblaetter/sucht/kaufsucht.shtml>.

smoking: <http://www.ift-nord.de/ift/jbsf/index.php?where=mdt;>, <http://www.rauchfrei-info.de/index.php?id=3>.

Swiss Center for Alcohol and Other Drug Problems ("Schweizerische Fachstelle für Alkohol- und andere Drogenprobleme" [SFA-ISPA]): <http://www.sfa-ispa.ch>. This nongovernmental organization focuses on prevention and research concerning problems with alcohol, illegal drugs, and tobacco. The website provides informational services (e.g., up-to-date epidemiological data of Swiss addiction problems), brochures (<http://www.sfa-ispa.ch/DocUpload/alkohol_wieviel/pdf>), and publishes the journals *Abhängigkeiten* (*Dependences*) and *Standpunkte* (*Standpoint*).

Swiss Online Information System ("Infoset Direct"): <http://www.infoset.ch>. This website provides extensive up-to-date information (via newsletters) concerning addiction policies and treatment in Switzerland and abroad.

Talk about ("Talk about - ein Präventionsprojekt zur Verringerung des Alkoholkonsums bei Jugendlichen"): <http://www.talkabout.org>. As a result of a Swiss project, this website presents a list of ideas regarding ways to sensitize youth to alcohol and how to self-limit consumption.

Finland

Alcohol or other substance problems: <http://www.paihdelinkki.fi>.

France

Everything you have always wanted to know about alcohol and alcoholism: <www. alcoweb.com>.

Italy

DrogaNet: <http://www.droga.net>. This website provides news, links, and discussions about drugs.

Gruppo Abele: <http://www.gruppoabele.it>. This website is a nexus of information on alcohol, drugs, and other social problems and offers various kinds of recovery methods.

Osservatorio sul tabacco - Istituto Italiano Tumory: <http://www.istituto-tumori.mi.it./osservatorio>. This website offers different solutions to quit smoking.

Why and how to give up smoking: <http://www.legatumori.it>. This website makes available the Fagerström Test as well as suggests four steps to quit smoking.

Sweden

Catalogue of links covering the psychosocial aspects of addiction: <http://www. sposit.se>. This website also has a listserve forum at <psyk@socialt>.

National Institute of Public Health: <http://www.fhi.se/lankar>. This website offers links to websites with facts and advice about drinking, smoking, and gambling.

Swedish Council for Information on Alcohol and Other Drugs: <http://www. can.se>. This website provides links to a number of relevant organizations and authorities, publishes topical facts on alcohol and drugs, and has a rather extensive addiction library.

Mexico

Centrov de Servicios Psicológicos ("Guillermo Dávila"): <http://www.psicol. unam.mx/ServiciosPsicologicos/servicios.htm>.

Spain

Adios Tabaco: <http://www.adiostabaco.com.ar> (Argentinean website).

Agència de Salut Pública de Barcelona: <http://www.elalcoholytu.org/elalcoholytu. php>.

Atención Farmacéutica del Tabaco, del Col·legi de Farmacèutics: <http://www. farmaceuticonline.com/cast/familia/familia_tabac_c.html>.

HCM Métodos Sistemas de autoayuda y autohipnosis: <http://www.hcm-auto ayuda.com/ cProduct/alcoholismo/399?PHPSESSID=cc9c9f6250293541eaa7 e04ca31f5e75>.

Ilustraciones: Sònia Ribas. Espais Telemàtics: <http://www.stop-tabac.ch/sp/ welcome.html>.

Instituto para el estudio de las adicciones: <http://www.lasdrogas.info/index.php>.

Manual de autoayuda para dejar de fumar: <http://www.usal.es/~retribucion esysalud/ssalud/prev_riesgos/no_fumar.pdf>.

Psicología online: Comprende tú alcoholismo: <http://www.psicologia-online. com/autoayuda/alcoholismo/cambio.htm>.

Additional Addiction Self-Change Resources Available Online by Request

Be Smart - Don't Start: <http://www.smokefreeclass.info>. A widespread program for schools in Europe to prevent children from smoking. All materials can be ordered from <http://www.ift-nord.de/ift/be>.

Bundeszentrale für gesundheitliche Aufklärung. (2001). Alles Klar? Tipps und informationen für den verantwortungsvollen Umgang mit Alkohol. Köln: BZgA. This resource provides a 30-item alcohol self-test and recommendations for moderate or abstinent drinking. The 61-page manual can be downloaded for free at <http://www.bzga.de>.

Bundeszentrale für gesundheitliche Aufklärung. (2005). Ja, ich werde rauchfrei. Köln: BZgA. This 104-page manual to quit smoking can be downloaded for free from <http://www.bzga.de>.

Deutsche Hauptstelle für Suchtfragen (Hrsg.). (2004). Umgang mit Alkohol. Informationen, Tests und Hilfen in 5 Phasen. Hamm: DHS. This resource offers systematic recommendations for changing one's drinking habits using DiClemente and Prochaska's stages of change theoretical model as its underpinnings. Free downloads are available at <http://www.dhs-intern.de/pdf/umgang_mit_alkohol.pdf>.

Drugs - Just Say Know (2004). This resource provides 22 cards to foster and promote knowledge about safer drug use for current users. The products can be ordered from <http://www.eve-rave.net/abfahrer/download/eve-rave/bericht115.pdf>.

Gehring, U. & Projektgruppe kT. (2003). Trainer-Manual für das "Ambulante Einzelprogramm zum kontrollierten Trinken" (EkT) und Teilnehmer-Handbuch. Heidelberg: GK Quest Akademie. This 114-page manual is similar to the AkT one, except it concentrates on individual treatment. The book can be ordered by e-mailing <info@gk-quest.de>.

Just be smokefree: This program to quit smoking targets young people. The manual can be ordered at <http://www.ift-nord.de/ift/jbsf>.

Körkel, J. (2005). 10-Schritte-Programm zum selbstständigen Erlernen des kontrollierten Trinkens (3rd ed.). Heidelberg: GK Quest Akademie. This bibliotherapeutical, behavioral self-control training focuses on controlled drinking. The 150-page book includes 10 steps, tables for standard units, and is preceded by a self-test addressing choice of self-change goals (i.e., abstinence or controlled drinking). The possibility of online counseling is also available if professional help is needed. The book can be ordered by e-mailing <info@gk-quest.de>.

Körkel, J. & GK Quest Academy. (2006). KISS-Trainer Manual und KISS-Teilnehmer-Handbuch (3rd ed.). Heidelberg: GK Quest Akademie. This provides a trainer's manual and accompanying participant's handbook for the KISS program (for the controlled use of drugs). This 100-page manual can be ordered by e-mailing <info@gk-quest.de>.

Körkel, J. & Projektgruppe kT. (2001). Trainer-Manual für das "Ambulante Gruppenprogramm zum kontrollierten Trinken" (AkT) und Teilnehmer-Handbuch. Heidelberg: GK Quest Akademie. This resource offers a professional's manual and accompanying participant's handbooks for the AkT program (group treatment approach with the goal of controlled drinking). The book can be ordered by e-mailing <info@gk-quest.de>.

References

Allen, J. P., Litten, R. Z., Fertig, J. B., & Babor, T. (1997). A review of research on the Alcohol Use Disorders Identification Test (AUDIT). *Alcoholism: Clinical and Experimental Research, 21*, 613–619.

Allen, J. P., & Wilson, V. (2003). *Assessing alcohol problems* (2nd ed.). Rockville, MD: National Institute on Alcohol Abuse and Alcoholism.

American Psychiatric Association. (2000). *Handbook of psychiatric measures.* Washington, DC: Author.

Annis, H. M., & Graham, J. M. (1988). *Situational Confidence Questionnaire (SCQ 39): User's guide.* Toronto: Addiction Research Foundation.

Berman, A., Bergman, H., Palmstierna, T., & Schlyter, F. (2005). Evaluation of the Drug Use Disorders Identification Test (DUDIT) in criminal justice and detoxification settings and in a Swedish population sample. *European Addiction Research, 11*, 22–31.

Breslin, F. C., Sobell, L. C., Sobell, M. B., & Agrawal, S. (2000). A comparison of a brief and long version of the Situational Confidence Questionnaire. *Behaviour Research and Therapy, 38*, 1211–1220.

Bush, K., Kivlahan, D., McDonell, M., Fihn, S., & Bradley, K. (1998). The AUDIT Alcohol Consumption Questions (AUDIT-C): An effective brief screening test for problem drinking. *Archives of Internal Medicine, 158*, 1789–1795.

Cherpitel, C. J. (1997). Brief screening instruments for alcoholism. *Alcohol Health & Research World, 21*, 348–351.

Cunningham, J. A., Sobell, L. C., Sobell, M. B., Agrawal, S., & Toneatto, T. (1993). Barriers to treatment: Why alcohol and drug abusers delay or never seek treatment. *Addictive Behaviors, 18*, 347–353.

Cyr, M. G., & Wartman, S. A. (1988). The effectiveness of routine screening questions in the detection of alcoholism. *Journal of the American Medical Association, 259*, 51–54.

Fagerström, K.-O., & Schneider, N. (1989). Measuring nicotine dependence: A review of the Fagerström Tolerance Questionnaire. *Journal of Behavioral Medicine, 12*, 159–182.

Fleming, M., & Manwell, L. B. (1999). Brief intervention in primary care settings: A primary treatment method for at-risk, problem, and dependent drinkers. *Alcohol Health & Research World, 23*, 128–137.

Fleming, M. F., Manwell, L. B., Barry, K. L., Adams, W., & Stauffacher, E. A. (1999). Brief physician advice for alcohol problems in older adults: A randomized community-based trial. *Journal of Family Practice, 48*, 378–384.

Garner, D. M., Olmsted, M. P., & Polivy, J. (1983). Development and validation of a multidimensional eating disorder inventory for anorexia nervosa and bulimia. *International Journal of Eating Disorders, 2*,15–34.

Gual, A., Segura, L., Contel, M., Heather, N., & Colom, J. (2002). AUDIT-3 and AUDIT-4: Effectiveness of two short forms of the Alcohol Use Disorders Identification Test. *Alcohol & Alcoholism, 37*, 591–596.

Heather, N. (1990). *Brief interventions strategies.* New York: Pergamon.

Heatherton, T. F., Kozlowski, L. T., Frecker, R. C., & Fagerström, K.-O. (1991). The Fagerström Test for Nicotine Dependence: A revision of the Fagerström Tolerance Questionnaire. *British Journal of Addiction, 86*, 119–127.

Korotitsch, W. J., & Nelson-Gray, R. O. (1999). An overview of self-monitoring research in assessment and treatment. *Psychological Assessment, 11*, 415–425.

Lesieur, H. R., & Blume, S. B. (1993). Revisiting the South Oaks Gambling Screen in different settings. *Journal of Gambling Studies, 9*, 213–233.

López Viets, V. C., & Miller, W. R. (1997). Treatment approaches for pathological gamblers. *Clinical Psychology Review, 17*, 689–702.

Marlatt, G. A., & Donovan, D. M. (2005). *Relapse prevention (2nd ed): Maintenance strategies in the treatment of addictive behaviors.* New York: Guilford Press.

Marlatt, G. A., & Gordon, J. R. (1985). *Relapse prevention: Maintenance strategies in the treatment of addictive behaviors.* New York: Guilford Press.

May, R. K., Whelan, J. P., Steenbergh, T. A., & Meyers, A. W. (1998, November). *The Situational Confidence Questionnaire for gambling: An initial psychometric evaluation.* Paper presented at the 32nd Annual Meeting of the Association for Advancement of Behavior Therapy, Washington, DC.

McLellan, A. T., Kushner, H., Metzger, D., Peters, R., Smith, I., Grissom, G., et al. (1992). The fifth edition of the Addiction Severity Index. *Journal of Substance Abuse Treatment, 9*, 199–213.

Miller, W. R., & Rollnick, S. (2003). *Motivational interviewing: Preparing people to change* (2nd ed.). New York: Guilford Press.

Pomerleau, C. S., Pomerleau, O. F., Majchrzak, M. J., Kloska, D. D., & Malakuti, R. (1990). Relationship between nicotine tolerance questionnaire scores and plasma cotinine. *Addictive Behaviors, 15*, 73–80.

Rollnick, S., Butler, C. C., & Stott, N. (1997). Helping smokers make decisions: The enhancement of brief interventions for general medical practice. *Patient Education and Counseling, 31*, 191–203.

Rollnick, S., Morgan, M., & Heather, N. (1996). The development of a brief scale to measure outcome expectations of reduced consumption among excessive drinkers. *Addictive Behaviors, 21*, 377–387.

Rounsaville, B. J., Tims, F. M., Horton, A. M., Jr., & Sowder, B. J. (1993). *Diagnostic source book of drug abuse research and treatment.* Rockville, MD: National Institute on Drug Abuse.

Rumpf, H.-J., Hapke, U., Hill, A., & John, U. (1997). Development of a screening questionnaire for the general hospital and general practices. *Alcoholism: Clinical and Experimental Research, 21*, 894–898.

Samet, J. H., Rollnick, S., & Barnes, H. (1996). Beyond CAGE: A brief clinical approach after detection of substance abuse. *Archives of Internal Medicine, 156*, 2287–2293.

Saunders, J. B., Aasland, O. G., Babor, T. F., De La Fuente, J. R., & Grant, M. (1993). Development of the Alcohol Use Disorders Identification Test (AUDIT): WHO collaborative project on early detection of persons with harmful alcohol consumption— II. *Addiction, 88*, 791–804.

Skinner, H. A. (1982). The Drug Abuse Screening Test. *Addictive Behaviors, 7*, 363–371.

Sklar, S. M., & Turner, N. E. (1999). A brief measure for the assessment of coping self-efficacy among alcohol and other drug users. *Addiction, 94*, 723–729.

Sobell, L. C., Ellingstad, T. P., & Sobell, M. B. (2000). Natural recovery from alcohol and drug problems: Methodological review of the research with suggestions for future directions. *Addiction, 95*, 749–764.

Sobell, L. C., Kwan, E., & Sobell, M. B. (1995). Reliability of a Drug History Questionnaire (DHQ). *Addictive Behaviors, 20*, 233–241.

Sobell, L. C., & Sobell, M. B. (2000). Drug abuse. In A. E. Kazdin (Ed.), *Encyclopedia of psychology* (pp. 93–97). Washington, DC and New York: American Psychological Association and Oxford University Press.

Sobell, L. C., & Sobell, M. B. (2005). Identification and assessment of alcohol problems. In G. P. Koocher, J. A. Norcross, & S. S. Hill III (Eds.), *Psychologist's desk reference* (2nd ed., pp. 71–76). New York: Oxford University Press.

Sobell, L. C., Sobell, M. B., Leo, G. I., Agrawal, S., Johnson-Young, L., & Cunningham, J. A. (2002). Promoting self-change with alcohol abusers: A community-level mail intervention based on natural recovery studies. *Alcoholism: Clinical and Experimental Research, 26*, 936–948.

Sobell, L. C., Sobell, M. B., & Toneatto, T. (1992). Recovery from alcohol problems without treatment. In N. Heather, W. R. Miller, & J. Greeley (Eds.), *Self-control and the addictive behaviours* (pp. 198–242). New York: Maxwell MacMillan.

Sobell, L. C., Sobell, M. B., Toneatto, T., & Leo, G. I. (1993). What triggers the resolution of alcohol problems without treatment? *Alcoholism: Clinical and Experimental Research, 17*, 217–224.

Sobell, L. C., Toneatto, T., & Sobell, M. B. (1994). Behavioral assessment and treatment planning for alcohol, tobacco, and other drug problems: Current status with an emphasis on clinical applications. *Behavior Therapy, 25*, 533–580.

Sobell, M. B., & Sobell, L. C. (1998). Guiding self-change. In W. R. Miller & N. Heather (Eds.), *Treating addictive behaviors* (2nd ed., pp. 189–202). New York: Plenum Press.

Substance Abuse and Mental Health Administration. (1993). *Screening and assessment of alcohol and other drug-abusing adolescents* (Treatment Improvement Protocol Series, 3). Rockville, MD: U.S. Department of Health and Human Services.

Substance Abuse and Mental Health Administration. (1995). *Assessment and treatment of patients with coexisting mental illness and alcohol and other drug abuse* (Treatment Improvement Protocol Series, 9). Rockville, MD: U.S. Department of Health and Human Services.

Substance Abuse and Mental Health Administration. (2002). *Enhancing motivation for change in substance abuse treatment* (Treatment Improvement Protocol Series, 35). Rockville, MD: U.S. Department of Health and Human Services.

Taj, N., Devera-Sales, A., & Vinson, D. C. (1998). Screening for problem drinking: Does a single question work? *Journal of Family Practice, 46*, 328–335.

Tate, J. C., & Schmitz, J. M. (1993). A proposed revision of the Fagerström Tolerance Questionnaire. *Addictive Behaviors, 18*, 135–143.

Woodruff, R. A., Clayton, P. J., Cloninger, R., & Guze, S. B. (1976). A brief method of screening for alcoholism. *Diseases of the Nervous System, 37*, 434–435.

Index

Printed in the United States
119536LV00001BB/4-33/A

9 780387 712864